Electronic Health Records

second edition

Byron R. Hamilton

Ozark Technical Community College, Springfield, Missouri
CEO, Med-Soft National Training Institution, BA, MA

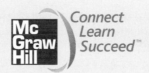

Connect
Learn
Succeed™

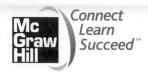

The McGraw·Hill Companies

Mc Graw Hill

Connect
Learn
Succeed™

ELECTRONIC HEALTH RECORDS

Published by McGraw-Hill, a business unit of The McGraw-Hill Companies, Inc., 1221 Avenue of the Americas, New York, NY, 10020. Copyright © 2011 by The McGraw-Hill Companies, Inc. All rights reserved. Previous edition © 2009. No part of this publication may be reproduced or distributed in any form or by any means, or stored in a database or retrieval system, without the prior written consent of The McGraw-Hill Companies, Inc., including, but not limited to, in any network or other electronic storage or transmission, or broadcast for distance learning.

Some ancillaries, including electronic and print components, may not be available to customers outside the United States.

This book is printed on acid-free paper.

2 3 4 5 6 7 8 9 0 DOW/DOW 1 0 9 8 7 6 5 4 3 2 1 0

ISBN   978-0-07-747755-4
MHID   0-07-747755-3

Vice president/Editor in chief: Elizabeth Haefele
Vice president/Director of marketing: John E. Biernat
Publisher: Kenneth S. Kasee Jr.
Sponsoring editor: Natalie J. Ruffatto
Director of development, Allied Health: Patricia Hesse
Developmental editor: Bonnie Hemrick
Editorial coordinator: Parissa DJangi
Executive marketing manager: Roxan Kinsey
Lead media producer: Damian Moshak
Media development editor: Marc Mattson
Director, Editing/Design/Production: Jess Ann Kosic
Project manager: Kathryn W. Mikulic

Senior production supervisor: Janean A. Utley
Senior designer: Srdjan Savanovic
Lead photo research coordinator: Carrie K. Burger
Media project manager: Cathy L. Tepper
Cover design: Daniel Krueger
Interior design: Pam Verros, PV DESIGN INC
Typeface: 10.5/12.5 Palatino
Compositor: MPS Limited, A Macmillan Company
Printer: R. R. Donnelley
Cover credits: thermometer: © D. Hurst/Alamy; pills in bottle: © Corbis; tablet: © Comstock/PunchStock; x-ray: © Royalty-Free/Corbis; test tubes: © GlowImages/Alamy.

Photo Credits: Chapter openers: 1: © Photomondo/Getty RF; 2: © Comstock Images/PictureQuest RF; 3: © Peter Scholey/Photographer's Choice/Getty Images; 4: © Comstock Images/Jupiter RF; 5: © Comstock Images/Jupiter RF; 6: © Comstock/PictureQuest RF; 7: © Comstock Images/Jupiter RF; 8: © Digital Vision/PunchStock; 9: © Flying Colours/Getty RF; 10: © Chad Baker/Ryan McVay/Getty RF; 11: © Comstock Images/Jupiter RF; 12: © Comstock Images/Alamy RF.

Copyright Notice: Screen captures of SpringCharts™ Electronic Health Records software are reprinted with permission from Spring Medical Systems, Inc. All rights reserved.

Library of Congress Cataloging-in-Publication Data

Hamilton, Byron, 1958–
    Electronic health records / Byron R. Hamilton.—2nd ed.
       p. ; cm.
    Includes bibliographical references and index.
    ISBN-13: 978-0-07-337439-0 (alk. paper)
    ISBN-10: 0-07-337439-3 (alk. paper)
    1. Medical records—Data processing. I. Title.
    [DNLM: 1. Electronic Health Records—Problems and Exercises. WX 18.2 H217e 2011]
R864.H32 2011
610.285—dc22
                                                                        2009047500

The Internet addresses listed in the text were accurate at the time of publication. The inclusion of a Web site does not indicate an endorsement by the authors or McGraw-Hill, and McGraw-Hill does not guarantee the accuracy of the information presented at these sites.

www.mhhe.com

about the author

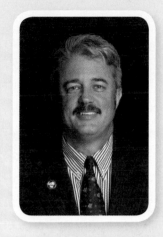

Byron R. Hamilton received a BA in Education from the College of Advanced Education in Australia, and taught for several years in both private and public institutions. He earned an MA in Biblical Literature in Springfield, Mo., and is currently teaching EHR as part of the Continuing Education Department at Ozark Technical Community College in Springfield, Missouri.

In 1997, Byron and his wife, Leesa, established *MedTech Medical Management Systems*, a medical billing and consulting company for both practice management software and electronic medical records. For the following decade they were involved with medical billing, supervision of health-care information management, medical consultation, and training. Byron has been involved with electronic health record systems from the inception of the industry.

In 2004, he launched *Med-Soft National Training Institute*, (MNTI), a software training group conducting onsite and online training on medical software, including Medisoft™ PMS and SpringCharts™ EHR, both nationally and internationally. He has written the product training manuals for several PMS and EHR programs and has authored numerous articles for professional magazines. MNTI, also provides strategies for health-care organizations in the selection, implementation and project management of electronic health records.

Byron is a national speaker at career college workshops, business college associations, and medical professional groups. ≫

brief contents

table of contents

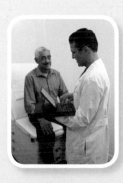

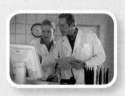

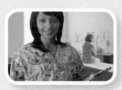

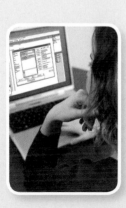

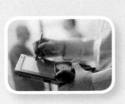

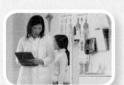

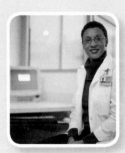

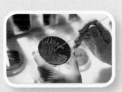

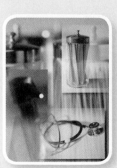

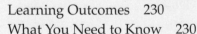

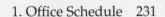
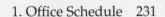
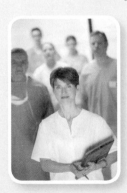

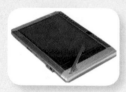

INTRODUCTION

Health Information Technology continues to expand rapidly across the entire spectrum of the medical community. Affordability in computer technology and medical software is now exerting a major influence on physicians in private practice groups of eight or fewer doctors to adopt electronic medical records. This enclave of medical professionals makes up nearly 78 percent of all medical practices in the United States. The availability and reliability of wireless computer networks, the public concern for patient safety, and the affordability of health information technology are being met with the federal government's involvement in coordinating and setting technical standards and implementing time tables for electronic medical records. These converging forces are bringing about a virtual explosion in the electronic health-care business, leading industry experts to concur that in less than five years 90 percent of small- to medium-sized practices will be utilizing an electronic health records system. Currently, it is estimated that only 20 percent of independent physicians utilize an electronic medical record system.

The remarkable surge of interest in electronic health records (EHR) is leading to further development in comprehensive clinical decision support that will continue to enhance computerized knowledge management systems and create even more robust EHRs. Through the EHR, medical consumers have become the beneficiary of improved medical care, greater patient safety, and increased control over medical records and are able to make important contributions to their health care.

With the forming of government agencies that now give guidance to the electronic health-care industry and set standards for feature development among health information vendors, the EHR elements are becoming uniform with clinical guidelines, protocols and care plans embedded into the programs. Templates, standard reports, medical database analysis, and clinical alerts have now become automated through most EHR programs. The electronic health record has matured and is poised to become the foundation for a national health information infrastructure.

KEY FEATURES

- **The CCHIT-certified SpringCharts™ premium EHR program is available with each text at no additional cost to the student or school.** Students learn EHR documentation through this industry-standard software. It combines the right mix of rich functionality and intuitive ease of use to enable rapid and complete clinical and clerical documentation.
- An abundance of screen captures and menu icons from SpringCharts™ EHR software provide step-by-step instructions for easy reference and application.
- Concept Checkups follow each topic and break down learning outcomes into manageable subject material.

- Focal Points and key term definitions appear in the margins throughout the text to spotlight critical data necessary to master end-of-chapter review quizzes.
- A **Certificate of Training** is available on McGraw-Hill's Online Learning Center (OLC) for each student completing the course.

TEXTBOOK OVERVIEW

This textbook, *Electronic Health Records*, arose from the need to train medical support personnel for the anticipated phenomenal growth of electronic health records in the health-care field. Understanding of and practical knowledge of electronic health records is essential to all medical professionals and support staff entering the workforce. Successful preparation in education is the seedbed for a successful career.

In *Electronic Health Records* we provide a detailed history of the EHR from the inception of the electronic medical record in the 1960s, tracing the influence of several federal agencies and private-sector organizations from the Health Insurance Portability and Accountability Act of 1996 to the Certification Commission of Health Information Technology formed in 2004 to the Medicare Improvements for Patient and Providers Act of 2008. *Electronic Health Records* devotes an entire 10 chapters to practical, hands-on experience with *SpringCharts EHR™*, a popular electronic health records program used by a wide range of medical specialties and health-care professionals both nationally and internationally. At the completion of this course you will receive a Completion Certificate acknowledging your successful training as a *SpringCharts* user.

In **Chapter 1** the student is introduced to a concise history of the EHR, and we unravel the multiple nomenclatures surrounding the development of the EHR. We also explore the perceived obstacles that have prevented medical professionals from speedily embracing the electronic patient chart and then discuss the benefits that many are now seeing in the adoption of electronic medical records.

Chapter 2 covers the history of the standards surrounding the EHR and looks at the influence that legislation and agencies like the Health Insurance Portability and Accountability Act, Consolidated Health Informatics, Institute of Medicine, and Certification Commission for Healthcare Information Technology have had on feature development in the EHR industry.

Chapter 3 covers an introduction to SpringCharts EHR and the system preferences that enables the program to function uniquely for each user. The student is taught the basic data setup of new patients, insurance companies, and clinical addresses.

In **Chapter 4** the student will learn how to function in an administrative role within the clinic by utilizing several managerial features of SpringCharts, including patient scheduling, tracking patient activity, and sending and receiving reminders, messages, and e-mails.

The electronic patient chart is discussed in detail in **Chapter 5.** Here the student will learn how to build the patient's electronic face sheet; order tests; document phone calls, excuse notes, and order forms; create letters; chart a patient's vitals, and import documents and images into the patient's chart.

Chapter 6 introduces the medical student to the comprehensive office visit note. The trainee will build a realistic medical note from a patient encounter, learn how to work with other clinical staff in document-ing portions of an office visit, add a new diagnosis and drug to the system database, create various reports from the patient encounter, work with several online medical databases, add an addendum note, and create a routing slip for billing purposes.

Clinical tools are addressed in **Chapter 7.** The student will learn how to evaluate electronic charts for wellness screenings, build a super-bill unique to the needs of a medical clinic, create and administer a patient instruction sheet, conduct a drug/allergy reaction check, and explore the clinical draw program.

Chapter 8 introduces the student to the flexibility of the electronic tem-plate and pop-up text. These two robust features enable medical staff to speedily document both clinical and clerical processes with a click of the mouse. The trainee will learn how to build templates and pop-up text and then utilize this information throughout the program.

Practical learning continues in **Chapter 9** with the creation, ordering, and processing of medical tests. The student will learn how to create, edit and use procedure and diagnosis codes.

Chapter 10 takes the medical student through the common clinical functions located in the *Productivity Center*. Here the trainee will work with the electronic bulletin board, send and receive electronic faxes, use the built-in time clock feature, access customized websites, archive unused electronic patient records, and analyze the medical database to create form letters and reports.

Chapters 11 provides the student with advanced exercises that will apply the knowledge gained from studying specific elements of the program and incorporate this information into practical multitasks.

Chapter 12 supplies the trainee with real medical source documents from which patient and medical data can be created in the electronic health record.

The purpose of *Electronic Health Records* is to provide a practical bridge to span the gap between how medical records have been kept for the past several centuries and how they are kept today. By making available a hands-on text-book, doctors, physician assistants, nurses, medical assistants, and clinical and medical clerical staff will make a comfortable journey across that bridge arriv-ing with practical expertise with EHRs.

WHAT'S NEW IN THE SECOND EDITION OF EHR?
ARRA

The American Recovery and Reinvestment Act of 2009, commonly known as the Stimulus Package, contains approximately $20 billion to promote the adoption of EHRs across the country. Up to $65,000 is being made available to physicians to invest in Health Information Technology, ensuring that every citizen has ac-cess to electronic medical records by 2014. This program and its impact upon the future allied health workforce is discussed in the second edition.

MIPPA

The Medicare Improvements for Patients and Providers Act of 2008 and its impact on e-prescribing in EHR programs is discussed. The current increased reimbursement incentives to physicians from CMS is outlined.

E-prescribing

By 2015 e-prescribing will be mandated; patients will no longer receive a written prescription for medication. A national clearing house is already in place to receive electronic prescriptions from multiple physicians into a single database for each patient. Details of e-prescribing are discussed in this edition.

New Four-Color Design

The second edition of *Electronic Health Records* has a new four-color design, making screen shots easier to read and the textbook more visually engaging to the student.

New Features to SpringCharts

SpringCharts EHR has gone through five upgrades since the first edition of *Electronic Health Records*. Students will now be working on version 9.7. Some of the additional features of this new version are outlined in the second edition of *EHR*.

- Digital signature—allows user to save a signature into the program that will print on letters, prescriptions, and anywhere an electronic signature is available. Only the user may use his digital signature; it is not available to other users. A Tablet PC must be in place to use this feature.
- Added capability to convert one type of note to an OV note—useful when a patient enters the office to have a blood pressure check but then needs to see the doctor.
- Vitals—right click on vitals fields to enter values without typing.
- Added an addendum feature for charted messages—messages that have been charted may now have an addendum, similar to the OV addendum.
- All text areas now have right-click support for adding date, time, and initials.
- Added right/left-hand orientation for new OV screen—moves the tabs to the left side for left-handed users and to the right side for right-handed users.
- Added font and margin choices to printing—a new print dialog was created to allow the user to define margins, font, and font size when printing documents.
- Overhauled face sheet—the multicolored boxes on the left half of the patient chart have been replaced with a more aesthetically pleasing face sheet. This design change also allows for easy future expansion of the face sheet.
- New office visit form—the office visit form has been redesigned to allow large screen users an always-visible face sheet and the tabs have been moved to the sides.
- Added automatic chart evaluations and pending/completed test lists to the face sheet—chart evaluations are now automatically processed on opening a chart and are shown on the new face sheet. Pending and completed tests are now shown on the face sheet instead of in the former pop-up window.
- Added right-click support to face sheet—right-click each face sheet item to view or edit that item.
- Added face sheet to all types of chart notes—the new face sheet was added to Nurse notes, Encounter notes, Rx Refill notes, TC notes, and Vitals Only notes.

- Overhauled Nurse note, TC note, Rx Only note, Encounter note, and Vitals note—these screens have been redesigned to follow the pattern of the new office visit form.
- Overhauled immunization window—can now be sorted by date or name.
- Added a lock icon to signed chart notes—a new icon identifies which items in a chart have been signed.
- Added drug search by generic name—prescription drug choices may now be searched by brand name or generic.
- Changed 'Referred by' to 'Other Providers'—more useful to specialist practices.
- Added tests to the OV templates—users may now enter tests to be included in each template.
- Added pop-up text to the notes sections of all tests (lab, imaging, med).
- Added NPI to routing slip.

WHAT IS CONNECT *PLUS+*?

McGraw-Hill Connect *Plus+* is a revolutionary online assignment and assessment solution, providing instructors and students with tools and resources to maximize their success.

Through Connect *Plus+*, instructors enjoy simplified course setup and assignment creation. Robust, media-rich tools and activities, all **tied to the textbook learning outcomes,** ensure you'll create classes geared toward achievement. You'll have more time with your students and spend less time agonizing over course planning.

Connect *Plus+* Features

McGraw-Hill Connect *Plus+* includes powerful tools and features that allow students to access their coursework anytime and anywhere while you control the assignments. Connect *Plus+* provides students with their textbook and homework, **all in one accessible place.**

- **Simple Assignment Management**
  - Creating assignments takes just a few clicks, and with Connect Plus+, you can choose not only which chapter to assign, but specific learning outcomes. **Videos, animations, quizzes,** and many other assignments and activities bring **active learning** to the forefront.

- **Smart Grading**
  - Study time is precious and Connect *Plus+* assignments **automatically provide feedback** to you and your students. You'll be able to conveniently review your class's or individual student's knowledge of concepts and assignments in an online environment.

- **Connect *Plus+* eBooks**
  - McGraw-Hill has seamlessly **integrated eBooks** into their Connect *Plus+* solution with **direct links to the homework, activities, and tools**—students no longer have to search for content and so they spend more time learning.

McGRAW-HILL HIGHER EDUCATION ONLINE LEARNING CENTER

Access the Online Learning Center at **www.mhhe.com/HamiltonEHR2e.**
- Quizzes for each chapter supplement the end-of-chapter reviews in the textbook.
- Flashcards containing key terms and definitions taken from each chapter enable the student to self-test throughout the course.
- A thorough PowerPoint® slide presentation for every chapter, containing teaching notes keyed to learning outcomes, makes the teaching and learning experience exciting and is available to students for the visual learner to be able to pace him/herself through the text material.

- An Instructor's Manual contains a course overview, chapter summaries, answer keys, and instructions for installing the SpringCharts EHR software.
- McGraw-Hill's EZ-Test Test Generator is an electronic testing program that allows instructors to create tests from book-specific items. It accommodates a wide range of question types, and instructors may add their own questions. Multiple versions of the test can be created, and any test can be exported for use with course management systems such as WebCT, BlackBoard, or PageOut. EZ-Test Online is a new service that gives you an place to easily administer the exams and quizzes you create with EZ-Test. The program is available for Windows and Macintosh environments.

DOWNLOADING SPRINGCHARTS IS EASY!

Overview

SpringCharts EHR is an electronic medical records software suite based on the latest industry standard Java technology. It requires a very modest network system for installation. SpringCharts is available in two different system configurations: Single Computer and Network Option.

> Note: Before you can begin working on the exercises in *Electronic Health Records*, you will need to access and download both the SpringCharts EHR software and the *EHR Material* folder located on the OLC at www.mhhe.com/HamiltonEHR2e. The *EHR Material* folder contains images, documents, and files to give students real scenarios for EHR documentation throughout the course.

Please follow the instructions below to download Java Runtime Environment, SpringCharts EHR program, and the EHR Materials folder onto your computer. If you encounter problems with the download, contact any of the support teams listed below.

Support

- McGraw-Hill Higher Education technical support team: 1-800-331-5094
  - 8 a.m.–11 p.m. CST, Monday–Thursday
  - 8 a.m.–6 p.m. CST, Friday
  - 6 p.m.–11 p.m. CST, Sunday
- www.mhhe.com/support
- Med-Soft National Training Institute textbook support: questions@spring-medical.com

Single Computer Version

The single computer version of SpringCharts will need to be installed onto each student's computer in the classroom. We recommend that SpringCharts be installed to and run from a 2GB flash drive; see further instructions below. This will eliminate the need for the students to back up and restore their data on a daily basis. The use of a flash drive enables a portable application of SpringCharts that can be used at home or any other computer that will accept the flash drive and will enable the students to continue their work outside the classroom. The single computer version of SpringCharts is not networked; therefore the instructor will not be able to view the students' exercises online. Exercises will need to be printed out and turned in or the instructor will need to view the completed exercises from the desktop of the students' computers.

Network Version

The network version of SpringCharts EHR comes in two applications; SpringCharts Server and SpringCharts Client. The downloadable network version of SpringCharts EHR will be provided to you via a personalized link. Open the zipped file and save to your computer.

> Note: The file is large and may take 15 minutes or more to download.

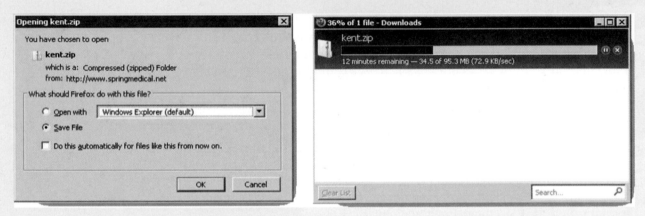

Figure 1 Saving file to computer windows.

SpringCharts Server will need to be installed on the server in the network and SpringCharts Client will need to be installed on all the computer workstations in the network. Because the instructor and the students will be on the same network, viewing of completed exercises can be done across the network. The limitation of the local network version is that students cannot work on exercises outside of the classroom.

The optimum network configuration is installing SpringCharts Server and SpringCharts Client versions in the same local computer lab. Because the system requirements for SpringCharts EHR are very conservative, a local computer can be designated as the server and the other work stations pointed to this server within the SpringCharts Client program.

System Requirements

The minimum requirements for SpringCharts **Single** Computer Version are

- An 800 MHz, or faster, processor.
- 400 MB of available disk space.
- 1 GB of memory.

- A computer running one of the following operating systems: Windows 2000 or above, Mac OS 10.4 (Tiger) or above, or Linux Red Hat Version 7 or above.

To complete all exercises in this text you will need to have access to a network printer and the Internet.

The minimum requirements for the **SpringCharts Server** network option are

- Pentium 4, or faster, processor (Xeon preferred).
- 150 GB of available disk space (after loading the JRE). This is primarily for the File Cabinet and local backups.
- 2 GB of memory.
- Computer running the following operating systems: Windows 2000 or above, or MacOS Tiger (10.4) or above. (The network computers do not need to be running the same operating system.)

The minimum requirements for the **SpringCharts Client** network option are

- 800 MHZ, or faster, processor.
- 25 MB of available disk space.
- 1 GB of memory.
- Work station computers running the following operating systems: Windows 2000 or above, or MacOS Tiger (10.4) or above. (The network computers do not need to be running the same operating system.)

Operating Environment Notice

SpringCharts is an online system that requires uninterrupted access to a minimum level of system resources. As a result, it is recommended that SpringCharts Server be located on a dedicated computer when possible.

It is also recommended that highly resource-intensive programs and/or programs that may intermittently use up the majority of system processing capacity or network bandwidth *not be run at the same time as SpringCharts*. Examples of these types of programs are

- Virus scans of the entire hard drive (scans of individual files are acceptable).
- Music streaming programs.
- Certain backup programs (when activated).

Single Computer Installation
Installing Java Runtime Environment (JRE) 1.6

JRE 1.6.0_17 must be installed on your computer before you run this version of SpringCharts EHR. The JRE version cannot be any higher than update 17 to run successfully.

- On your Internet browser type in the following address: www.java.com.
- Click the *Do I have Java?* link to test your system for the correct version of Java.
- If your computer has JRE 1.6, you do not need to upgrade.
- If your system does not meet the requirements of JRE 1.6, you will need to download JRE 1.6.0_17. **Do not download the latest version of JRE from the java website.**

Running SpringCharts from a Flash Drive

If you are working in a computer environment that uses a product like Deep Freeze™ to return the computer to its baseline configurations each day, all your work in SpringCharts will be eradicated when the computer is reset to its original state. To bypass the need to backup and restore SpringCharts data on a daily basis the SpringCharts program can be run from a flash drive that is placed into the computer's USB port daily. **You will need a 2GB flash drive.** However, if your school requires an administrative password to run programs from a flash drive you may not be able to utilize this method. Please consult with your IT department before proceeding.

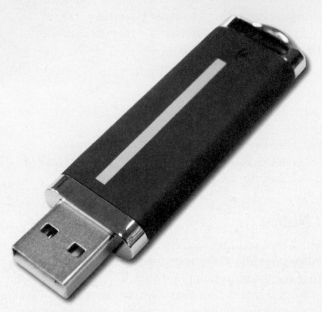

A flash drive is a portable device for memory storage. It can also referred to as a jump drive or a thumb drive. Flash drives will fit into any USB (universal serial bus) port on a computer.

Simply install JRE 1.6.0_11, SpringCharts EHR, and the *EHR material* folder as outlined in the next sections; however, **install the Java Runtime (JRE) onto the computer**, and the SpringCharts program and *EHR Material* folder to the flash drive. When installing SpringCharts you will be presented with an option to change the default location of installation (see Figure 2). To install SpringCharts to your flash drive, select this option and locate *My Computer* then choose the USB port where your flash drive is located. Once installed, a SpringCharts icon will appear on your desktop. To access SpringCharts, place your flash drive into the computer's USB port and double-click on this icon. If this icon has been removed, you will need to locate the flash drive and double-click the SpringCharts icon in the SpringCharts folder.

> Note: You will not need to backup and restore SpringCharts data when SpringCharts is operating from your flash drive.

When you close down the SpringCharts program you will be given the option to back up. If you are utilizing a flash drive simply select **No** at this point. You will also be able to place your flash drive in any computer's USB port and continue to work the exercises in this text.

Installing SpringCharts EHR on a Single Computer

The SpringCharts installation procedure has just a few easy steps. Remember, the JRE needs to be installed on your computer before SpringCharts EHR will run.

- On your Internet browser type in the following address: www.mhhe.com/HamiltonEHR2e.
- Click the *SpringCharts* link in the left-hand menu.
- Locate the *Downloading and Installing SpringCharts EHR* portion of the page.
- Click either the *SpringCharts PC Demo installer zip file* link or the *SpringCharts Mac Demo installer stuffed file* link depending on your operating system.
- Download the installer file to your computer desktop.
- Decompress the downloaded file (use a file program such as Winzip or StuffIt.)
- Double click either the **SpringChartsDEMOSetup.exe** or **SCDemoSetupMac** installation applications (depending on your operating system).
- Follow the directions offered by the installer. You will see a screen similar to the one displayed in Figure 2.

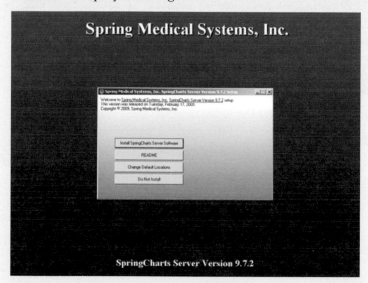

Figure 2 SpringCharts installation window.

- SpringCharts program files will be installed in the default location of C:\Program Files\SCDemo. This is the recommended installation location for a computer. To accept this default, simply click on the **Install SpringCharts Demo Software** button. However, if you are installing SpringCharts to a flash drive you will select the **Change Default Locations** button and select the appropriate drive.
- Accept the license agreement and the installation will begin.
- After the files have been successfully installed, the final installation completion screen will appear, seen in Figure 3.
- Click on the **Thanks!** button and the installation is complete.
- Close any open window and you will see a shortcut icon to SpringCharts on your desktop. Double-click on the SpringCharts icon to open the program. A *Log On* window appears, illustrated in Figure 4. The user name and password is hardcoded in. Simply select the **Log on** button.

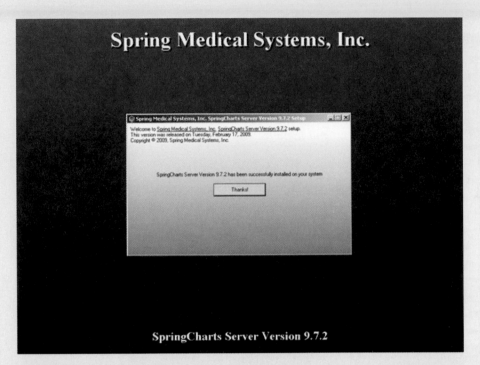

Figure 3 SpringCharts installation completion window.

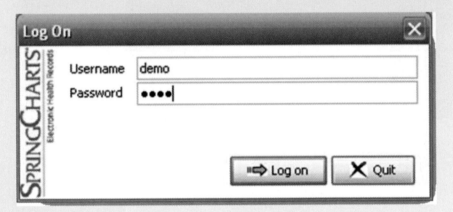

Figure 4 SpringCharts log on window.

Downloading The EHR Material Folder

There are several files that you will need to import into your SpringCharts program to complete many of the exercises in the textbook. These files are contained in the folder titled *EHR Material* on the McGraw-Hill OLC at **www.mhhe.com/ HamiltonEHR2e**.

- Access this website via your browser.
- Click the *SpringCharts* link in the left-hand menu.
- Locate the *Downloading the EHR Material folder* portion of the page.
- Click the *EHR Material* link.
- Download the zip file to your computer desktop.
- Decompress the downloaded file (use a file decompression program such as Winzip or StuffIt.)
- Once the folder has been copied to your desktop or flash drive you may close the web browser window.

Installing SpringCharts Network Option
Installing SpringCharts Server

The SpringCharts installation procedure has just a few easy steps:

1. Verify hardware requirements (see above).
2. Ensure the JRE is at the correct version (see above)
3. Install SpringCharts Server on the server.
4. Install SpringCharts Client on all the client computers.
5. Set the IP address of SpringCharts Server in SpringCharts Client version.

When these steps are completed successfully, you may begin using SpringCharts.

> Note: Download the SpringCharts program via the provided link. The zipped file contains the Server folder, Client folder, supplemental docs folder, and text file.

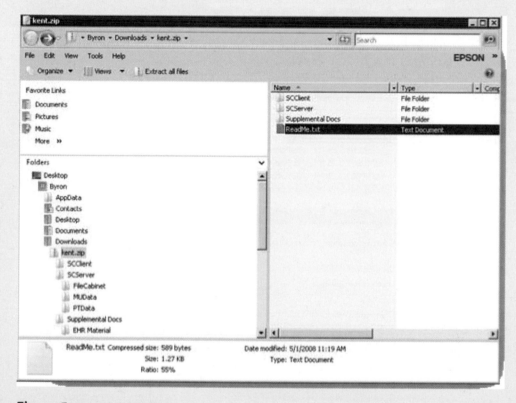

Figure 5 Downloaded file.

Double-click on SCServer where you will see the following files: FileCabinet folder, MUData folder, PtData folder, and the compressed executable file **SpringChartsServer.exe.** Double-click on the executable program and extract the files to the *Program Files* folder on the C: Drive (or other designated drive). (See *INSTALLING SPRINGCHARTS IN WINDOWS VISTA* below for installation within the Vista operating system.)

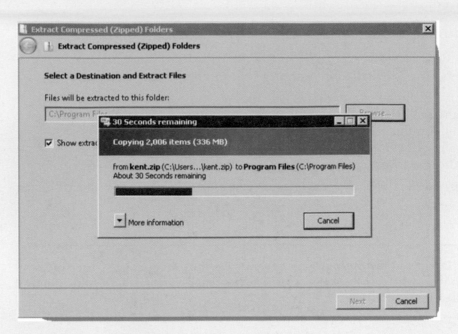

Figure 6 Extracting zipped SpringCharts program files.

An SCServer folder and an SCClient folder will be created in the *Program Files* folder containing the above-mentioned folders, and an SCServer folder will be placed on the desktop. Double-click on **SpringCharts Server.exe** in this folder to launch the installation program.

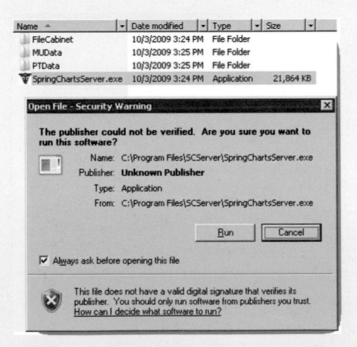

Figure 7 Installing SpringCharts Server.

> Note: The SpringCharts Server program must be running at all times for the SpringCharts Client program to access the database.

To locate the IP address of SpringCharts Server, click on the *File* menu and select *SpringCharts Info*. The *Program Information* window contains the IP address that you will need when activating each SpringCharts Client program for the first time. Write this address down.

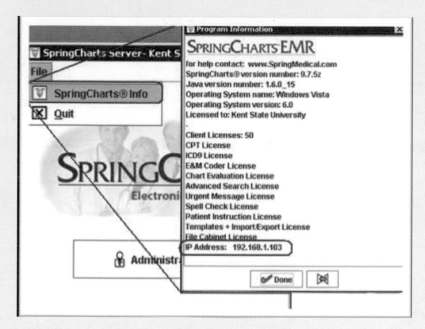

Figure 8 Locating SpringCharts Server IP address.

Installing SpringCharts Client

The SCClient folder on the server can now be copied across the network and installed in the *Program Files* folder on the C: Drive (or other designated drive) of each work station. (See *INSTALLING SPRINGCHARTS IN WINDOWS VISTA* below for installation within the Vista operating system.)

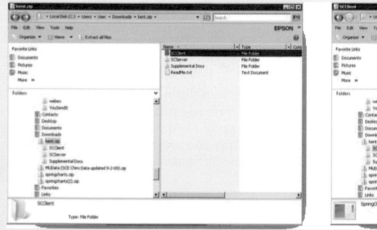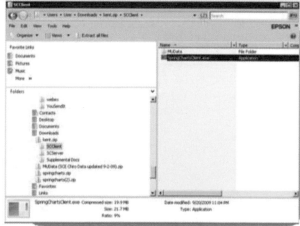

Figure 9 Installing SpringCharts Client program.

Double-click on the **SpringCharts Client.exe** in this folder to launch the installation program. You will be presented with *Log On* window; enter the following **Username:** *demo* and **Password:** *demo*.

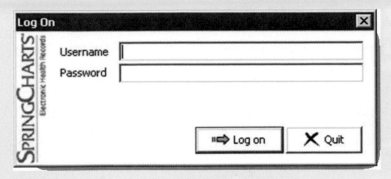

Figure 10 Logging on to SpringCharts Client program.

You will then be asked for the IP address of SpringCharts Server. Enter the IP address that you noted in the *Program Information* window of SpringCharts Server.

Loading The EHR Materials Folder

Contained within the *Supplemental Docs* folder that was downloaded, you will find the *EHR Materials* folder. The *EHR Materials* folder will need to be copied across the network and placed on each workstation. Students will access this folder and retrieve files to complete various exercises.

Adding Additional Users

The network version of SpringCharts EHR that accompanies the *Electronic Health Record* textbook by Hamilton comes loaded with 50 user accounts and the accompanying pop-up text for each user. Each user account is set up on SpringCharts Server under the **Users** button. If you require additional simultaneous users operating in SpringCharts it will be necessary to add additional user accounts. Locate the **Adding Additional Users and PopUp Text. pdf** file in the *Supplemental Docs* folder of the downloaded file and follow the instructions.

Installing SpringCharts EHR on a Windows Terminal Server

SpringCharts can run on a Microsoft Windows Terminal Server in one of two fashions. The choice depends on the hardware resources that are available and the number of concurrent users that are expected to access SpringCharts during peak usage. In either case, the installation procedures are the same whether you are installing the SpringCharts Server or the SpringCharts Client.

Single Server Method

If resources are not an issue, then the Single Server Installation (Figure 11) might be a good choice.

- Set up Terminal Services as instructed by Microsoft, and create a user account for each student that will be accessing SpringCharts.
- Install SpringCharts Server (see Installation Guide for instructions).
- Install SpringCharts Client to the folder of your choosing (see Installation

> Note: the folder where you installed the SpringCharts Server needs to have modified permissions for all users.

Guide for instructions). Run the SpringCharts Client once, in order to configure the client with the Server's IP address.

- Copy the SpringCharts Client folder to each user's home directory, giving each user a copy of the SpringCharts Client.
- Set the login script to run SpringCharts Client whenever the user logs in (this is optional), or simply put a shortcut on each user's desktop for his SpringCharts Client.

System Requirements

The minimum requirements for running SpringCharts on a single terminal server are

- (2) Dual Core 2.8 GHz Xeon Processors or comparable.
- 24+ GB RAM (1 GB per user plus 2 GB for the SpringCharts Server).
- 10 GB of Free Disk Space.

This configuration should support 20 to 30 concurrent SpringCharts Client users, with the amount of physical memory being the deciding factor.

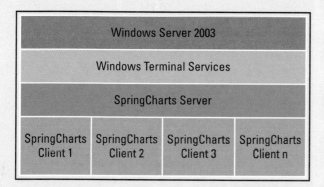

Figure 11 Running SpringCharts on a single terminal server.

Multiple Server Method

Another option is to install SpringCharts over multiple servers (Figure 12). This option would be preferable if hardware is limited and you want to spread users over multiple resources.

- Set up Terminal Services as instructed by Microsoft, and create a user account for each student that will be accessing SpringCharts.
- Install SpringCharts Server (see Installation Guide for instructions).

> Note: the folder where you installed the SpringCharts Server needs to have modified permissions for all users.

- Install SpringCharts Client to the folder of your choosing (see Installation Guide for instructions). Run the SpringCharts Client once, in order to configure the client with the Server's IP address.

- Copy the SpringCharts Client folder to each user's home directory, giving each user a copy of the SpringCharts Client.
- Set the login script to run SpringCharts Client whenever the user logs in (this is optional), or simply put a shortcut on each user's desktop for his SpringCharts Client.

System Requirements
The minimum requirements for running SpringCharts on multiple servers are

SERVER:
- Dual Core Pentium 2 GHz or higher
- 4 GB RAM (2 GB for SpringCharts Server and 2 for the OS)
- 10 GB of Free Disk Space

CLIENTS:
- (2) Dual Core 2.8 GHz Xeon Processors or comparable
- 24+ GB RAM (1 GB per user plus 2 GB for the SpringCharts Server)

This configuration should support 20 to 30 concurrent SpringCharts Client users, with the amount of physical memory being the deciding factor. As an option, you can lower your server requirements for each Client server by splitting the clients over multiple terminal servers.

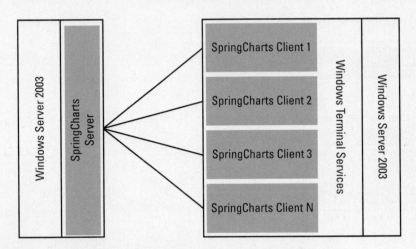

Figure 12 Running SpringCharts on multiple terminal servers.

Backing Up Your Files

If you are working in a computer environment that uses a product like Deep Freeze™ to return the computer to its baseline configurations each day, all your work in SpringCharts will be eradicated when the computer is reset to its original state. It is important that you backup SpringCharts at the close of your session. **You will need a 2GB flash drive.**

> Note: If you are running SpringCharts from your own flash drive, you will not need to perform a backup of the program files. See earlier section titled *RUNNING SPRINGCHARTS FROM A FLASH DRIVE* for details.

The SpringCharts application automatically activates the system backup each time you shut down the program. The process may take several minutes. The MUData and PtData folders from the SpringCharts directory are included in the backup.

Use the following steps to back up and restore your data.

1. Click on the main *File* menu option in the *Practice View* window.
2. Click on the **Quit** submenu option to exit the program. The following window opens.

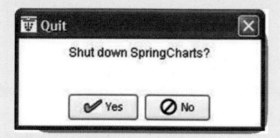

Figure 13 Shut down SpringCharts confirmation window.

3. Click on the **Yes** button to close the program. The following window opens.

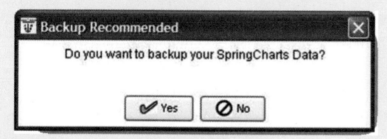

Figure 14 Backing up SpringCharts Data option window.

4. Click on the **Yes** button to start the backup process. The following window opens.

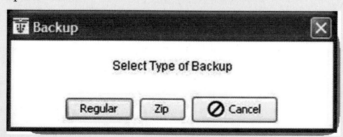

Figure 15 Regular or Zip backup option window.

5. Click on the **Zip** button. The following window opens.
6. Click on *My Computer* in the left side column. Select the USB drive into which you have placed your USB flash drive. The drive name appears in the **File Name** field.
7. Click on the **Backup To This Folder** button to start the backup process. The following window appears while the program backs up the data.

The program automatically shuts down when the backup is complete. Remove your flash drive.

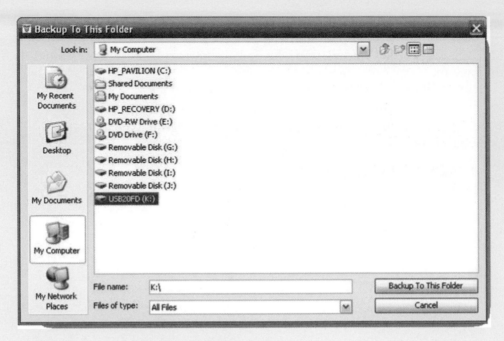

Figure 16 Backup destination window.

Restoring Your SpringCharts Files

You will only need to restore your SpringCharts data if you are working in a computer environment that removes all added data to the program and restores the computer to its original configuration each day. To restore your data follow these steps.

1. Open your SpringCharts program.
2. Click on the *Administration* menu. Select the *Restore Data From Zip Backup* option.

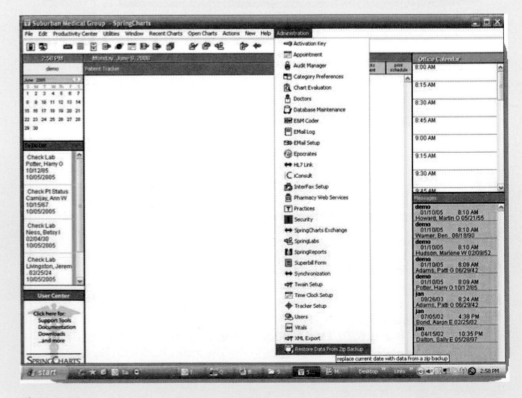

Figure 17 Locating the Restore Data window.

3. In the subsequent *Restore from this zip file* window, click on *My Computer* in the left side column. Double-click on the USB drive into which you have placed your USB flash drive. The next window will display all the files on your flash drive. Select the backup zip file. The file name appears in the **File name** field.

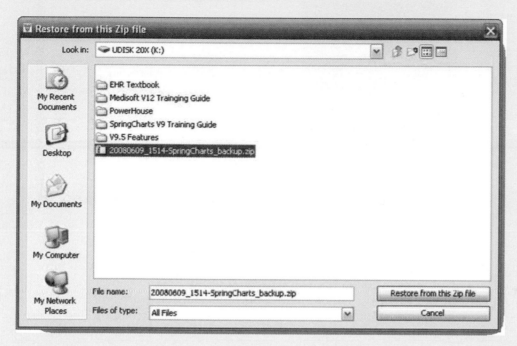

Figure 18 Locating the Restore Data file window.

4. Click on the **Restore from this Zip file** button in the lower right corner.

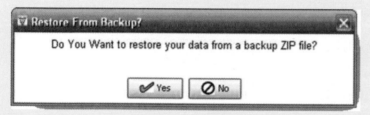

Figure 19 Restore backup confirmation window.

5. Confirm that you want to restore data from your backup zip file. SpringCharts will automatically shut down in order to perform the restoration process.

6. Once the restoration of the backup data is completed, you will need to restart the SpringCharts program.

Installing SpringCharts in Windows Vista

SpringCharts is compatible with Microsoft Windows Vista; however, because of the added security features it is **not** recommended that SpringCharts be installed to the normal default location of *Program Files*. In order to configure SpringCharts Client or SpringCharts Single Computer Version to run on a Windows Vista computer, the steps below will need to be followed.

1. Turn off User Access Control (UAC). The easiest way to disable UAC is through the User Account Control Panel shown in Figure 20.

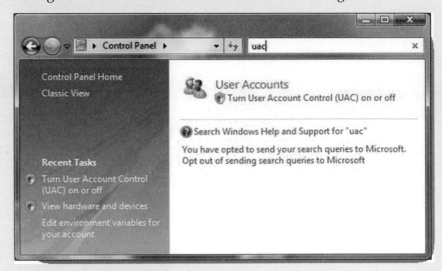

Figure 20 Turning off User accounts.

2. Make sure that the SpringCharts Client folder (SCClient) or Single Computer Version folder (SCharts) is located in the Root folder (C:). If SpringCharts Client or Single Computer Version is already installed on the computer, simply cut and paste the corresponding folder to the C: drive. If this is a new installation, you can change the location of the installation by clicking on *Change Default Location* on the first screen of the installation program.

3. Finally, change the permissions on the folder to Modify Access for Users and Everyone. This is done by right-clicking on the folder and clicking on Properties. Then, click on the tab labeled Security. In this panel, make sure that Users and Everyone have modify access.

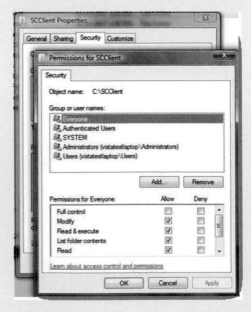

Figure 21 Changing permission accounts window.

Acknowledgments

Electronic Health Records is dedicated to my wife Leesa and daughter Kelsey, whose inspiration, love, patience, and understanding allowed me the countless hours for preparing this text when I could not play, and whose faith provided motivation when my own was dwindling.

Electronic Health Records is dedicated to Gregory Barton who has worked side by side with me for more than a decade in the ever-changing medical community. We have labored together in medical billing, medical management and supervision, and medical consultation and training. His contribution in research has provided the historical backdrop for this text. Greg continues to bring dynamic training across the country, both onsite and online, to medical practices with his expertise in medical billing software and electronic health records.

Electronic Health Records is also dedicated to my good friend and fellow EHR trainer, Steve Burnich, who painstakingly extracted hundreds of review questions from the text.

My appreciation is extended to Jack B. Smyth, President and CEO of Spring Medical Systems Inc. and Ken Santoro, Director of Support and Operations at Spring Medical Systems Inc. for the contribution of the *SpringCharts EHR* program for every student. The incorporation of this full-featured, popular electronic health record software has taken the medical student from a sterile, abstract setting to a dynamic, realistic learning environment. This hands-on experience will successfully equip each student with the knowledge and confidence necessary to contribute to the electronic health records in the medical office.

For insightful reviews, criticisms, helpful suggestions, and information, we would like to acknowledge the following:

Second Edition Reviewers

Hooshiyar Ahmadi, MD, DC
Remington College Dallas
  Campus

Gail Albert, CMA (AAMA)
Berks Technical Institute

Yvonne Beth Alles, MBA
Davenport University

Mary Ann Alspaugh,
RETS College

Cynthia Boles, BS, MBA, CMA
Bradford School

Robin K. Choate, LPN, CHI
Pennsylvania Institute of
  Technology

Tracie Fuqua, B.S., CMA (AAMA)
Wallace State Community College

Daniel F. Gant, BS, MDiv
Savannah River College

Vonda R. Godette, RN, MSN,
  CMA (AAMA)
Carteret Community College

Randi Haight, CPC
Sanford Brown Institute

Salesi F. Havili, DSM, DPed
Eagle Gate College

Elizabeth Hoffman, MA Ed., CMA
  (AAMA), CPT (ASPT)
Baker College

Jody Kirk, BS, CCA
Cambria-Rowe Business College

Leigh Ann Long, RN
Brookstone College of Business

Tabitha Lyons, NCMA
High-Tech Institute
TCI Education

Robin Maddalena
Branford Hall Career Institute

Annette Martijn, BS
Remington College

Teresa Montgomery, CMA
Brookstone College

Quang Myers-Stallings, BS, MBA
SBI

Lisa Nagle, CMA (AAMA), BS ed
Augusta Technical College

Kathleen M. Olewinski, MS,
RHIA, NHA, FACHE
Bryant & Stratton College

Angela Parmley-Williams, MBA
Sanford Brown Institute

Becky Rodenbaugh, CMA
(AAMA), MBA
Baker College

Shelley C. Safian, MAOM/HSM,
CCS-P, CPC-H
Berkeley College

Rose Scaringella, BA
Hunter Business School

Amy Semenchuk, RN, BSN
Rockford Career College

Lynn G. Slack, BS CMA
Kaplan Career Institute – ICM
Campus

Catherine A. Teel, AST, RMA,
CMA
McCann School of Business and
Technology

Marilyn M. Turner, RN, CMA
(AAMA)
Ogeechee Technical College

Marta E. Urdaneta, PhD
Keiser University

Katrina Varner, BS
Centura College

Lori A. Warren, MA, RN, CPC,
CPC-I, CCP, CLNC
Spencerian College

Stacey F. Wilson, CMA, MT, MHA
Cabarrus College of Health
Sciences

Barbara Worley
King's College

Lori D. Wright, AS
Cambria-Rowe Business College

Jane Yakicic, CMA, CCA
CRBC

Janet M. York, BS
TN Technology Center

First Edition Reviewers

Marty Bachman, PhD, RN
Front Range Community College

Beth Anne Batturs, MSN
Anne Arundel Community
College

Kim Bell, RHIA
Edgecombe Community College

Norma Bird, MEd, BS, CMA
Idaho State University College of
Technology

Lauralyn K. Burke, MS, RHIA,
CHES
Florida A&M University
Division of Health Information
Management

Barbara Desch, LVN, CPC, AHI
San Joaquin Valley College, Inc.

Jane W. Dumas, MSN
Remington College

Catherine Gierman-Riblon, RN,
MEd
Career Education Corporation

Cheri Goretti, BS, MA
Quinebaug Valley Community
College

Grethel Gomez, AS
Florida Career College

James N. Hader, BS
Bryant & Stratton College

Tiffany Heath, CMA, CS, AHI
Sanford Brown Institute

Beulah A. Hofmann, BSN, MSN,
CMA
Ivy Tech Community College

Susan Horn, AAS, CMA
Indiana Business College

Dawn W. Jackson, MAEd, RHIA
Eastern Kentucky University

Josephine Jackyra, MLT, CMA
The Technical Institute of Camden
County

Carol Lee Jarrell, MLT
Brown Mackie College

Cindy Johnson, BS, M.Ed.
Arapahoe Community College

Crystal Kitchens, CMT, MA
Richland Community College

Jennifer Loddo, L.P.N.
Sanford Brown Institute

Sandy Ludwig, RN, MSN, NNP
Eastern Arizona College

Christine Malone, MHA
Everett Community College

Michael Meyer, DO, CCS, CPC
Florida Memorial University,
DeVry University, and Herzing
College

Jeffrey Rivera, RN, BSN, MBA
Florida Memorial University

Cynthia Thompson, RN, BS, MA
Davenport University

Barbara Tietsort, M.Ed.
University of Cincinnati

Marilyn M. Turner, RN, CMA
Ogeechee Technical College

Marianne Van Deursen, BS, CMA
Warren County Community
College

Dana Woods, AAS, BS
Southwestern Illinois College

walkthrough

Chapter Openers

Every chapter opens with Learning Outcomes, Key Terms, and a What You Need to Know section that prepares the student for the chapter they are about to read.

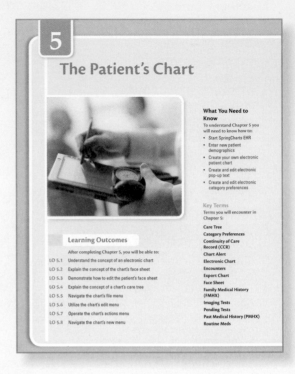

5

The Patient's Chart

What You Need to Know
To understand Chapter 5 you will need to know how to:
- Start SpringCharts EHR
- Enter new patient demographics
- Create your own electronic patient chart
- Create and edit electronic pop-up text
- Create and edit electronic category preferences

Key Terms
Terms you will encounter in Chapter 5:

Care Tree
Category Preferences
Continuity of Care Record (CCR)
Chart Alert
Electronic Chart
Encounters
Export Chart
Face Sheet
Family Medical History (FMHX)
Imaging Tests
Pending Tests
Past Medical History (PMHX)
Routine Meds

Learning Outcomes

After completing Chapter 5, you will be able to:

LO 5.1 Understand the concept of an electronic chart
LO 5.2 Explain the concept of the chart's face sheet
LO 5.3 Demonstrate how to edit the patient's face sheet
LO 5.4 Explain the concept of a chart's care tree
LO 5.5 Navigate the chart's file menu
LO 5.6 Utilize the chart's edit menu
LO 5.7 Operate the chart's actions menu
LO 5.8 Navigate the chart's new menu

Learning Outcomes Tags

Each section heading, Concept Checkup box, practice exercise, and review question is tied directly to the chapter's learning outcomes. This tagging allows instructors to move students from general theory to application in a step-by-step, logical manner through a variety of activities and exercises tied to the learning outcomes of the chapter.

2 Chapter One

Focal Point
Improvement to the quality of patient medical care and safety has always been the catalyst for the development of the electronic health record concept.

Electronic Health Record (EHR)
Electronic health records is the most commonly accepted term for software with a full range of functionalities to store, access, and use patient medical information.

LO 1.1 THE ELECTRONIC HEALTH RECORD HISTORY

The concept of a patient's medical information stored electronically instead of on paper is not a new one. In the 1960s, as medical care became more complex, doctors realized that in certain situations the patient's complete health history would not be accessible to them. The availability of comprehensive medical information when needed brought the innovation of storing the patient's information electronically. Improvement of patient medical care was and is the catalyst for the **electronic health record (EHR)**.

The Mayo Clinic in Rochester, Minnesota, and the Medical Center Hospital of Vermont were some of the first clinics to utilize an electronic medical record system. Their systems were developed in the early 1960s. Over the next two decades, more information and functionalities were added to the electronic medical record system in order to improve patient care. Drug dosages, side effects, allergies, and drug interactions became available electronically to doctors, enabling that information to be incorporated into electronic health-care systems. Electronic diagnostic and treatment plans, which gave doctors information for patient care, proliferated and were integrated into electronic medical record systems. More academic and research institutes developed their own computerized medical record systems as tools to track patient treatment. Overall, the utilization and growth of these computer models was to increase the quality of patient care.

LO 1.2 METHODS OF DATA ENTRY

As computer technology continues to rapidly develop, the versatility of the EHR becomes greater. Access through the EHR to patient information, medi-

Focal Points

Focal Point
The message center in SpringCharts enables the user to send and receive messages from coworkers or e-mail messages from out of the office.

Focal Points appear throughout the text as marginal inserts spotlighting critical data necessary to master end-of-chapter review quizzes.

Key Term Definitions

Key Term definitions appear in the margin every time a new Key Term is introduced for quick and easy reference.

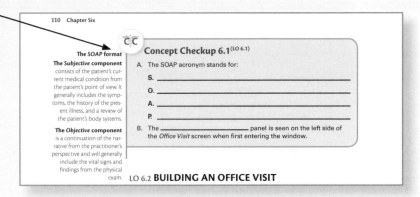

142 Chapter Seven

Chart Evaluation
Used to define criteria to search patient charts for health needs in order to support disease management, routine preventive services, and wellness health-care standards.

Wellness Screenings
Periodic medical checkups to test for or inoculate against significant diseases. Wellness screenings are preventive services given before the onset of chief complaints.

LO 7.1 CHART EVALUATION

SpringCharts' **chart evaluation** feature allows users to define preventive health criteria and then assess patients' charts by these criteria. This enables the physician to be proactive in the **wellness screenings** of patients. In order to set up chart evaluations, the administrator will select *Chart Evaluation* from the *Administration* menu, seen in Figure 7.1. (In a networked environment the *Administrator* panel is accessible on SpringCharts Server.) From this window the user can access the *National Guideline Clearinghouse* (NGC) through the Internet to evaluate medical standards for wellness screenings. This information from NGC can then be set up within SpringCharts to provide ongoing chart evaluations.

Selecting the [New] button presents the *Evaluation Item* window for setting up evaluation criteria, illustrated in Figure 7.2.

In the setup window, users will define criteria specifications by:

1. *Gender*—Select whether a criterion is specific to male, female, or either one.
2. *Age*—Select the age within which the criteria should be met.
3. *Actions*— Indicate the *Test*, *Procedure*, or *Encounter* required to meet the criteria.

Concept Checkups

Concept Checkups follow each topic, breaking down learning outcomes into manageable subject material.

110 Chapter Six

The SOAP format
The *Subjective* component consists of the patient's current medical condition from the patient's point of view. It generally includes the symptoms, the history of the present illness, and a review of the patient's body systems.

The *Objective* component is a continuation of the narrative from the practitioner's perspective and will generally include the vital signs and findings from the physical exam.

C C

Concept Checkup 6.1 (LO 6.1)

A. The SOAP acronym stands for:

S. _____

O. _____

A. _____

P. _____

B. The _____ panel is seen on the left side of the *Office Visit* screen when first entering the window.

LO 6.2 BUILDING AN OFFICE VISIT

Chapter Review

Each chapter ends with a review including Using Terminology, Checking Your Understanding, fill in the blank, and multiple choice questions to reinforce the learning outcomes that were presented in the chapter.

chapter 7 review

Name _____ Instructor _____ Class _____

USING TERMINOLOGY

Match the terms on the left with the definitions on the right.

_____ 1. Superbill
_____ 2. Wellness screenings
_____ 3. Care plans
_____ 4. Chart evaluations
_____ 5. E&M coder
_____ 6. Patient instruction manager
_____ 7. NGC
_____ 8. NewCrop RX
_____ 9. Well woman visit
_____ 10. Encounters
_____ 11. Draw program
_____ 12. RTF

A. Determines the correct evaluation and management CPT code for office visit encounters.[LO 7.5]
B. In this feature patient instructions can be modified and new ones created.[LO 7.5]
C. A comprehensive database of evidence-based practice guidelines known as the National Guidance Clearinghouse.[LO 7.4]
D. The drug interaction and allergy checking feature is a SpringCharts interface with this web-based company.[LO 7.5]
E. Practice guidelines are specific documents that provide a "road map" to guide all who are involved with a patient's care.[LO 7.6]
F. Chart evaluation summaries are automatically recorded in the care tree under this category.[LO 7.1]
G. Periodical medical checkups to test for or inoculate against significant diseases.[LO 7.3]
H. A feature in the *Tools* menu of the *office* visit screen that enables the provider to illustrate procedures on built-in templates.[LO 7.6]
I. A SpringCharts feature used to establish criteria for medical checkups and appraise patients' charts for needed health screenings and test.[LO 7.1]
J. When a new patient instruction is needed it must be created in this format to save into SpringCharts.[LO 7.5]
K. An annual pap smear would be included in this encounter and recorded in an office visit note.[LO 7.3]
L. In SpringCharts this panel contains additional codes that can be added to the routing slip for the purposes of billing.[LO 7.4]

CHECKING YOUR UNDERSTANDING

Write "T" or "F" in the blank to indicate whether you think the statement is true or false.

_____ 13. Patient instructions can be created in SpringCharts then accessed in the *Office Visit* screen to print or e-mail the patient.[LO 7.5]

_____ 14. The customized superbill may display procedures and codes such as vehicle-punctures, shunts, and other billable and non-billable items.[LO 7.4]

_____ 15. Some key words in the E&M coder are: review of systology, examine body crustaceans, and organic systems.[LO 7.5]

_____ 16. You cannot set up chart evaluations on SpringCharts Server in a network environment.[LO 7.1]

164

1

An Introduction to Electronic Health Records

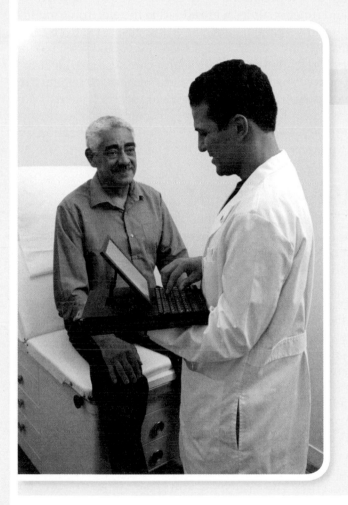

Learning Outcomes

After completing Chapter 1, you will be able to:

LO 1.1   Explain a brief history of Electronic Health Records (EHRs)

LO 1.2   Identify the methods of entering information in an EHR program

LO 1.3   List the acronyms for EHRs

LO 1.4   Explain the barriers to EHR use

LO 1.5   Describe the benefits of EHR

LO 1.6   Discuss the current EHR incentives

What You Need to Know

To understand Chapter 1 you will need to know:

- The concept of a patient's chart in a medical office

Key Terms

Terms and abbreviations you will encounter in Chapter 1:

Ambulatory EHR

American Recovery and Reinvestment Act (ARRA)

Application Server Provider (ASP)

Continuity of Care Record (CCR)

Centers for Medicare and Medicaid Services (CMS)

Electronic Health Record (EHR)

Evaluation and Management (E&M) Code

Electronic Medical Record (EMR)

Encrypted

Interoperability

Intranet Technologies

Local Area Network (LAN)

Personal Health Record (PHR)

Point of Care

Return on Investment (ROI)

Tablet PC

LO 1.1 THE ELECTRONIC HEALTH RECORD HISTORY

The concept of a patient's medical information stored electronically instead of on paper is not a new one. In the 1960s, as medical care became more complex, doctors realized that in certain situations the patient's complete health history would not be accessible to them. The availability of comprehensive medical information when needed brought the innovation of storing the patient's information electronically. Improvement of patient medical care was and is the catalyst for the **electronic health record (EHR)**.

The Mayo Clinic in Rochester, Minnesota, and the Medical Center Hospital of Vermont were some of the first clinics to utilize an electronic medical record system. Their systems were developed in the early 1960s. Over the next two decades, more information and functionalities were added to the electronic medical record system in order to improve patient care. Drug dosages, side effects, allergies, and drug interactions became available electronically to doctors, enabling that information to be incorporated into electronic health-care systems. Electronic diagnostic and treatment plans, which gave doctors information for patient care, proliferated and were integrated into electronic medical record systems. More academic and research institutes developed their own computerized medical record systems as tools to track patient treatment. Overall, the utilization and growth of these computer models was to increase the quality of patient care.

LO 1.2 METHODS OF DATA ENTRY

As computer technology continues to rapidly develop, the versatility of the EHR becomes greater. Access through the EHR to patient information, medical alerts, warnings, drug information, and disease management is now at the **point of care** for the health-care provider in a more user-friendly form. Modes of data entry into the EHR have progressed. Traditionally, a keyboard was the only source for data entry. However, the need for convenience, efficiency, and speed has mandated other methods. Voice recognition systems adapt to a person's voice and speech patterns so that the computer inputs data directly into the EHR program as the operator speaks. Electronic handwriting recognition is also now available. These two methods of data input are not commonly used because they require that the user repeat the same verbiage each time the data is needed. More commonly, large bodies of preset text known as "templates" can be easily selected to input into the patient's record. Instead of significant amounts of typing, health-care providers can enter data and access data through a few taps of a stylus pen on a touch screen or the click of a mouse. Touch screens are utilized on such devices as a Notebook Tablet or a **Tablet PC**, making the EHR portable and accessible for easy data entry. The ease of use and speed of the "Tap&Go"™ feature with the Tablet PC has made EHRs more desirable. Traditionally, a stationary computer workstation in each exam room has been cost-prohibitive for the independent physician, or a desktop computer may not be available at the point of care, resulting in delayed data entry, thus patient information is not readily available to other physicians and medical support staff. However, in recent years the increased use of laptops, Tablet PCs, and wireless connectivity has brought greater mobility and lower costs to the health-care provider.

Networks have advanced in security and reliability to enable both flexibility and mobility of the EHR. A **Local Area Network (LAN)** enables computers to communicate together and utilize a main server for the database. The LAN system is very customizable, according to the office needs. This network system may consist of wired connections and/or utilize a wireless network as

Focal Point

Improvement to the quality of patient medical care and safety has always been the catalyst for the development of the electronic health record concept.

Electronic Health Record (EHR)
Electronic health records is the most commonly accepted term for software with a full range of functionalities to store, access, and use patient medical information.

Point of Care
Point of care is the time and place of care being given to the patient from the health-care provider.

Tablet PC
A portable, handheld computer with the ability to document directly on the screen with a stylus pen.

Local Area Network (LAN)
A wired and/or wireless connection of computers on a single campus or facility.

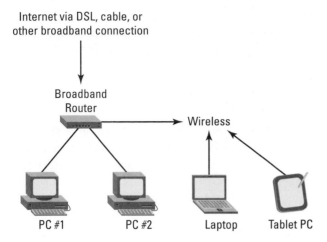

Internet via DSL, cable, or other broadband connection

Broadband Router

Wireless

PC #1   PC #2   Laptop   Tablet PC

Figure 1.1 Hardwired and wireless LAN system.

illustrated in Figure 1.1. The wireless LAN networks enable health-care providers full or open access to their EHRs from anywhere within their office.

Internet and **intranet technologies** have increased the availability of medical databases that can be shared and accessed across large distances. This remote access gives health-care providers entrance to their EHR from such remote locations as nursing homes, a home office, or hospitals through an Internet connection. These networks are secure and access is limited. Data flowing on the network is also **encrypted** for security.

Another network option for a medical practice is the web-based EHR or **Application Server Provider (ASP)**. The EHR is accessed by the health-care provider via the Internet. In this model, the medical practice does not house the software on a computer server at the medical office. Maintenance, updates, and backups are conducted remotely by the EHR web-hosting company. High-speed

Concept Checkup 1.1 (LO 1.1, LO 1.2)

A. _____
was the initial reason, and continues to be the reason, for the development of electronic health records (EHRs).

B. Several modes of data entry into the EHR programs exist. Some of these methods of data entry are:

1. _____

2. _____

3. _____

4. _____

C. What two types of technologies have increased the availability of medical databases and access to the EHR?

1. _____

2. _____

Focal Point
The affordability of both hardware and software, and the reliability of intranet technology and wireless connectivity have enabled many independent physicians to take advantage of the EHR in recent years.

Intranet Technologies
Intranet technology is a privately maintained computer network that provides secure accessibility to authorized persons, especially members or employees of an organization, enabling the sharing of software, database, and files.

Encrypted
When computer data is changed from its original form to be transmitted securely so as to be unintelligible to unauthorized parties and then decrypted back into its original form for use.

Application Server Provider (ASP)
This enables a doctor's office to access an EHR via the Internet; the EHR software and database are housed and maintained by a separate company in a remote location.

Internet connectivity is required in this situation. However, concerns can be the security of the EHR, the speed of downloading and uploading images or large files, and ensuring that the Internet connectivity is always available.[1]

LO 1.3 ACRONYM ALPHABET SOUP

An alphabet soup of acronyms surrounds electronic health records (EHRs). Some of these definitions have been flexible and reveal an evolution of terms and meanings to government agencies and independent associations influencing the field of electronic health records. The differences are not just semantics; the terms have evolved with more and more distinct definitions. They disclose some of the history in the progression of the electronic health record. However, although the following terms and meanings are supplied to help with clarity, the various acronyms can all still be used to describe the concept of an electronic health record.

Electronic Medical Record (EMR)
The term for software that lacks a full range of higher-end functionalities to store, access, and use patient medical information.

Interoperability
Interoperability is the ability of a software program to accept, send, or communicate data from its database to other software programs from multiple vendors.

Continuity of Care Record (CCR)
A core set of provider-oriented health data reflecting the most relevant and timely facts about a patient's health care. It is vendor and technology neutral, enabling the access of patient information between health-care providers.

EHR - Electronic Health Record: Currently, this term is the most commonly accepted and used term for storing and accessing patient medical information electronically. EHR encompasses a full range of functionalities and information including patient demographics, progress notes, problems, medications, vital signs, past medical history, immunizations, laboratory data, radiology reports, scheduling, transcription, e-prescribing, evaluation and management (office visit level) coding, care alerts, chief complaints, evidence-based decision support, and health maintenance. In the future, an EHR will include a continuity of care record (CCR) and the personal health record (PHR); standards for these functionalities are still being developed.

EMR - Electronic Medical Record: This term was widely used as the terms migrated away from the computer-based patient record. As definition of terms became clearer, **EMR** came in second to the fully functional EHR. An EMR does not offer certain high-end functionalities such as health maintenance and disease management, care alerts, the CCR (continuity of care record), personal health record functions, or interconnectivity with providers outside the practice.

CPR - Computer-Based Patient Record: This term was one of the first used to conceptualize the idea of an EHR. A computerized patient record is a lifetime patient record that includes all information from all specialties (even dentistry and psychiatry) and is available to all providers (potentially internationally). Because the CPR requires full **interoperability** between EHRs, the CPR is not realistic in the foreseeable future. In the early 1990s there was an initiative to use the CPR; however, the concept evolved into the EMR and EHR.

EPR - Electronic Patient Record: EPR is similar to the CPR but does not necessarily contain a patient's lifetime record and does not include dental, behavioral, or alternative care. It focuses on the patient's relevant medical information.

CCR - Continuity of Care Record: The **CCR** is health-provider-oriented and defines a core set of data reflecting the most relevant and timely facts about a patient's health care. The CCR would be a subset of the EHR. Typically it includes patient information, diagnoses, recent procedures, allergies, medications, and future treatment plans. It should be accessible to all care providers whenever needed. The electronic CCR is designed to be vendor and technology neutral, that is, accessible and readable by other electronic systems. The CCR should be updated by the practitioner at the close of a patient encounter or upon the transfer of data from one caregiver to another, whether inpatient-, outpatient-, or community-based.

PHR - Personal Health Record: The **PHR** allows the patient to become an interactive source of health information and health management through an Internet-based connection to the practice website. Through a secure connection, patients may schedule appointments, request medication refills, access lab or radiology results, and ask questions about their health. Some PHRs enable patients to complete or update family or social histories or even read their medical records and notify providers of incorrect or missing information.

Concept Checkup 1.2 (LO 1.3)

A. What is most commonly accepted term for storing and accessing patient medical information electronically? _____

B. What term was one of the first used to conceptualize the idea of an electronic health record (EHR)?

_____

Personal Health Record (PHR)

PHRs allow the patient access via the Internet to store and update personal medical information and make inquires to the patient's health-care provider about prescriptions, appointments, or concerns.

LO 1.4 BARRIERS TO THE EHR

Although Electronic Health Records (EHRs) bring tremendous benefits to patient care and to the health-care provider, use of the **ambulatory EHR** instead of the paper chart did not become widespread among the independent physicians during the 1990s. Even though the motivation of improved patient care and availability of medical data was present, health-care providers were hesitant to begin using this medical tool. Specific reasons have been hypothesized for the lack of EHR implementation, and they are outlined below.

A Lack of Standards for EHR Systems

The content within the systems did not have uniformity for compatibility or interoperability. Various programs offered different features and the exchange of data was not possible. Also, standards for the security of confidential information through encryption or data integrity had not been set. The quality of EHR programs and computer networks was not sufficiently reliable to prevent downtime, thus resulting at times in the lack of access to patient information or medical information. Data for clinical protocols, management of patient care, and decision support through algorithms were not yet standard for EHRs.

Unknown Cost and Return on Investment

Health-care providers found it difficult to accurately calculate costs and **Return on Investment** (**ROI**) with the use of an EHR. The full cost of an EHR includes the software purchase price, additional computer hardware, implementation including the training of staff, customization of the system, ongoing technical support, system maintenance, and future program upgrades. Measuring ROI

Ambulatory EHR

The word *ambulatory* indicates the ability to walk from one place to another. When referring to EHR programs it indicates those used in physicians' offices as contrasted with EHR programs used in inpatient settings.

Return on Investment (ROI)

The measure, expressed as a percentage, of the amount that is earned on a company's total purchase or investment calculated by dividing the total capital into earnings or financial benefits.

includes intangible, immeasurable, and nonfinancial information, such as improved patient care, patient safety, and more efficient processes. Measurable financial ROI includes increase in income from more accurate coding, greater time efficiency as a result of rapid chart documentation, expanded patient load because of this efficiency, and reduced office supply costs such as paper, charts, and printing supplies. It was difficult to accurately calculate costs and ROI with the use of an EHR.

Difficult to Operate

Doctors perceived that it took more time for data entry than handwriting. A physician order form may have been simpler to handwrite than to process through a computer system. Learning where the information should be entered or accessed was complicated and computers were not always accessible at the point of care. System warnings and medical alerts containing vital information had not been developed. The long-term benefits were difficult for some health-care providers to value over the perceived difficulties of operation.

Significant Changes in Clinic Processes

Although an EHR can be customized for specific medical practices, there is always some process change required by the provider and medical staff. An EHR may bring a more rigid structure for entering information than flipping through a paper chart. Adapting to new standards of operation for entering and locating information can be difficult initially. Some EHRs have specifications or specific routines for practicing medicine that the provider may not adapt to easily. The health-care provider may not be able to address and analyze problems in the same ways that may have been done in the past, even though the information in an EHR is more thorough and instantly available. New tools for improved patient care require retraining, new processes, and changes in the medical practice culture.

Lack of Trust and Safety

A concern for the security of the medical record stored electronically instead of on paper is common. Health-care providers may be concerned that the electronic medical record could be altered without their consent or knowledge. Providers must have the assurance that the medical records are safely stored for future accessibility. Power outages, computer "crashes," viruses, concerns about adequate backup, and so on are issues providers must overcome to be confident in using an EHR.

Use of EHR programs, particularly in the small- to medium-sized practices, is expanding rapidly. Nearly 78 percent of physicians in private practice are within this market group of eight or fewer doctors. With the explosive growth of EHR implementation in this segment of the medical community, a great need has been generated for both clerical and clinical support staff that have professional training and exposure to the EHR. Concerns about the transition from traditional paper charts to EHRs are now being overcome. Many of the concerns expressed about EHRs have been addressed more fully in recent years. Although the motivations vary from a practice wanting to simply "become paperless" to another practice wanting to improve patient care, medical clinics are quickly recognizing the incredible tool the EHR is bringing to the medical practice.

Focal Point

A lack of feature uniformity and affordability, and change to clinical processes were some of the barriers to the adoption of ambulatory EHRs in the 1990s.

Concept Checkup 1.3 (LO 1.4)

A. List the five perceived barriers to the adoption of an EHR.

1. _____

2. _____

3. _____

4. _____

5. _____

B. What is the most rapidly expanding segment of the medical community in terms of EHR implementation?

_____

LO 1.5 BENEFITS OF THE EHR

The promotion of the EHR concept by many organizations is because of the benefits EHRs bring to health care. The Institute of Medicine (IOM) recognized these benefits and in 1991 called for EHRs to be implemented with the elimination of paper-based patient records by 2001. In his 2004 State of the Union address, President George W. Bush stated, "By computerizing health records, we can avoid dangerous medical mistakes, reduce costs, and improve care."[2] President Bush created a sub-Cabinet-level position for a national health information coordinator at the Department of Health and Human Services. In April of 2004, he outlined a plan "to ensure that most Americans have electronic health records within the next 10 years."[3] From that plan, government agencies have been able to promote the use of and overcome barriers for the EHR. Subsequent to the president's plans, Hillary Clinton, then a U.S. Senator, announced a proposal to introduce legislation to encourage development of a national health information infrastructure, including the adoption of EHRs. Although the Bush administration empowered the HHS Department to promote EHRs, the advocacy toward electronic medicine occurred mainly in the private sector.

In 2008, the concerns over reducing costs and improving patient care were echoed by presidential candidate Barack Obama. Mr. Obama promised to sponsor the adoption of EHRs through a sizable government financial commitment as part of a broader economic stimulus package. In its economic recovery plan of 2009, President Obama's administration outlined strategies to spend $19 billion to accelerate the use of computerized medical records in doctors' offices over the coming years.

> "Our recovery plan will invest in electronic health records and new technology that will reduce errors, bring down costs, ensure privacy, and save lives," President Obama stated in his speech to Congress in February 2009.[4]

Industry analysts have identified some major benefits that are motivating physicians toward clinical automation.

Better Clinic Information and Accessibility

EHRs bring better clinical information to the health-care provider. Access to the patient's medical information is not limited to the location of the paper chart, but is available at the patient point of care. The health-care provider can easily be informed of past medical history, family medical history, immunization records, and so on. Up-to-date information such as test results, routine and current medications, and allergy information are crucial for informed medical decision making. With the EHR, this information is easily accessible when decisions need to be made. For example, if a patient calls with an issue concerning a current medication, the health-care provider can instantly access the patient's chart on the EHR (even if the provider is not in the medical office), make an informed decision, create a prescription, and document the consultation rapidly with a few mouse clicks or with the Tap&Go™ feature on a Tablet PC. In addition, accessible within the EHR is information regarding drug interactions with current and routine medications, dosage information for the prescription being created, and instant alerts with allergy warnings. With a paper chart environment some information is not retrievable or the provider may not have access to the chart and the process is more complicated and time-consuming.

Patient Safety

The challenge of reading handwritten notes, orders, and prescriptions has been eliminated with the EHR. Patients' chart information is clear and legible. Reports and letters to other specialists and patients are comprehensive, professional, and easy to create. Chart information is always accessible and found in the same place. Paper charts, on the other hand, can become cluttered with a lot of necessary but misplaced information.

EHRs provide routine information and reminders for the health-care provider. Health maintenance screenings can be tracked automatically by patient age, gender, past diagnoses, past medical procedures, or even family medical history, which enables the provider to be proactive in patient care. The EHR can evaluate the patient information and alert the practitioner regarding tests, procedures, or screenings that are due. With automated medical analysis the health-care provider can offer more consistent patient care. For example, an influenza vaccination alert may be offered to all patients, whereas a mammogram may be advised because of the patient's gender and age. A routine colonoscopy may be recommended by the EHR because the patient is younger than 50 years old and has a family history of colon cancer. Support for medical decision making is accessible to the health-care provider through an EHR. Decision-making support gives information about medications, tests, and care plans. The practice of medicine has become more and more complex because medical procedures, drugs, and treatment plans have continued to evolve. There are over 2,000 "best practice guidelines" that have been developed by reputable medical organizations.[5] The Illinois State Medical Society, for example, states that:

> "Practice guidelines, based on 'evidence-based medicine,' often are very complex, with what is best for a patient with a particular condition depending on a variety of factors, including the patient's history, the patient's family history, other conditions of the patient and patient medications, and the availability of different modes of treatment in a community. No physician is able to keep up with all the latest practices and apply them to the particular conditions of each of his or her patients."[6]

The national debate and exposure to patient safety is driving the medical industry toward drastically reducing errors through e-prescription writing and e-medical orders. EHR programs now offer physicians detailed summaries of past medical records, family medical history, and allergy information to re-inform medical staff about treatment choices, clinical decisions, and diagnoses.

Better Patient Care

Another benefit driving the use of EHRs is better patient care. Improved patient care is a direct result of the availability of more thorough clinical information. Because the EHR provides the health-care practitioner with alerts or notices to better practice guidelines, patients receive the most current standard of care consistently. Patient records in most EHRs have treatment protocols available and recommendations of tests that better inform the health-care provider.

Kaiser Permanente of Ohio saw the following practice guidelines compliance improvements after implementing a medical automated record system and adding reminders at the point of care:

- Aspirin use in patients with coronary artery disease increased from 56 percent to 82 percent in 27 months, while lipid-lowering agents increased from 10 percent to 20 percent in 7 months.
- ACE inhibitor use in patients with congestive heart failure increased from 54 percent to 66 percent.
- Stratification (staging) for patients with diabetes mellitus and asthma increased to 76 percent in 26 months and 65 percent in 29 months, respectively. In addition, referrals to podiatry for medium- and high-risk diabetics increased from 14 percent to 66 percent in 12 months.
- Percentage of hypertensive patients taking nonrecommended medications decreased from 16 percent to 12 percent in 12 months.
- Percentage of patients older than 64 years of age who were offered an influenza vaccination during a primary care visit increased from 56 percent to 69 percent in 36 months.[7]

Patients can also receive patient instruction sheets specifically concerning their diagnosis or the planned treatments. These instructions are easily accessed in the EHR by the provider and either printed out or emailed to the patient. The EHR reports and records the processing of treatment plans, the instructions for procedural preparation, or post-treatment care for the patient to safeguard the health-care provider against liabilities.

The EHR will access pertinent patient information and the most current practice guidelines, thus providing the health-care practitioner with the best tools for improved medical decision making.

Drug recalls are much more proficiently handled. Reports generated through an EHR can document which patients are currently taking specific medications. Form letters can be quickly generated, alerting patients to the recall and requesting an office visit appointment to discuss future plans. The alternative process in a paper chart environment is time-consuming and open to errors. A staff member would have to review all paper charts looking for the specific prescriptions or a letter would need to be generated to all patients informing them of the drug recall. These options are costly processes to a medical practice trying to provide good patient care.

EHRs reduce the repetition of labs and tests because all medical test information is clearly displayed and readily accessed. Lost or delayed test and/or lab results are not as common with EHR programs, resulting in a quicker diagnosis and treatment plan for the patient.

> **Focal Point**
>
> Immediate access to all patient medical information promotes informed medical decisions. Automated medical alerts and the reduction in handwriting promote patient safety.

Efficiency and Savings

A major motivation for widespread use of an EHR is both efficiency and financial savings. One obvious savings is the elimination of the paper-based chart, storage costs, and retrieval costs. One study cites "that a chart pull costs $20 at Scott and White Memorial Hospital, Clinic, and Health Systems in Temple, Texas. Their electronic chart solution reduced electronic chart pulls to less than $1 apiece."[8]

Electronic messaging systems built into an EHR enable speedier communication among staff members. Communication to the health-care provider concerning diagnoses, drug refills, pre-authorizations for treatments, and general patient concerns is expedited and simplified. Electronic communication among the office staff regarding referral setup, patient phone call documentation, and letters to patients and other professionals are accelerated and the items are automatically saved into the patient's chart.

Time savings for clinicians is significant, as their job processes are streamlined and become more efficient. Studies by Dassenko and Slowinski reported a reduction in nurse intake time from 35 minutes to 20 minutes for initial office visits and from 35 minutes to 15 minutes for return visits at the University of Wisconsin Hospital and Clinics. The elimination of repeatedly collecting and entering information and the addition of the enhanced display of the patient's history, vital signs, weight, and medical problems were attributed to the greater efficiency and time savings through the adoption of the EHR.[9]

Reporting to public health organizations is expedited and eased with the reporting capabilities of EHRs. The simplification of this process for medical offices is another example of time savings that translates into cost savings. Charts are easily accessed and patient data sorted by diagnoses, treatments, or care plans and then sent to the appropriate agencies.

When health-care providers complete their documentation on an EHR, the need for a transcriptionist is often eliminated. This efficiency has generated an estimated savings of $300 to $1,000 or more per month per physician. In one six-provider practice, transcription took 150 hours per week. After implementing an EHR, that time was decreased by one-third. The turnaround time of the transcription went from 7 days to 1 day. The time and money savings enabled the practice to add two additional providers.[10]

EHRs' coding programs give health-care providers confidence and support for coding **Evaluation and Management (E&M)** encounters with patients. Often, undercoding occurs by medical providers. However, with an EHR, more accurate level-of-care coding is based on documentation from the review of systems and examination within the office visit assessment. EHRs help recover lost revenue for the practice.

Malpractice insurance carriers are considering or currently giving discounts to their insured when an EHR is utilized. The more thorough documentation and improved patient care have warranted a reduction in rates.

The Illinois State Medical Society reported the ROI of a Chicago-area hospital that implemented a $40 million-plus EHR.

> "The hospital estimates that it will save $10 million annually. The new system is substantially enhancing patient care. The turnaround time for obtaining test results has fallen significantly, with mammograms now taking a day compared to up to three weeks, and cardiographics reports dropping from as long as 10 days to one day. Entire categories of medication errors and potential errors have been eliminated,

Evaluation and Management (E&M) Code

This code is a five-digit Current Procedural Terminology (CPT) code used by a physician to report evaluation and management services with a patient. The E&M encounter may include documenting a patient's medical history, a physical examination, and medical decision making. An E&M encounter may be with an inpatient, an outpatient, or a consultation and may occur in any number of medical settings.

Focal Point

The availability of care plans and practice guidelines increase the accuracy of patient care. Rapid documentation and accurate coding has reduced costs and increased reimbursement as a result of the implementation of EHRs.

including transcription errors, errors due to misunderstood abbreviations and mix-ups due to look-alike drug names. In addition, delayed administration of patient medications has decreased 70 percent while omitted administration of medications has dropped 20 percent across the organization due to the electronic medication administration records and system tools that alert nurses of new patient orders and of overdue medications."[11]

Concept Checkup 1.4 (LO 1.5)

A. In April of 2004, President George W. Bush outlined a plan "to ensure that most Americans have electronic health records" by what year? _____

B. List the four perceived benefits of implementing an EHR program.

1. _____

2. _____

3. _____

4. _____

LO 1.6 EHR INCENTIVES

On February 17, 2009, President Obama signed the **American Recovery and Reinvestment Act (ARRA)** into law. The ARRA provided $787 billion to accelerate the nation's economic recovery. It was designed to stimulate the economy through investments in infrastructure, unemployment benefits, transportation, education, and health care. The Health Information Technology for Economic and Clinical Health (HITECH) Act, as part of this stimulus package, included over $19 billion to aid in the development of a health-care infrastructure and to assist providers and other entities in adopting and using health information technology, including EHRs. Money has been made available as incentives through the Medicare and Medicaid reimbursement systems to assist providers in adopting EHRs.

For financial remuneration from the ARRA program, physicians will need to use a "certified" EHR. Based on meeting certain requirements, doctors would receive a bonus or incentive payment from the **Centers for Medicare and Medicaid Services (CMS)** at the beginning of the year following participation. The first year of possible involvement is 2010.

A provider who fully complies with the requirements in 2010 will be eligible for payment at the beginning of 2011. Payments can be substantial starting at $18,000 in 2011, with an accumulation of $44,000 over the life of the program for Medicare assigned providers. On the other hand, physicians can opt for reimbursement as a Medicaid participating provider for up to $65,000 starting in 2011 based on state-defined guidelines.

Table 1.1 details total potential payments to physicians under the Medicare program.[12]

The government incentives are designed to encourage the adoption and "meaningful use" of EHRs to promote medical information accessibility, better patient care and safety, greater efficiency, and financial savings.

American Recovery and Reinvestment Act (ARRA)
Commonly known as the stimulus package, the ARRA was passed by Congress in 2009 to stimulate the economy through investments in infrastructure, unemployment benefits, transportation, education, and health care.

Centers for Medicare and Medicaid Services (CMS)
Formerly known as the Health Care Financing Administration (HCFA), CMS is a federal agency responsible for administering Medicare, Medicaid, HIPAA, CLIA and several other health-related programs.

Table 1.1	Potential Payments to Physicians
Payment Year	**Incentives**
First Payment Year	• $18,000 if the first payment year is 2011 or 2012 • $15,000 if the first payment year is 2013 • $12,000 if the first payment year is 2014
Second Payment Year	$12,000
Third Payment Year	$8,000
Fourth Payment Year	$4,000
Fifth Payment Year	$2,000

*for providers in a health professional shortage area (HPSA), payment amounts will be increased by 10%

Name _____ Instructor _____ Class _____

USING TERMINOLOGY

Match the terms on the left with the definitions on the right.

_____ 1. EHR

_____ 2. CPR

_____ 3. CCR

_____ 4. PHR

_____ 5. ASP

_____ 6. Power outage

_____ 7. Better patient care

_____ 8. Health maintenance screenings

_____ 9. Tablet PC

_____ 10. Remote access

A. An Internet-based connection that allows the patient to become an interactive source of health information and health management.(LO 1.3)

B. A concern a provider may have about EHRs.(LO 1.4)

C. A portable means of entering information in an EHR utilizing the Tap&Go™ method.(LO 1.2)

D. Enables the health-care provider to work on the EHR from a nursing home, home office, or hospital.(LO 1.2)

E. A benefit of EHRs.(LO 1.5)

F. The most commonly accepted and used term for storing and accessing patient medical information electronically.(LO 1.3)

G. Tracked by patient age, gender, past diagnoses, past medical procedures, or family medical history.(LO 1.5)

H. Health-provider-oriented and defines a core set of data reflecting the most relevant and timely facts about a patient's health care and is accessible and readable by other electronic systems.(LO 1.3)

I. The EHR is stored, maintained, and updated off-site by an EHR web-hosting company for the doctor.(LO 1.2)

J. Contains all patient information for the patient's lifetime and includes medical information from all specialties and is fully interoperable.(LO 1.3)

CHECKING YOUR UNDERSTANDING

Write "T" or "F" in the blank to indicate whether you think the statement is true or false.

_____ **11.** Voice recognition systems cannot be used with electronic health records systems.(LO 1.2)

_____ **12.** LAN technology provides a wireless network for the Tablet PC.(LO 1.2)

_____ **13.** A high-speed Internet connection is necessary for an ASP.(LO 1.2)

_____ **14.** Decision-making support gives information about medications, tests, and care plans.(LO 1.5)

_____ **15.** The implementation of an EHR does not bring process changes to the medical office.(LO 1.4)

_____ **16.** The challenge and danger of handwritten prescriptions is non-existent with an EHR.(LO 1.5)

_____ **17.** Better patient care is a direct result of more thorough and detailed clinical information.(LO 1.5)

_____ **18.** An EHR does not enhance the provider's coding for billing.(LO 1.5)

Answer the question below in the space provided.

19. List three main benefits of EHRs and provide an example of each benefit.^(LO 1.5)

a) _____

_____

b) _____

_____

c) _____

_____

20. List three cost savings of using an EHR rather than paper-based charts.^(LO 1.5)

a) _____

b) _____

c) _____

Choose the best answer and circle the corresponding letter.

21. The time and place where the concept of an electronic health record was first developed and utilized was:^(LO 1.1)
   a) 1950 at University of California
   b) 1980s at Mayo Clinic
   c) 1960s at Medical Center Hospital of Vermont and the Mayo Clinic
   d) This information can not be ascertained

22. For security, data on a wireless network is:^(LO 1.2)
   a) Encrypted
   b) Scrambled
   c) Coded
   d) Blocked

23. Which acronym was one of the first terms used to conceptualize the idea of storing medical information electronically?^(LO 1.3)
   a) EHR
   b) PHR
   c) CPR
   d) BYO

24. Measuring the ROI of an EHR includes:^(LO 1.4)
   a) Cost of training
   b) Reduced cost of office supplies
   c) Cost of future upgrades
   d) All of the above

25. The IOM called for elimination of paper-based patient records by the year:(LO 1.5)
    a) 1998
    b) 2001
    c) 2008
    d) 2010

26. With an EHR, the health-care practitioner provides more consistent care for the patient because the information is:(LO 1.5)
    a) More accessible and better utilized with care plans and alerts
    b) Reviewed with the patient
    c) More clearly written and stored in a consistent place for future reference
    d) Backed up electronically on a regular basis

27. The stimulus package of 2009 is officially known as:(LO 1.6)
    a) Centers for Medicare and Medicaid Services (CMS)
    b) American Recovery and Reinvestment Act (ARRA)
    c) Health Information Technology for Economic and Clinical Health (HITECH)
    d) Troubled Asset Relief Program (TARP)

28. The elimination of a paper-based chart does not eliminate the cost for:(LO 1.5)
    a) Receptionists
    b) Chart storage space
    c) Paper costs
    d) Chart retrieval

2

Standards for Electronic Health Records

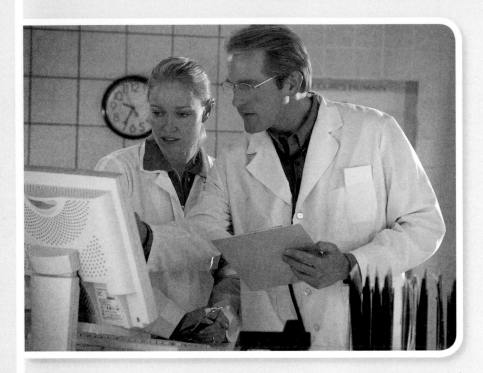

Learning Outcomes

After completing Chapter 2, you will be able to:

LO 2.1   Describe the standards history for the EHR

LO 2.2   Identify the basic HIPAA regulations for an EHR

LO 2.3   List the basic CHI regulations for an EHR

LO 2.4   Explain the IOM's core functions of an EHR

LO 2.5   Summarize the basic CCHIT standards for an EHR

LO 2.6   Evaluate the effect of MIPPA incentives on EHR adoption

What You Need to Know

To understand Chapter 2, you will need to know:

• The concept of an electronic health record
• The history of an electronic health record

LO 2.1 THE ELECTRONIC HEALTH RECORD STANDARDS HISTORY

With the premise that EHRs can improve the quality of health care, the U.S. government and other institutions like the **Institute of Medicine (IOM)** have been promoting the use of EHRs for the last decade. Obstacles such as cost, organization, standards, functionality, and interoperability have slowed the progress of the EHR. Committees, reports, and standards from independent associations and the federal government have served as stepping stones to facilitate wider use of EHRs.

Health Insurance Portability and Accountability Act (HIPAA) began in 1996 to establish standards for accountability and criteria for the protection and confidentiality of health information that was transported electronically. The HIPAA standards, which initially regulated Practice Management Systems, played an important role in affecting the early development of EHRs. Several associations and government departments called for further action to help promote and set baselines for the EHR. The next significant step was conducted by **Consolidated Health Information (CHI)**, which released EHR standards in 2003. In 2005, the U.S. Department of Health and Human Services (HHS) commissioned the nongovernment organization known as the **Certification Commission for Health Information Technology (CCHIT)** to credential EHR programs. Other government agencies have continued to promote the use of EHRs and guide health-care providers toward utilizing these programs to promote better patient care.

Concept Checkup 2.1 (LO 2.1)

A. The government regulation known as the _____ played an important role in the early development of the EHR.

B. What year did the federal government commission CCHIT to credential EHR programs?

Institute of Medicine (IOM)
An organization that gives advice and information about government policies that affect human health.

Health Insurance Portability and Accountability Act (HIPAA)
Passed in 1996, this act enforces standards for electronic patient health, administrative, and financial data.

Consolidated Health Informatics (CHI)
A federal government initiative that seeks to provide adoption of health information interoperability standards for health vocabulary and messaging.

Certification Commission for Health Information Technology (CCHIT)
An independent nongovernment organization that seeks to accelerate the adoption of EHRs with a credible certification program.

LO 2.2 HEALTH INSURANCE PORTABILITY AND ACCOUNTABILITY ACT OF 1996

HIPAA regulations affect EHRs because of the portability of the patient's **Protected Health Information (PHI)**. These regulations are multiple and complex and affect many areas of the health-care industry. HIPAA's core regulations for an EHR are as follows:

Password Management

Policies and procedures are necessary for password management. EHRs must provide clinics with the ability to create, change, and safeguard passwords for the program. Password length formats of eight or more characters with a combination of alpha, numeric, and special characters are recommended, although not required. Default passwords are to be eliminated and a password

Protected Health Information (PHI)
Regulated under HIPAA that covers the protection of any past, present, or future medical and mental health condition whether in oral or recorded form or other medium.

expiration period of 90 to 120 days is recommended. Log-in attempts are to be monitored for auditing as well.

Unique User Identification

Each user of the EHR must be assigned a unique name and/or number for identifying and tracking user activity within the program. Modifications made to patients' demographics and charts are to be audited along with a user's log-in and log-out history.

International Classification of Diseases (ICD) codes
The international standard diagnostic classification for all medical data dealing with the incidence and prevalence of disease in large populations and for other health management purposes.

Access Authorization

Electronic PHI is protected by specifying access levels to individually identifiable health information. Users must be assigned appropriate security access level based on minimal data necessary to perform their jobs. Specific assignable security levels will not be able to access, modify, delete, or transmit certain information. For example, the receptionist may not be able to view lab results and the EHR can track who viewed or modified this information. Also, an EHR should be able to limit user access because of the nature of an office visit; for example, mental health and substance abuse. Access may also be regulated to certain reports or tests such as HIV or other PHI.

Accounting of Disclosures of Protected Health Information (PHI)

An accounting of health information disclosures from a patient's medical record must be provided for a period of 6 years prior to the date on which the accounting is requested. By allowing users to insert notes, track modifications to PHI, and include date and time stamps, EHR software enables covered entities to provide individuals with an accounting of health information disclosures. Also, patients are to have access to their electronic medical records. EHRs are required to either print or electronically transmit the patient's medical information to the patient or other health-care provider.

Current Procedural Terminology (CPT) codes
Five-digit codes developed by the AMA and adopted by insurance carriers and managed care companies as the means to identify common medical procedures.

Security and Data Backup and Storage

A retrievable, exact copy of electronic PHI should be accessible from a backup of the medical database. Security measures are required to be enacted to reduce the risks and vulnerabilities to electronic PHI. These include controlled access, administrative passwords, server firewalls, and so on. The database and backup storage units must be in a secure location.

Auditing Abilities

Prevention of intentional or unintentional disclosures and modifications to PHI is accomplished by tracking user access. Administrative audit reports are necessary to examine deletion and modification activities in the information systems that contain the electronic PHI.

Healthcare Common Procedure Coding System (HCPCS) codes
Codes used by CMS (Medicare & Medicaid) to indicate medical supplies such as durable medical equipment and other medical procedure codes; coding supplies ensures uniformity for billing and financial reimbursement.

Code Sets

The EHR must use the national standard code sets such as **International Classification of Diseases (ICD) codes, Current Procedural Terminology (CPT) codes,** and **Healthcare Common Procedure Coding System (HCPCS) codes** when storing and transmitting information.

Concept Checkup 2.2(LO 2.2)

A. Name the seven HIPAA regulations that affect the development of features within the EHR.

1. _____

2. _____

3. _____

4. _____

5. _____

6. _____

7. _____

B. What does the acronym PHI stand for?

_____

HITECH

The American Recovery and Reinvestment Act (ARRA) became law in February 2009. Besides non-economic related items, ARRA funds target the rebuilding of infrastructure, the expansion of unemployment benefits, social welfare provision, and education expansion. As part of this law, the Health Information Technology for Economic and Clinical Health (HITECH) Act was passed which governs development within the health-care industry. In this bill the Department of Health and Human Services (HHS) issued guidance specifying the technologies and methodologies that render protected health information unusable and indecipherable to unauthorized entities.

The HITECH Act expands HIPAA's coverage by increasing compliance obligations, increasing privacy regulations, and strengthening enforcement penalties as it relates to a patient's health records in PMS and EHR programs.

HITECH introduces the first federally mandated "data breach notification requirement" that expands the reach of HIPAA data privacy and security requirements to include "business associates." Business associates are companies like accounting firms, billing agencies, and so on that are in relationship with and provide services to medical facilities, pharmacies, and health-care providers; entities that were already covered under HIPAA.

Traditionally, a business associate (e.g., billing company) that failed to properly protect patient information was liable only to the covered entity (e.g., medical office) via the service contract between the two entities. Under the HITECH Act, these support entities are now directly accountable to HIPAA security and privacy requirements, as well as to the same civil and criminal penalties that health-care providers, hospitals, pharmacies, and other HIPAA-covered entities face for violations.

These changes became effective one year after the enactment of ARRA, in February 2010.

LO 2.3 CONSOLIDATED HEALTH INFORMATICS STANDARDS

Consolidated Health Informatics (CHI) standards were initiated by the Office of Management and Budget (OMB) under the auspices of the HHS so that the approximately 20 federal agencies involved in health care and health-related missions could be interoperable, i.e. effectively share electronic information. Some of those agencies include the Department of Veterans Affairs, Department of Health and Human Services, the Department of Defense, and the Social Security Administration. Standards would include common clinical vocabularies and standard methods for transmitting health information. The first set of standards was announced in March 2003 and included five regulations. In May 2004 the second set of fifteen standards was adopted. These 20 criteria became the benchmark to standardize how the information would be coded or termed for use in exchanging data to or from an EHR.

CHI standards are not required by law. However, vendors doing business with the federal government voluntarily adopt these standards. The federal government, as the largest purchaser of health-care services, uses these standards to promote interoperability between EHR systems. Some of these adopted standards are as follows:

Health Level Seven (HL7)
An international computer language by which various health-care systems can communicate. HL7 is currently the selected standard for the interfacing of clinical data between software programs in most institutions.

Health Level Seven (HL7) is a computer messaging and vocabulary standard for demographic information, units of measure, immunizations, clinical encounters, and Clinical Document Architecture for text-based reports. Practically, it is the communication standard for the coordinated care of patients for scheduling, orders, tests, admittances, discharges, and transfers. HL7 enables clinical systems to communicate with each other (a.k.a. "interface") when they receive new information. HL7 is currently the selected standard for the interfacing of clinical data in most institutions.

National Council on Prescription Drug Programs (NCPDP) creates and promotes standards for the transfer of data to and from retail pharmacy services. NCPDP standards are focused on prescription drug messages and the activities involved in billing pharmacy claims and services, rebates, pharmacy ID cards, and standardized business transaction between pharmacies and the professionals who prescribe medications.

Telehealth
The use of electronic and communication technology to deliver medical information and services over large and small distances through a standard telephone line.

Institute of Electrical and Electronics Engineers 1073 (IEEE—pronounced as *eye-triple-e*) is an international organization for the advancement of technology related to electricity. The 1073 format is the *Point of Care Medical Device Communication Standards*, which addresses the interoperability of medical devices. It sets electronic standards to allow connection of medical devices to information and computer systems, allowing health-care providers to monitor information from such places as ICUs and from **telehealth** services, specifically on Native American reservations.

Digital Imaging and Communications in Medicine (DICOM)
This standard was created to aid in the distribution and viewing of medical images, such as CT scans, MRIs, ultrasound, and x-rays.

Digital Imaging Communications in Medicine (DICOM) enables images and associated diagnostic information to be accessed and transferred from various manufacturers' devices as well as medical staff workstations.

Laboratory Logical Observation Identifier Name Codes (LOINC) set standards for the electronic transfer of clinical laboratory results.

Systematized Nomenclature of Medicine Clinical Terms (SNOMED-CT) provides a common language that enables a consistent way of capturing, sharing, and aggregating health data across specialties and sites of care. It provides standard terminology for laboratory result contents, anatomy, diagnosis, medical problems, and nursing.

HIPAA's Transaction and Code Sets are the standards for electronic exchange of information for billing and administration.

Food and Drug Administration (FDA) sets medication standards for medication names, codes for ingredients, manufactured dosage forms, drug products, and medication packages. The description of clinical drugs and drug classifications are set by the National Library of Medicine's RxNORM.

The Human Gene Nomenclature (HUGN) sets standards for the transfer of information about the role of genes in biomedical research.

Environmental Protection Agency (EPA) sets standards are for nonmedicinal chemicals that are important to health care through the Substance Registry System.

Concept Checkup 2.3 (LO 2.3)

A. By 2004, the CHI had set 20 criteria to regulate EHRs for the purpose of

_____

_____

_____

B. List the 10 standards and/or organizations that regulate the standards used to promote interoperability between EHR systems.

1. _____

2. _____

3. _____

4. _____

5. _____

6. _____

7. _____

8. _____

9. _____

10. _____

LO 2.4 INSTITUTE OF MEDICINE'S CORE FUNCTIONS OF AN EHR

In May 2003, the U.S. Department of Health and Human Services (HHS), a government agency, requested the Institute of Medicine (IOM) to provide guidance on the key capabilities of an electronic health record (EHR) system. The IOM gives information and advice about government policies that affect public health. The IOM's Committee on Data Standards for Patient Safety identified the following eight key capabilities that should accompany an EHR.

Health Information and Data—Complete patient data must be present. This is not a function as much as a quality of an EHR. Simply, the EHR must contain pertinent patient data so that the provider of care has all the information easily accessible for sound clinical decisions. For example, past medical information, narratives, and diagnoses must be present. Patient allergies and drug interactions need to be clearly available. Past laboratory results should be present to prevent redundant or unnecessary tests being ordered. Also, the information needs to be well displayed so that the end user is not inundated with information.

Patient Support—Home monitoring of patients, patient education, and telehealth. This functionality improves care quality and reduces medical costs. Computer-based patient instructions and treatment plans are available to the patient. Home monitoring or self-testing of patients in their homes provides valid medical information for the provider about the patient. Telemonitoring allows the patient's current health status, symptoms, and activities to be monitored around the clock on a daily basis.

Results Management—Management and ordering of lab tests results and radiology results. Computerized results can be accessed more easily by the provider at the time and place they are needed. The electronic results of labs are available much quicker. The reduced lag time increases both office efficiency and patient safety by allowing for speedier recognition, detection of abnormalities, and treatment of medical problems.

Administrative Processes—Scheduling, billing, medical claims, authorizations, and referrals. These features provide clearer information about insurance eligibility (including completing the verification process online) and matching up referrals and authorizations to services. Supporting documentation for medical claims to insurance companies is easily accessible through EHRs.

Order Entry/Management—Entry of orders and prescriptions. Computerization of orders for labs and tests improves the work processes and eliminates lost orders, ambiguities, handwriting discrepancies, duplication of orders, and pre-printed forms. Financial benefits are evident by greatly reducing clinical staff time on these orders and reducing errors.

Reporting and Population Health—Automated reporting to government agencies. Reporting is mandated for public health and health-care organizations on local, state, and national levels. Traditionally, this data has been manually collected from paper charts and reported. Standardized terminology and automation make this information easily accessible with greater accuracy and reduces provider or staff time for reporting.

Medical Decision Support—Drug prescribing and dosage, disease screening, diagnosis and treatment, and care quality improvement. Information can be accessed through the EHR for prescription details, drug interaction, allergies, dosing information, diagnoses, management of diseases and symptoms, disease outbreak, and adverse reactions or events. This information significantly improves health care and is a major reason for the promotion of EHR use. Studies have shown that more appropriate clinical decisions were made by physicians using an EHR than by physicians in the same practice using traditional paper charts.

Electronic Communication and Connectivity—Accessing information between specialists, primary care physicians, radiology, laboratories, and pharmacies. This functionality is currently still in the research and development stage; it is often termed *interoperability*. Ambulatory EHR credentialing and standards will include this feature in coming years. However, the numerous EHR software systems that exist make this transfer of information difficult at best. (The issue of what information should be accessed is also in question.) Electronic **connectivity** can be essential in creating and populating EHR systems, especially for those patients with chronic conditions who characteristically have multiple providers in a number of settings who need to coordinate care plans. The absence of interoperability presents possible harmful situations and its presence can be critical to the quality of medical care for some patients.

Connectivity
The ability to make and maintain a connection between two or more points in a telecommunications system. It allows for the viewing and/or transfer of data from one computer system to another.

Concept Checkup 2.4(LO 2.4)

A. Name the eight core features determined by the Institute of Medicine (IOM) for EHRs.

1. _____
2. _____
3. _____
4. _____
5. _____
6. _____
7. _____
8. _____

B. One of the functions of the IOM is to give _____ _____ that affect public health.

LO 2.5 CCHIT—CERTIFICATION COMMISSION FOR HEALTH INFORMATION TECHNOLOGY

CCHIT®, The Certification Commission for Health Information Technology, was organized in July 2004 with support from the American Health Information Management Association (AHIMA), the Healthcare Information and Management Systems Society (HIMSS), and the National Alliance for Health Information Technology (NAHIT). These three organizations committed resources during the organizational phase to create the independent, nonprofit organization called the *Certification Commission*. It is composed of 21 commissioners who now guide approximately 300 work group members who are charged with the Commission's development work. These volunteers represent the scope of Health Information Technology (HIT) stakeholders—including providers, payers, vendors, consumers, and government agencies—and are recruited in an open call for applications.

The Certification Commission states its mission is "to accelerate the adoption of health information technology by creating an efficient, credible and sustainable product certification program."[1] In September 2005, the U.S. Department of Health & Human Services (HHS) awarded the Commission a three-year contract to develop certification criteria, evaluate these standards, and create the inspection process for HIT. The three specific HIT areas are (1) ambulatory EHRs for the office-based physician or provider, (2) inpatient EHRs for hospitals and health systems, and (3) network components through which they interoperate and share information. The Certification Commission is "the recognized certification body for electronic health records and their networks, and an independent, voluntary, private-sector initiative."[2] Each year, the Commission develops and announces new criteria and features for EHRs. EHR companies must pay approximately $25,000 to go through the inspection process for their ambulatory EHR product for a three-year term of certification. Vendors who wish to annually recertify their subsequent product releases to meet the new criteria must go through the certification inspection process again.

The Certification Commission brings an official recognition and approval that has been requested from both the private sector and from government agencies. Such industry standards–based criteria for EHRs will promote their use and a confidence in utilizing them. In the past, the lack of uniform requirements and standards was a considerable hurdle to the extensive use of EHRs. When HHS awarded the contract to the Certification Commission, this obstruction was specifically being addressed to promote the use of an EHR by physicians, hospitals, home health-care providers, and other organizations. As stated by Mike Leavitt, the HHS secretary, "The seal of certification removes a significant barrier to widespread adoption of electronic health records. It gives health-care providers peace of mind to know they are purchasing a product that is functional, interoperable, and will bring higher quality, safer care to patients."[3]

The creation of harmonized standards upon which criteria are based is primarily developed by the Health Information Technology Standards Panel (HITSP), a federally contracted standards development organization. The Commission evaluated these standards as part of their development of conformance criteria and test scripts, and published the first set of 300 proposed ambulatory EHR criteria in May 2006. Approximately 150 of these criteria became the Commission-approved baseline for certification testing in 2006. By July of the same year, 22 ambulatory EHR products had completed the initial certification process and were "CCHIT Certified®." CCHIT certification means the product has met basic requirements for:

- Functionality—ability to carry out specific tasks.
- Interoperability—compatibility and communication with other products.
- Security—ability to keep patients' information safe.

Each year, additional criteria and test steps are added to the requirements for CCHIT certification. EHR companies developing subsequent version releases of their ambulatory EHR products, and who desire the CCHIT Certified® stamp of approval, will be required to undergo the CCHIT certification process for the current year. When marketing their product, EHR companies are required to list the year of their CCHIT certification.

The following are some of the Certification Commission criteria categories set for all aspects of ambulatory EHRs:

- Access to scheduling
- Clinical task assignments and routing
- Data availability
- Document storage and retrieval
- Generation of patient instructions
- Health record definition
- Test results handling
- Management of authorizations and consents
- Medication adverse reaction
- Patient demographics
- Patient medical history
- Prescriptions
- Provide criteria for disease management
- Secure communication between providers

- Insurance eligibility verification and determination of coverage
- Allergy lists
- Data archiving and destruction
- Data retention
- Drug interaction
- Guidelines and protocols
- Immunization records
- Medical coding assistance
- Standard care plans
- Medication lists
- Patient information access audit
- Pharmacy communications
- Problem lists
- Report generation
- Test orders
- Wellness and preventive criteria

Regulations, agencies, and recognized certification bodies will continue to influence the EHR industry, bringing the medical field to a higher level of patient care and greater efficiency in the medical office. These national requirements become very practical in the functionality and ease of use of an EHR. The features, the way information is presented by code or terminology, and how information is presented or shared are directly related to the regulations by Consolidated Health Informatics (CHI), HIPAA, and the voluntary certification by CCHIT.

Because most EHRs will follow the criteria, credentialing, and regulations reviewed in this chapter, the distinguishing factor between different software will not be functionality. Certified EHRs will have similar functionalities or capabilities. However, each EHR will be unique in data layout, ease or complexity of use, and accessibility to functions by the user.

LO 2.6 MIPPA—MEDICARE IMPROVEMENTS FOR PATIENT AND PROVIDERS ACT OF 2008

On July 15, 2008, the **Medicare Improvements for Patients and Providers Act of 2008 (MIPPA)** was enacted by Congress and became law. Besides important changes that increase Medicare benefits to low-income beneficiaries, MIPPA provides positive incentives for practitioners who use **e-prescribing** in 2009 through 2013. Electronic prescribing is intended to bring greater safety to patients by providing for automatic drug and allergy interaction checking and the elimination of medication errors due to poor handwriting. E-prescribing is designed also to bring a greater efficiency to the prescribing process for providers. It will dramatically decrease communication from pharmacies requesting clarification of prescriptions.

MIPPA defines e-prescribing as the ability to transmit prescriptions electronically and conduct all alerts. Alerts include: *automated prompts that offer information on the drug being prescribed and warn the prescriber of possible undesirable or unsafe situations such as potentially inappropriate dose or route of administration of the drug, drug-drug interactions, allergy concerns, or warnings/cautions.*[4]

Eligible providers who successfully reported e-prescribing in 2009 were eligible to receive an additional incentive payment equal to 2 percent of all of their

Focal Point

EHR vendors are required to display the term "CCHIT Certified®" and the year of certification when marketing their software.

Medicare Improvements for Patient And Providers Act (MIPPA)
Passed in 2008, this act reestablishes Medicare reimbursement for providers, reduces racial and ethnic disparities among Medicare recipients, and reins in certain rapidly-growing Medicare supplemental insurance policies.

E-prescribing
Electronic prescribing is the use of computerized tools, usually embedded in an EHR program that create and sign prescriptions for medicines. E-prescribing replaces handwritten prescriptions and is sent to pharmacies over the Internet via clearinghouses.

Medicare Part B
That part of the Medicare insurance program that covers physicians' supervision, outpatient hospital care, diagnostic tests, ambulance services, and other ambulatory services. Part A of Medicare covers hospitals, skilled nursing facilities, home health agencies, and other nonambulatory services.

Medicare Part B allowed charges for services furnished during the reporting year. This 2 percent bonus continues for successful e-prescribing throughout 2010. In 2011 and 2012 the incentive drops to 1 percent. The measure also imposes penalties of minus 1 percent in 2012, minus 1.5 percent in 2013, and minus 2 percent in 2014 and beyond for physicians who do not e-prescribe. MIPPA law prohibits the application for financial incentives and penalties to those who write prescriptions infrequently, and permits the Secretary of Health and Human Services to establish a hardship exception to providers who are unable to use a qualified e-prescribing system.

Providers are required to report that they are successfully utilizing e-prescribing by using specified "G" codes when submitting Medicare claim forms. These G codes must appear on at least 50 percent of Medicare Part B claim forms for the reporting year.

The e-prescribing incentive provision is designed to move providers toward the adoption of EHR programs for clinical activity.

Surescripts is the national clearinghouse for e-prescribing. The company connects a network of thousands of physicians, pharmacists, and payers nationwide enabling them to exchange health information and prescribe without paper.

By adopting the NCPDP standard for data transfer, Surescripts collaborates with national EHR vendors, pharmacies, and health plans to support physicians using EHR software. With this network in place health-care providers are able to electronically access prescription information from pharmacies, health plans, and other providers to see the patient's total prescription history from all sources. Currently, prescribers are able to send e-prescriptions to any of 51,000 retail pharmacies and six of the largest mail-order pharmacies.

Through e-prescribing, EHRs are providing meaningful improvements in cost, quality, and patient safety.

C&C
Concept Checkup 2.5 (LO 2.5, LO 2.6)

A. The mission of CCHIT is to:

_____

_____

_____

B. In the year _____ the first group of EHRs was certified by CCHIT.

C. Electronic prescribing brings greater patient safety and efficiency because of the following:

1. _____

2. _____

3. _____

It is important in today's medical environment that both clerical and clinical staff and providers be familiar with the functionality of EHRs and have "hands-on" experience. Medical offices will find potential workers with this training valuable and necessary. This textbook specifically covers the functionality and practical use of SpringCharts® EHR in the following chapters.

Name _____ Instructor _____ Class _____

USING TERMINOLOGY

Match the terms on the left with the definitions on the right.

_____ 1. HL7

_____ 2. DICOM

_____ 3. Functionality

_____ 4. Interoperability

_____ 5. HIT

_____ 6. Access authorization

_____ 7. HUGN

_____ 8. Administrative processes

_____ 9. SNOMED - CT

_____ 10. Medical decision support

A. Assignment of appropriate access levels to minimum necessary information.(LO 2.2)

B. Information for drug prescribing and dosage, disease screening, diagnosis and treatment, and care quality improvement.(LO 2.4)

C. Compatibility language with other software programs.(LO 2.3)

D. Scheduling, billing, medical claims, authorizations, referrals, and so on.(LO 2.4)

E. Standards for Digital Imaging Communications transferable between devices.(LO 2.3)

F. Ability to carry out specific tasks.(LO 2.5)

G. Messaging standards of communication between clinical systems for health information.(LO 2.3)

H. Standards of terms for laboratory result contents, anatomy, diagnosis, medical problems, and nursing.(LO 2.3)

I. Human Gene Nomenclature(LO 2.3)

J. Health Information Technology(LO 2.5)

CHECKING YOUR UNDERSTANDING

Write "T" or "F" in the blank to indicate whether you think the statement is true or false.

_____ 11. CCHIT is composed of 21 commissioners.(LO 2.5)

_____ 12. CCHIT was organized in July 2004 with support from the following organizations: AHIMA, HIMSS, and HIPAA.(LO 2.5)

_____ 13. CHI standards are required by law.(LO 2.3)

_____ 14. CHI standards were created to promote interoperability between EHR systems.(LO 2.3)

_____ 15. Passwords are not recommended to have alpha, numeric, and special characters to meet HIPAA standards.(LO 2.2)

_____ 16. Reporting of public health information is an IOM core function of an EHR.(LO 2.4)

Answer the question below in the space provided.

17. List the three tasks that in September of 2005 the U.S. Department of Health & Human Services (HHS) awarded CCHIT a 3-year contract to do: (LO 2.5)

1. _____

2. _____

3. _____

18. List four core functions of an EHR as determined by the IOM and a description of each: (LO 2.4)

1. _____

_____

2. _____

_____

3. _____

_____

4. _____

_____

Choose the best answer and circle the corresponding letter.

19. Standards by this organization were created so that approximately 20 government agencies could share health-care and health-related information:(LO 2.3)
    a) HIPAA
    b) CHI
    c) AHIMA
    d) SNOMED-CT

20. Who or what directed the IOM to establish key capabilities of an EHR?(LO 2.4)
    a) Department of Health and Human Services
    b) President George W. Bush
    c) CHI
    d) HIPAA

21. The first set of 300 CCHIT ambulatory EHR criteria was published in:(LO 2.5)
    a) March 2005
    b) July 2005
    c) May 2006
    d) November 2006

22. CCHIT is an acronym for:(LO 2.5)
    a) Credentialing Certification for Healthcare Information Technology
    b) Certification Criteria for Health Impaired Technicians
    c) Certification Commission for Health Information Technology
    d) Certification Committee for Health Information Technology

23. HIPAA is an acronym for:^(LO 2.2)
    a) Health Information Portability and Accountability Act
    b) Health Information Problems and Answers Act
    c) Health Insurance Portability and Accountability Act
    d) Health Insurance Portability and Accessibility Act

24. MIPPA is an acronym for: ^(LO 2.6)
    a) Medical Improvements Per Patient Annually
    b) Medicaid Improvement for Patients Act
    c) Medicare Improvement for Patients and Providers Act
    d) Medicare Installments for Patients Pay Plan Act

25. MIPPA provides positive incentives for physicians who use e-prescribing because: ^(LO 2.6)
    a) The government will be able to access any patient medical records
    b) Drug companies will have access to the database for advertising
    c) It makes patients safer by providing for automatic drug and allergy interaction
    d) Pharmacies won't need to clarify prescriptions because of teleosmosis

3

Introduction and Setup

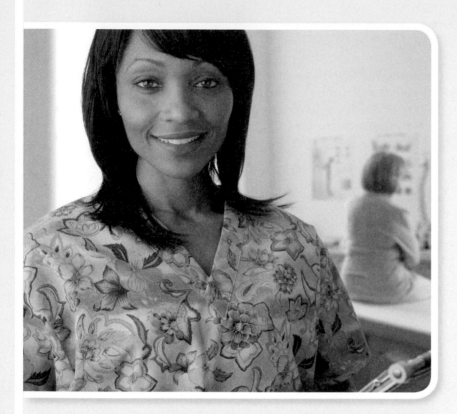

Learning Outcomes

After completing Chapter 3, you will be able to:

LO 3.1   Describe some basic features of SpringCharts EHR

LO 3.2   Discuss a brief history of SpringCharts EHR

LO 3.3   Set up user preferences

LO 3.4   Set up and edit addresses

LO 3.5   Set up and edit patients

LO 3.6   Set up and edit insurance companies

LO 3.1 SPRINGCHARTS FEATURES

The CCHIT certified *SpringCharts EHR*™ software has been chosen as the training tool for this textbook because of its ease of use, richness in features, and its ability to be customized to suit a wide range of medical specialties. SpringCharts is an international program and is used by over 1,000 physicians.

SpringCharts EHR software was designed by practicing physicians and technology executives to introduce easy-to-use, yet functional, technology to a large number of practitioners who remain dependent on paper charting systems and traditional clinical workflows. The program is largely focused on streamlining communications and documentation, and improving workflows in both the administrative and clinical practice areas.

SpringCharts EHR was developed and implemented over a period of 10 years to provide physicians with a powerful and intuitive software solution for the clinical side of the office. The program is designed to manage all *non-financial* activities of a medical practice. It combines robust clinical tools to enhance patient care, including a template-based electronic medical records system, a chart evaluation manager for proactive patient health-care maintenance, an evaluation and management (E&M) coder for automatic and accurate E&M coding, plan-of-care practice guidelines, and real-time drug and allergy interaction. These clinical features are incorporated with integrated patient tracking, integrated e-mail, messaging, reminders, a time clock, and template-based clerical tools designed to speed and streamline office communication and documentation. SpringCharts EHR makes available a one-click link to many powerful medical, pharmaceutical, and utility websites providing integrated access to industry-standard drug formularies (i.e., listings of pharmaceutical substances and formulas for making medicinal preparations), dosage information, patient education instructions, and electronic faxing.

LO 3.2 SPRINGCHARTS HISTORICAL OVERVIEW

In 2004, NDCHealth Inc. and Spring Medical Systems Inc. (SMSI) launched a jointly developed software communication piece enabling the bidirectional flow of data between two popular Windows™ **Practice Management Software (PMS)** programs, Medisoft™ and Lytec™, and SpringCharts EHR. This communication model provides data exchange of patient demographics, insurance information, and transaction details. Since this time, over 50 links have been developed to many other popular Windows-based and Macintosh PMS programs.

In 2006, SMSI released *MacExchange*, an interface with the widely used Macintosh PMS program, MacPractice™. This module provides for the automatic transfer of patient data between SpringCharts and MacPractice.

In 2009, SpringCharts™ EHR Version 9.7 became SureScripts Certified®, enabling the delivery of electronic prescriptions and refills across the internet and making use of real-time clinical decision support tools including drug and allergy interactions, formularies, and dosage checking. Patients benefit through faster service and the highest levels of safety and security available.

Practice Management Software (PMS)
A software program that manages, among other things, financial transactions, both charges and payments, and the billing of insurance claims and patient statements

> Disclaimer: The Certification Commission for Healthcare Information Technology does not endorse the certified product named as an example in this textbook, SpringCharts™ EHR, and did not participate in the preparation of the material.

Version 10 of SpringCharts EHR was CCHIT Certified® in 2010 for Ambulatory EHRs. That means that SpringCharts EHR has met a comprehensive set of criteria for:

- Functionality—setting features and functions to meet a basic set of requirements.
- Interoperability—establishing basic functionality enabling standards-based data exchange with other sources of healthcare information in future versions of the product.
- Security—ensuring data privacy and robustness to prevent data loss.

Concept Checkup 3.1(LO 3.1, 3.2)

A. SpringCharts EHR was chosen as the instructional software for this textbook because of its:

1. _____
2. _____
3. _____

B. In what three areas did SpringCharts EHR qualify for CCHIT certification?

1. _____
2. _____
3. _____

LO 3.3 USER PREFERENCES

Preferences 1

User Preferences
Setup window in SpringCharts that enables each user to preset the default practice name, physician name, schedule, and various other features that will be displayed when the user logs into the program.

Graphic User Interface
Software program screen that can display icons, sub-windows, text fields, and menus designed to standardize and simplify the use of the computer program by typing in fields and by using a mouse to manipulate text and images.

SpringCharts enables the setting up of **user preferences** that will determine the default **graphic user interface** of several key areas of the program specific for each user. To set the user preferences, each user will need to access the main *File* menu and select *Preferences > User Preferences* (see Figure 3.1).

In the *Set User Preferences* window, each user will set:

1. the doctor's name that will appear as the default for the user on reports and letters. The list of doctors is based upon the providers who were set up as doctors in the administration panel of SpringCharts Server.
2. the practice name that will default for letterheads. Although the doctor and the practice name are chosen here as "default," they can be changed within the program at the time of creating various letters and reports. A clinic may have several practices set up in various locations but use the same database for SpringCharts via the Internet. This allows each practice unlimited access to any patient medical records regardless of location.
3. the default appointment schedule in a stand-alone SpringCharts system. Many appointment schedules can be set up in SpringCharts for different providers and therapy resources. Here the user will choose which schedule he/she wants to see as the main screen upon successful entry to SpringCharts' *Practice View* screen. When SpringCharts is being used

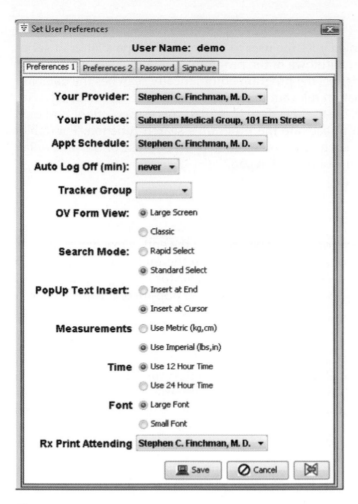

Figure 3.1 Set user preference window.

in conjunction with Medisoft™ or Lytec™ PMS, the server administrator has the option to display the PMS appointment schedule in SpringCharts instead. If this is the case then this field will be left blank.

4. the number of minutes of inactivity before SpringCharts closes down and only displays the login window.

5. the *Tracker Group* that will display the list of patients in the *Patient Tracker* window of the *Practice View* screen. Clinics that have several locations and work from the same patient database over the Internet are able to track the patients separately for each location. The various tracker groups are set up in the administrative panel of SpringCharts Server. *Show All* will display all patients in the *Patient Tracker* window from all locations. If the medical facility has only one location the Tracker Group field will be left blank.

OV Form View

The *Large Screen* view of the **Office Visit (OV)** window was an added feature to SpringCharts subsequent to the original *Classic* view. Its layout is more user-friendly and provides easier navigation. Although the OV text material is the same, the user will notice a different layout when editing an OV template (*Classic* view) and when creating a new OV (*Large Screen* view). It is recommended that all new users select the *Large Screen* View.

Office Visit (OV)
Used in SpringCharts to designate the graphic-user-interface window in which the encounter note is created.

Search Mode

The *Rapid Select* function enables the user to immediately type a letter or series of letters to many search windows in the program. When the user pauses after typing the desired characters, the program automatically searches the database and displays the information relevant to the letters selected. Alternatively, with *Standard Select* activated, the user needs to type in the necessary letters, and then click on the search icon to activate the program's search function. For Tablet PCs the *Standard Select* search mode is recommended because of the time delay in selecting letters from the onboard keypad.

Pop-Up Text Insert

The user can determine where additional pop-up text is added to existing pop-up text throughout the program. It can be added at the end of existing sentences or where the cursor is positioned, for example, in the middle of a sentence. It is recommended that all users select *Insert at Cursor* for the pop-up text insert option. This will become clearer when we study the pop-up text feature later in this text.

Measurements

Metric Units
Having to do with weights and measures relating to the metric system, which is mandatory in a large number of countries; also known as the International System of Units.

The measurements option allows the user to select the units of measure in which the vitals will be recorded, either **metric units** or **imperial units.** Most countries of the world use the metric system of weights and measures. The United States continues to use the imperial measurements in most cases. However, because this is a user-defined option, the program will adjust according to each user logged on.

Time

Imperial Units
Having to do with weights and measures that conform to the standards legally established in Great Britain. This measurement system is still widely used in the United States.

Time stamps are available in various places throughout the program. The user's selection here will determine whether notes and other documents are stamped in a 12-hour time style with a.m./p.m. or a 24-hour military style time.

Font

The font size used in the program can be determined for each user, either Arial 10 or Arial 12. After saving the user preferences information, the program will adjust its font based upon this selection.

> Note: The optimal screen resolution for SpringCharts is 1024 × 768 pixels, which can be set in the computer's *Control Panel > Display > Settings.* Monitors set at this resolution will allow SpringCharts the most favorable window display. If you prefer a lower screen resolution, for example, 800 × 600 pixels, then the smaller font size setting for the user preferences will be adequate.

Rx Print Attending

The selection of a practitioner in this field will print this name as the attending provider on the pharmacy prescription forms. See Figure 3.2 for illustration of

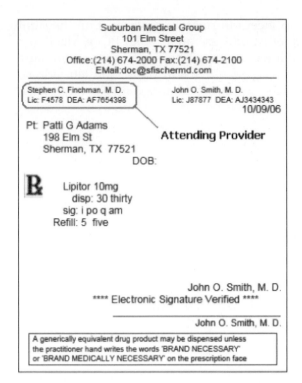

Figure 3.2 Prescription form with attending provider.

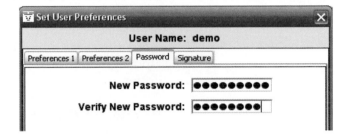

Figure 3.3 Password tab in set user preferences window.

a prescription form displaying an attending provider. Nurse practitioners and other providers may be required to indicate the attending provider when creating prescriptions.

Concept Checkup 3.2(LO 3.3)

A. SpringCharts provides each user the option to select the default _____ and _____, which will print on reports and letters.

B. The *Tracker Group* option is only used when the clinic has _____ _____.

C. How many appointment schedules can be set up in SpringCharts? _____

Preferences 2

The user has an option to choose either left or right orientation for the SpringCharts program. The point of reference affects the side that the navigation buttons appear in the *office visit* screen. The program defaults to "right." If the user selects "left," then the navigation button plane appears on the left side of the screen and the patient's face sheet information replaces it on the right side. This option allows for a greater ease of use on a Tablet PC or MacBook; right-handed users will prefer having the navigation panel on the right side of the *office visit* screen, while left-handed users will prefer the left side so that the user's arm does not block the screen when accessing the navigation buttons. Once the orientation preference has been chosen, the user will select the [Save] button.

Password

Passwords can be changed in the third tab of the *User Preferences* window. The user simply adds a new password, verifies password and clicks [Change Password]. Figure 3.3 illustrates the password tab in the *User Preferences* window. Passwords may be changed as often as needed when *Low Security* has been selected on the server administrator. However, when *High Security* has been selected on SpringCharts Server the program will enforce rigorous password rules, including minimum and maximum number of characters, and alphanumeric usage. Setting SpringCharts to high security is an administrative option.

Password High Security

SpringCharts EHR provides the medical clinic with the optional for high-security password management. When this feature is enabled it will obscure all passwords and requires users to reset passwords every 2 months. Some of the security elements of password management include:

- Encrypted passwords that are obscured from the user's view
- Automatic password reset every 60 days; users are prohibited from logging on until the password is changed
- Preset password length of eight to 16 characters
- Case-sensitive passwords
- Preset password guidelines that require at least one number, one character, and one special character (!@#$%&*)
- Administration-controlled replacement passwords, ensuring that users must request a new password if they forget
- Three strikes password protection; users get three tries before the program closes
- All user logins and logouts are recorded in the audit manager

Signature

SpringCharts allows for importing the user's digital signature which may then be used in various places throughout the program to stamp the user's real signature on letters, reports, prescriptions, and so on. There are three ways of setting up the users' signatures: 1. Creating a handwritten signature, scanning the image and saving it to the computer. Then by selecting the [Import] button, the user can navigate to the file and import it into the *User Preferences* window. 2. Using the stylus pen on a Tablet PC or MacBook to create the digital signature directly in the signature box. 3. Creating a signature in the field by signing an electronic signature pad that is connected to the computer via the USB port. The digital signature should be a maximum size of 2.3 x 0.75 inches.

After the signature has been placed in SpringCharts the user will select the [Save] button, return to the *Preferences 1* tab, and save all changes to the *Set User Preference* window.

Focal Point

HIPAA regulates the policies and procedures for password management in both PMS and EHR programs.

Focal Point

Each user of SpringCharts has the ability to customize various features and views of the program that will become the standard function for each specific user once logged on.

Concept Checkup 3.3 (LO 3.2)

A. With the high-security feature activated, users are required to change their password every _____ .

B. Also, passwords must contain at least:

1. _____   3. _____

2. _____   4. _____

Note: Before working Exercise 3.1, download and install SpringCharts EHR demo program from the Online Learning Center (www.mhhe.com/hamiltonehr2e). See pp. xxi–xxxvi for instructions on downloading, installing, and logging on to SpringCharts EHR. When the program initially opens, a tutorial launches. Please close this since you will not use it with this text.

Network Users

If you are operating SpringCharts on a network environment, your instructor will assign you a logon name and a password. Do not complete the exercises in each chapter. Exercises for network environments are located in Appendix C.

Exercise 3.1 Setting Your User Preferences (LO 3.2)

1. Double click on the SpringCharts icon on your desktop.

Note: This is the only time you will double click while using SpringCharts. Once the program is opened all functions are activated by a single click of the mouse.

2. SpringCharts is designed to allow each user the ability to change certain functions of the program. These preferences will adjust when the user logs on. Select the *File* menu on the main window and choose *Preferences > User Preferences.* Set up your preferences based on the items selected in the *Set User Preferences* window (see Figure 3.1.)

Note: Only change preferences under the *Preferences 1* tab. Do not change information under the *Preferences 2, Password,* and *Signature* tabs.

3. Click the [Save] button to save your material.

Additional Features

The optimal screen resolution for SpringCharts is 1024 × 768 pixels. To modify this setting, go to www.mhhe.com/hamiltonehr2e for details. SpringCharts has auto-formatting features: first and last names, middle initials, and addresses are automatically capitalized. Date of birth, phone numbers, and social security numbers are automatically punctuated once the user tabs off the data field. SpringCharts EHR is designed to automatically populate the city, state, zip code, and area code for a new patient via the setup of the medical practice. It assumes most patients will visit an area clinic. If the user enters patient information that differs from that area, he/she will backspace in these fields and type in the appropriate information. SpringCharts is preset with *Suburban Medical Group,* Sherman, Texas 77521 and the 214 area code.

LO 3.4 ADDRESS DATA SETUP

New Address

New addresses are added to SpringCharts through the *New* menu option in the main *Practice View* window. The *New Address* window is seen in Figure 3.4. **Patients are not added in the address book.** However, pharmacies, testing facilities, referring physicians, and vendors can be set up here. The address book can be accessed from various locations throughout SpringCharts.

The fields that must be completed for the new address to save are *Last Name* or *Company* and the *Category* fields. If users are recording information for a non-person entity, then the entry can commence on the *Company* line. If the user is recording information for a person, then at least the *Last Name* field must be completed; the *Company* field is optional in this case. The program will default in the city, state, and area code based upon the setup information of the practice. The required *Category* field displays a drop-down list of options that will enable SpringCharts to display specific addresses throughout the program based upon these groupings. For example, in the *Pending Tests* area, the [*Testing facility*] button will give the user a choice of facilities that have been assigned the classification of *Testing Facility* in the address setup window.

The *Category* and *Specialty* fields are populated from lists that have been set up on the SpringCharts Server. Figure 3.5 illustrates these two lists in the *Category Preferences* setup window on the server. If an additional item is needed on these lists, the administrator will need to add line entries in the *Category Preferences* window under the appropriate sections. The *Specialty* field is only used when adding a provider to the address book. Referring providers and consultants are added into the address book, not the providers within the clinic. In-house physicians are set up on SpringCharts Server as doctors. If an e-mail address is added to the profile, SpringCharts is able to access it through its integrated e-mail feature and send out messages, letters, reports, and so on from within the program. The window illustrated in Figure 3.6 appears

Figure 3.4 New address window.

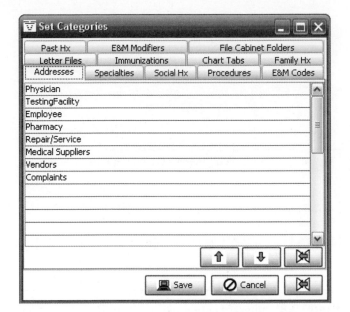

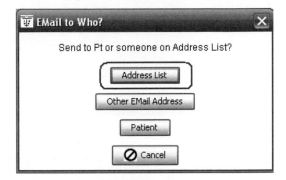

Figure 3.5 Address categories and specialties setup on SpringCharts Server.

Figure 3.6 E-mail address options within SpringCharts.

when a user clicks on the "send e-mail" option located in various places in SpringCharts.

The *Account* # field is for internal use and may be used to reference that address entity number in another program. The *Note* box is to record additional information that is not available in the provided field.

> Note: When entering a company name that has multiple locations in the *Company* field, users will need to indicate some defining information (such as location) in that same field. This extra information helps distinguish the different companies in the *Address Book* search window as seen in Figure 3.7.

The [Print] button in the *New Address* window will print the image and details of the address window. The [Print Card] option will allow the user to either print or fax the address information to a card-size image measuring approximately 1.75 × 4 inches, illustrated in Figure 3.8. This option may be useful when a patient needs an address and phone number for a physician or pharmacy.

Editing Addresses

The *Address Book* feature located in the *Productivity Center* is used to store, edit, and search for the address of supporting businesses, such as pharmacies, testing facilities, therapists, or outside physicians. The drop-down menu is used to search by name, company, specialty, or category. (This list of search criteria cannot be amended.) The first few letters of the name, company, specialty, or category are entered in the *Find* field and then the *Search* button is activated. A list of the addresses that match the search criteria is displayed.

The address information is displayed when the user double-clicks on a name; it can then be edited.

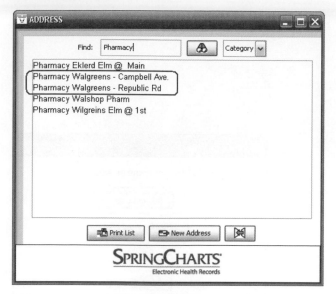

Figure 3.7 Address display for pharmacy category.

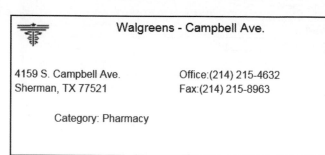

Figure 3.8 Print card option will print card-size information.

A new address can be added from the *Address Book* window by selecting the [New Address] button.

Exercise 3.2 Adding a New Address(LO 3.4)

1. In the *New* menu of the main screen select *New Address*.
2. Enter the name and demographics of your primary care physician. If you do not have one, please make up the information. In the *Category* field you will select *Physician*. Choose the medical specialty in the *Specialty* field. The *Account #* field is for internal use only; it could be used to reference the entry in another software program. Save the information.
3. Enter your name and demographics as a clinic employee. You will not fill in the *Company* and *Specialty* fields. Although SpringCharts users are set up as *Users* in the *Administration Panel* of SpringCharts Server, they need also to be entered in the *Address Book* as employees in order to capture the address and other information. Save the information.
4. Set up a pharmacy of your choice. You will start by entering information in the *Company* field. (You will not need to fill out the *name* information.) In this entry you will not fill out the *Specialty* field. Save the information.
5. Set up a Testing Facility: *MRI of the Ozarks, 103 E. Battlefield St., Springfield, MO 65807*. As with the pharmacy, you will not fill out the *name* information or choose a *Specialty* field. Be sure to use *Testing Facility* in the *Category* field so the program can display this entry in the appropriate place in SpringCharts. Add the other demographic details. Save the information.
6. Access the *Productivity Center* and the *Address Book* submenu. Locate each of your new addresses by searching under the *Category* option and typing the category in the *Find* field. As you open each address complete step 7.
7. Print out each of your addresses as a card size, write your name on the page, and submit to your instructor.

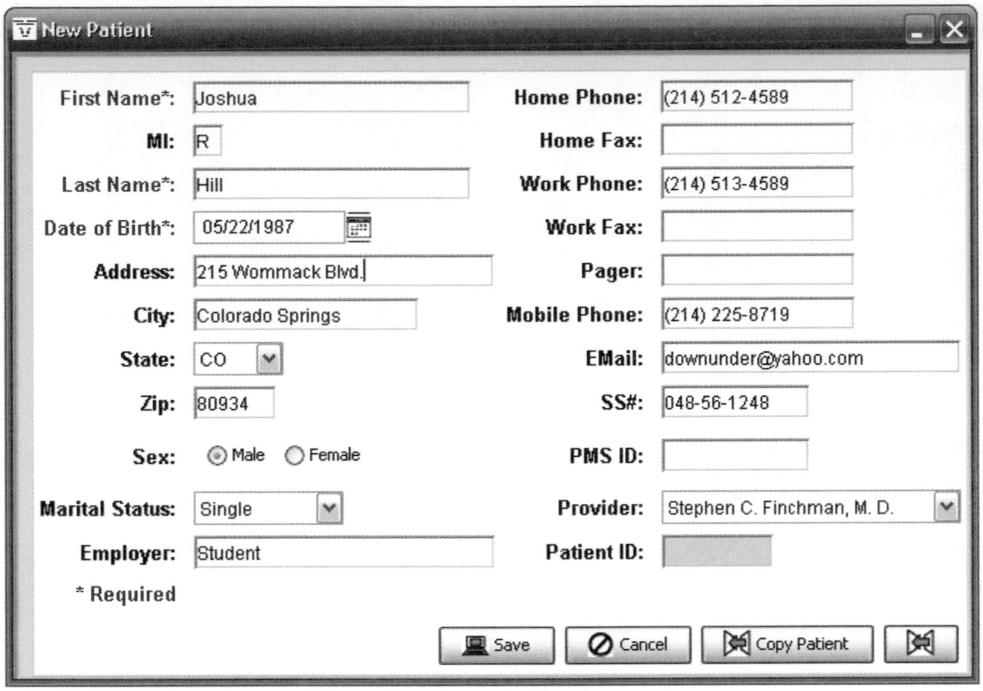

Figure 3.9 New patient setup window.

LO 3.5 PATIENT DATA SETUP

New Patient

The *New Patient* feature is used to create an electronic chart for a new patient. The front office personnel will click on the *New* menu option in the main *Practice View* window. A *New Patient* window will appear as seen in Figure 3.9.

Fields marked in red are required fields for the patient to be saved and a chart created. A patient's chart can be created rapidly by recording only the patient's first and last name and the date of birth. In a front office clerical environment this basic information can be received from the patient over the phone. The patient file can then be saved and the patient added to the schedule. On the scheduled appointment day, the remaining information can be added when the patient completes the Intake Forms. The *PMS ID* field is automatically populated with the patient unique identification code from a practice management system (PMS) if SpringCharts is interfaced with such a program. Otherwise this field is left blank. The *Patient ID* field is grayed out because the program will assign a unique consecutive ID number to the patient when the *new patient* information is saved. SpringCharts can store up to 1 million patient ID numbers.

Existing demographic information can be copied from a family member who is already set up in SpringCharts by selecting the [Copy Patient] button. In the *Choose Patient* window, the staff will enter the first few letters of the patient's last name and click on the search button then select the appropriate patient name. The last name, address, and phone number are copied into the *New Patient* window.

Editing Patients

When editing a patient record the clerical staff will select *Patients* under the main *Edit* menu. Patients can be located by selecting one of the criteria in the *Search* dropdown list: last name, zip code, social security number, home number, work number, patient number, birth date, and e-mail. Any of the demographic information can be modified once the desired patient is located.

Focal Point

Only the patient's first name, last name, and date of birth are necessary to create a new patient chart.

Focal Point

In order to create a patient chart, the patient information must first be entered into the program.

Focal Point

A duplicate patient alert is triggered in SpringCharts when the patient's first name, last name, and date of birth are entered a second time. This guards against a patient being set up in the program multiple times. The social security number (SSN) is not used to trigger a duplicate patient because some people will give their SSN with their personal information. The SSN is not a required identifier with medical records.

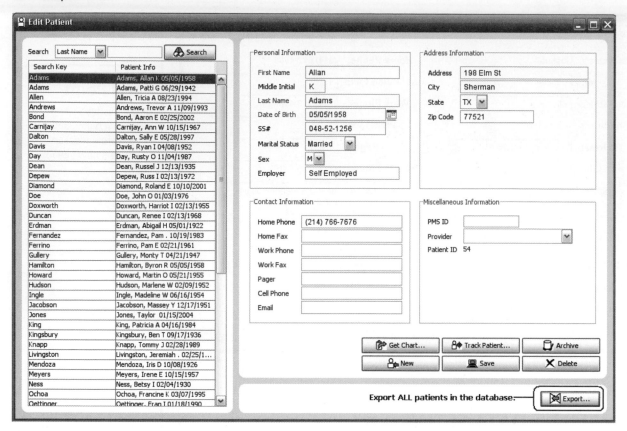

Figure 3.10 Edit patient window.

From the *Edit Patient* window one may: get the patient's chart, track the patient into the *Patient Tracker*, delete the selected patient or create a new patient. A patient can be removed from the active list and moved to an archived patient list by selecting the [Archive] button. (The archive feature of SpringCharts will be discussed in detail in Chapter 10.)

The entire list of patients can be viewed by clicking the [Search Button] without entering any data in the *Search* field, illustrated in Figure 3.10. To export the list of patients the administrator would select the [Export] button and choose either *Export Item* or *Export List* to export the specific highlighted patient or to export the entire database of patients. The standard options for exporting will be displayed for the user. (The universal export feature will be discussed in further detail in Chapter 10.)

Exercise 3.3 Adding a New Patient(LO 3.5)

1. Select the *New* menu on the main screen. Select the *New Patient* submenu and enter yourself as a patient. Note the first name is filled out first. Save the information.

Note: The date of birth can be entered by using the mmddyyyy format (without the punctuation) in the *Date of Birth* field. The punctuation will occur automatically after you tab off the field. Another method of selecting the patient's date of birth is by using the popup calendar to the right.

2. Once again, open a *New Patient* window and record a patient's first name, middle initial, and date of birth. Click the [Copy Patient] button and type *"adams"* in the *Choose Patient* window. Select *Patti Adams*. Note the family information that is copied from an existing patient. Complete the remaining information. The *Home Phone* will need to remain the same in order for these two patients to be linked in the same household list. Save the information.

3. Select the main *Edit* menu and then choose the *Patients* submenu. Select *Zip Code* as the *Search* criterion and type "77521" in the *Search* field and click the [Search] button. You will be provided a list of all the patients in the database having this specific zip code. Select *Patti Adams* and add a *Work Phone* to her demographics. Click the [Save] button.

4. Click the [Export] button and select *Export List*. Choose the [Open in Word Processor] option and SpringCharts will recreate the list of patients with a zip code of 77521 into your computer's default word processing program. In most cases this will be Notepad™. From here the list can be printed out, saved, and so on. You will notice that the date of birth is in the yyyymmdd format. Notepad defaults to the font size that was last used on the computer. If your text size appears abnormal, change the font under the *Format* menu in Notepad to 10 points.

5. Print out your list, write your name on the paper, and submit to your instructor.

LO 3.6 INSURANCE DATA SETUP

New Insurance

To add new insurance companies into SpringCharts, the clerical staff will select *Insurance* under the main *Edit* menu. Because SpringCharts is not a billing program, the insurance information is used to select the primary insurance for the patient, which is then stored in the face sheet of the patient's chart. The patient's primary insurance can also be added to an order form so that outside testing facilities are able to bill insurance companies for their work. Only the primary insurance is added to the patient's face sheet; most practitioners do not find secondary insurance information useful.

Once in the *Insurance* window the user will select the [New Insurance Company] button to record the insurance information and claim mailing address. The *Details* window enables the user to record additional information.

In the *Insurance* window the user can also select the [Get Patient's Insurance] button to view the details of a specific patient's insurance record. This feature is useful when examining other family members' insurance information for accuracy. When the *Patient Insurance Information* window is opened the user may select the [Edit] button to modify any of the insurance information that had been previously saved under that patient's profile.

Add new insurance button

View other patient's insurance button

Editing Insurance

To edit existing insurance information the user will select the specific insurance company in the left-hand column, illustrated in Figure 3.11. The [Edit] button will display the insurance details which can be modified. The entire insurance company can be deleted from the list by selecting the [Delete] button.

The linking of the primary insurance company to the patient's chart is discussed in Chapter 5.

Focal Point

Only the patient's primary insurance is stored in SpringCharts. This is used for reference material; insurance billing is typically handled by the PMS program.

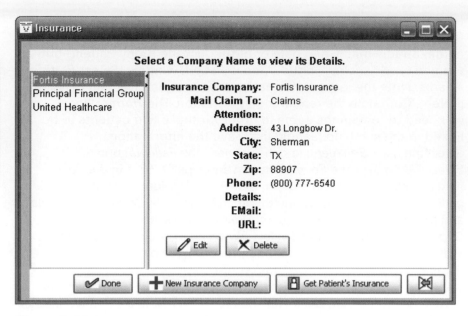

Figure 3.11 Insurance setup window.

Exercise 3.4 Adding a New Insurance(LO 3.6)

1. Click on the *Edit* menu on the main menu. Select the *Insurance* submenu. Click on the company name: Fortis Insurance. Click the [Edit] button and add your own contact person in the *Attention* field and an e-mail address. Save this information.
2. Click the [New Insurance Company] button and add a new insurance company to SpringCharts. If you have your own insurance card, you may want to record this information. If not, you can make up an insurance company and the demographics. Save the new insurance company.
3. Highlight the newly added insurance company and select the *Universal Export* button in the lower right corner. Select the [Open in Word Processor] button.
4. In the word processing program, type your name at the top of the insurance information.
5. Print the document and submit to your instructor.

Universal Export

Concept Checkup 3.4 (LO 3.4, 3.5, 3.6)

A. New patients are added into SpringCharts through which windows?

   1. *Address Book* window   **2.** *New Patient* window

B. In the address book, the *Specialty* field is only used when setting up a _____.

C. Only the _____ insurance is stored in the face sheet of the patient's chart.

Name _____ Instructor _____ Class _____

USING TERMINOLOGY

Match the terms on the left with the definitions on the right.

_____ **1.** 1024 × 768 pixels

_____ **2.** PMS

_____ **3.** Rapid select

_____ **4.** Measurements

_____ **5.** Drug formulary

_____ **6.** Bi-directional flow

_____ **7.** Standard select

_____ **8.** Time stamp

A. Listings of pharmaceutical substances and formulas for making medicinal preparations.(LO 3.1)

B. Will automatically insert a 12-hour time (a.m./p.m. style) or military 24-hour time at various locations in the program.(LO 3.3)

C. Selects what units of measure the vitals will be recorded in (imperial or metric).(LO 3.3)

D. The optimal screen resolution for SpringCharts.(LO 3.3)

E. Data exchange to and from two different software programs.(LO 3.1)

F. Type in the necessary letter(s) and then click on the search icon to activate the search function.(LO 3.3)

G. Practice Management Software.(LO 3.1)

H. A search function of SpringCharts that is activated once the user pauses after typing a few letters.(LO 3.3)

CHECKING YOUR UNDERSTANDING

Write "T" or "F" in the blank to indicate whether you think the statement is true or false.

_____ **9.** SpringCharts EHR makes available a one-click link to many clinical and pharmaceutical websites.(LO 3.2)

_____ **10.** In 2002 SMSI released MacExtraction, an interface with the Mcintosh PMS program, MacPractice.™ (LO 3.1)

_____ **11.** Clinics that have several locations can work from the same patient database over the Internet and can track the patients separately for each location.(LO 3.3)

_____ **12.** The term "OV" stands for the ovulation cycle of gynecology patients.(LO 3.3)

_____ **13.** There are two types of search modes in SpringCharts—"RealQuik Select" and "SloMo Select."(LO 3.3)

_____ **14.** The measurements option allows you to record vitals in either metered or imperative units.(LO 3.3)

Answer the question below in the space provided.

15. Name at least three advantages that SpringCharts EHR will bring to a clinic.(LO 3.2)

_____

_____

_____

Choose the best answer and circle the corresponding letter.

16. SpringCharts EHR was designed and implemented by:^(LO 3.1)
    a) Practicing physicians
    b) Technology executives
    c) Both a and b

17. The EHR program is designed to manage this side of a medical practice:^(LO 3.1)
    a) Financial
    b) Non-financial
    c) Both a and b

18. A practice that has several clinics in various locations has the ability to:^(LO 3.2)
    a) View complete patient medical records stored at the central office only
    b) View complete patient medical records at each location provided that the records are stored there
    c) View complete patient medical records for any of the clinics from any location

19. The tracker group options that displays the list of patients in the patient tracker window:^(LO 3.3)
    a) Can track patients in multiple locations
    b) Can track patients in a specific practice only
    c) Can track patients in competitors' offices also

20. In the United States, the typical units of measure in which the vitals will be recorded are:^(LO 3.3)
    a) Metric
    b) Imperative
    c) Imperial

21. The optimal screen resolution for SpringCharts is:^(LO 3.3)
    a) 800 × 600 pixels
    b) The maximum that your computer will allow
    c) 1024 × 768 pixels

22. Automatic capitalization and punctuation is a SpringCharts feature designed to:^(LO 3.3)
    a) Make front office staff lazy
    b) Speed the data entry process
    c) Be set up in the User Preferences window

23. A duplicate patient alert is triggered when the following patient information is duplicated:^(LO 3.5)
    a) Social Security number
    b) Date of birth, zip code, and area code
    c) First name, last name, and date of birth

24. Why is the *Category* field a required field when setting up a new address?^(LO 3.4)
    a) So the program can display specific addresses throughout the program based on these categories
    b) So more information can be stored for companies
    c) To provide an alternative to the *Specialty* field

25. The patient's primary insurance is stored in the patient's chart so that:^(LO 3.6)
    a) It can be used to bill insurance companies
    b) It can be added to an order form for testing facilities
    c) Patients can be reminded to file with their insurance companies

4

The Clinic Administration

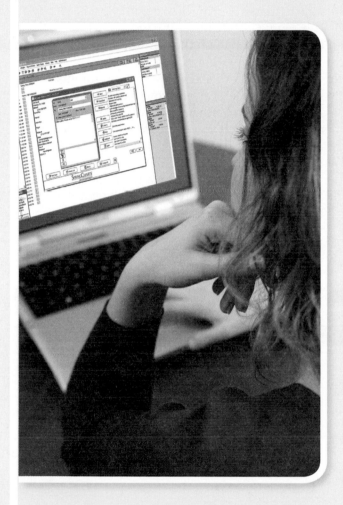

What You Need to Know

To understand Chapter 4 you will need to know how to:

- Start SpringCharts EHR
- Set your user preferences
- Set up new patients and demographics
- Set up new addresses

Key Terms

Terms you will encounter in Chapter 4:

Appointment Schedule

Message Archive

No Show

Patient Status

Patient Tracker

Pop-Up Text

Tracker Archive

Tool Bar

Urgent Message

LO 4.1 **OVERVIEW**

Most administrative and communicative work will be done from the practice view window of the SpringCharts Client program. This is the first screen displayed upon successful logon. The practice view screen provides an up-to-the-minute overview of all office activity. At-a-glance tools include:

- Calendar
- Appointment schedule
- Patient tracker with color coding
- ToDos with visual status indicators
- Detailed message list with patient identifiers

In most cases, when choosing an item in SpringCharts, simply click *once* with the left-click of the mouse. The *Tap-n-Go*™ feature utilized on a Tablet PC enables the user to tap once with the stylist pen on the desired item and move to the next one.

The practice view window, seen in Figure 4.1, shows appointments for the day in the middle section, with views of the 1) appointment calendar, 2) patient tracker, 3) ToDo/Reminders list, and 4) message list, surrounding the main window. The top left corner of the practice view screen displays the current time and the user presently logged on. The *Appointment Schedule* and the *Patient Tracker* are consistent for all users on the network; the *ToDo List* and the *Messages* are user-defined and will only show information relevant to the specific user logged on. Each of these four mini-programs is fully integrated with the patient charting feature of SpringCharts, enabling the user to access the chart from multiple locations within the program. The **Tool Bar,** illustrated in Figure 4.2, presents the most commonly used features accessed from the practice view screen.

Tool Bar

Offers a lineup of icons that give the user shortcut access to the most commonly used functions of the program.

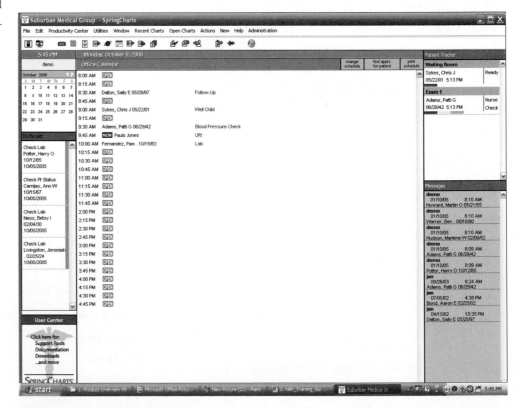

Figure 4.1 Practice view screen.

These universal icons enable speed selection, which is particularly useful when implementing Tap-N-Go™ computing on Tablet PCs.

Concept Checkup 4.1(LO 4.1)

A. List the four main elements of the practice view screen.

1. _____

2. _____

3. _____

4. _____

B. Which two elements of the practice view screen only display information specifically related to the user logged on?

1. _____

2. _____

Focal Point

SpringCharts functions by a single click of the mouse or a single tap of the stylus pen on a touch screen computer.

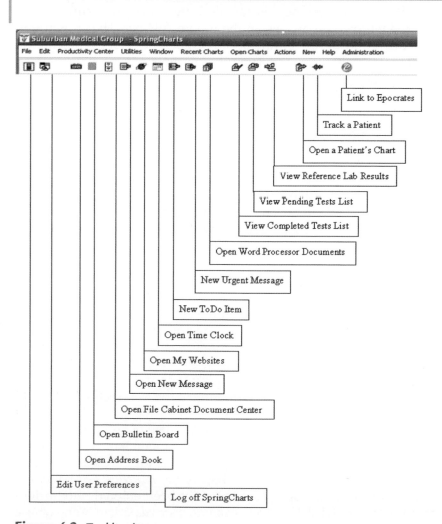

Figure 4.2 Tool bar icons.

Concept Checkup 4.2(LO 4.1)

A. The following three icons on the practice view toolbar correspond to opening what three tests? 🖊️ 📷 📠

   1. _____

   2. _____

   3. _____

B. Draw the icon that represents opening a patient's chart.

C. ⬛ This icon enables the user to _____ without shutting down the program.

Appointment Schedule

Displays past, current, and future appointments for patients. Multiple appointment schedules can be created in the one program to display patient appointments for medical providers and other resources. Appointment Schedules can show a variety of appointment length slots.

Office Calendar menu items

NEW

New patient identifier

Focal Point

Patients' names, scheduled breaks, and notes can be placed on the office schedule.

LO 4.2 APPOINTMENT CALENDAR

From the appointment calendar the user can navigate to prior or future months by clicking on the left or right arrows on the month title bar. The current day will always be displayed in red. Future schedules can be seen by clicking on the appropriate date of the calendar. The window opens to a smaller screen from where other office schedules for the same day can be viewed, edited, and printed.

From the **Appointment Schedule** the user can view other office schedules by clicking on [Change Schedule] on the office calendar menu bar (see margin illustration). The newly selected schedule will become the main window schedule. Appointments and breaks can be easily set by clicking on the appropriate time slot and filling out the required information in the *Edit Appointment* window. **Existing** patients are added to the appointment schedule by first selecting the [Choose Patient] button. Patients are chosen by typing the first few letters of the patient's last name in the *Choose Patient* window. To add a **new** patient only to the appointment schedule without adding the patient's name and demographics to the database, the user will simply type the patient's name in the *Patient* field of the *Edit Appointment* window shown in Figure 4.3. This will stamp the *New* symbol (see margin illustration) onto the schedule beside the patient's name after the [Done] button has been selected. This option is suited for clinics that want to wait until the new patient actually arrives for the appointment before entering the patient's name and demographics into SpringCharts database.

When blocking time, the administrator will select the [Block This Time] button rather than the [Choose Patient] button in this window. If the user would like to display the reason for blocked time, information in the *Note* section of the *Edit Appointment* window will need to be filled out.

Past and future appointments for patients can be viewed and printed by selecting [Find Appts for Patient] on the office calendar menu bar. Once selected, the user will be given the choice to view appointments for either *new* or *existing* patients in the search window (Figure 4.4). A *New/Unregistered* patient is a patient whose name and demographics have not been entered into Spring-Charts database, as described above. An *Existing/Registered* patient is one whose information has been set up in SpringCharts database. When searching for a

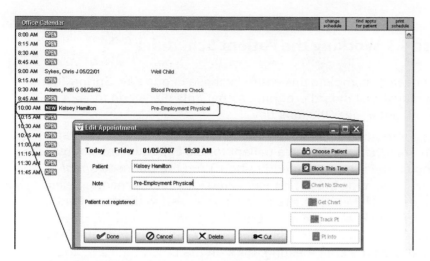

Figure 4.3 Adding a new patient to appointment schedule.

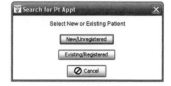

Figure 4.4 Searching for new or existing patient appointments option.

new/unregistered patient, simply type the patient's name in the *Find New Patient* field. When searching for an *Existing/Registered* patient, type the first few letters of the patient's last name in the *Choose Patient* window. The following printable appointment list will show all past and future appointments for the selected patient.

The current schedule displayed can be printed by selecting [Print Schedule] on the office calendar menu bar. (Set up of and modifying of the start and end time slots as well as the appointment length intervals is conducted in the administration panel of SpringCharts Server.) SpringCharts appointment grid can be used as a stand-alone scheduler or integrated with many Practice Management Software (PMS) systems so that the appointment schedule from the Practice Management Systems' scheduler is imported dynamically into SpringCharts. If the medical clinic is using a link to a PMS program it is recommended that all the scheduling be done in the PMS software. PMS schedulers typically are more robust, offering a wider range of reporting capabilities.

SpringCharts gives the clinic the ability to chart a **no show** for patients who do not show up for their appointments. If a patient missed a scheduled appointment, the receptionist would click on the patient's name in the office schedule. In the *Edit Appointment* window the [Chart No Show] button would be clicked. A note is added to the patient's chart documenting the no show.

No Show
Term used to indicate a patient missed a scheduled appointment without calling in advance to inform the clinic of his or her intentions and/or to reschedule.

Concept Checkup 4.3(LO 4.2)

A. To stamp the word: "New" beside the patient's name on the scheduler, one must type the patient's name in the *Patient* field rather than selecting the patient from the _____ button.

B. A *New/Unregistered* patient is a patient whose _____ _____ have not been entered into SpringCharts database.

C. To add a No show note in the patient's chart, click on the _____ _____ button in the *Edit Appointment* window.

Focal Point
The appointment schedule in SpringCharts can be used as a stand-alone feature or the schedule from a PMS program can be imported through an interface module.

Exercise 4.1 Working the Patient Scheduler (L.O. 4.2)

OPEN
Open Appointments

Note: You need to complete this entire exercise in one day. SpringCharts EHR is an industry-standard program, so patients placed on today's schedule will not appear the next day.

1. With your mouse in hand, left click on an "OPEN" icon on the appointment schedule. Assign a patient to this appointment slot by clicking on the [Choose Patient] button. With the *Choose Patient* window open, type in the first few letters of your last name. Select your name and then type a reason for your visit in the *Note* field. Add your initials after the note. Click the [Done] button.[(LO 4.1)]

2. Choose the last hour of the day where you will block out time from the schedule for a staff meeting. Click on the *OPEN* time slot and type *Staff Meeting* in the *Note* field. Click on the [Block this Time] button in the *Edit Appointment* window. Do this exercise three more times until the entire hour is blocked.[(LO 4.2)]

3. Click on another *OPEN* slot on the appointment schedule. Type a new patient's name in the *Patient* field then type in a reason for the visit in the *Note* field. Add your initials after the note. Click the [Done] button.[(LO 4.1)]

4. Add the established patients, Sally Dalton and Robert Underhagen, to the appointment schedule. Add the reason note "UTI" (urinary tract infection) to Sally and the reason note "Lab" to Robert. Remember to add your initials after the note for each patient that you add to the schedule.[(LO 4.1)]

5. Add two new patients to the appointment schedule along with appropriate reason notes.[(LO 4.1)]

6. Block out time for a half-hour staff meeting on the last Friday of each month for the next 6 months. Label the blocked time. Close the additional appointment windows.[(LO 4.2)]

7. Print the current patient schedule. Circle your name on the schedule and submit to your instructor.[(LO 4.3)]

8. Chart yourself as a No Show. Save the No Show documentation under the *Encounter* tab. The program will indicate the charting of the No show. Click on the [Get Chart] button in the *Edit Appointment* window. Click on the "+" sign to the left of the *Encounter* tab in the upper right panel of the patient's chart to view the no show entry. Clicking on the "No Show" entry will display the details in the lower window. The *No Show* note can be further modified by clicking on the [Edit] button.[(LO 4.4)]

LO 4.3 PATIENT TRACKER

Patient Tracker
Enables all users across the network to see at a glance the current location and the status of all patients in the clinic. It records the time each patient entered and left the clinic.

The *Patient Tracker* is located at the upper right side of the practice view window. This notable feature, illustrated in Figure 4.5, enables all users to see at a glance the current location and the status of all patients in the clinic.

Patients can be added to the *Patient Tracker* by clicking once on their name in the schedule. In the following *Edit Appointment* window (Figure 4.6) the user selects [Track Pt] and then chooses the appropriate location for the patient from the *Location* window. The patient is then added to the *Patient Tracker*. It is important to add patients to the *Patient Tracker* as soon as the patient arrives in the clinic. The program will time-stamp the tracker record when a patient is added. This information

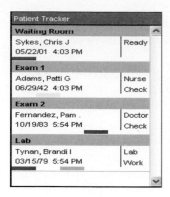

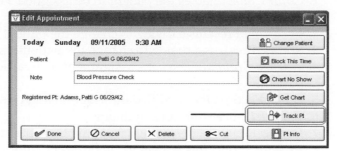

Figure 4.5 Patient tracker window.

Figure 4.6 Edit appointment window.

may be important at a later time when determining the time frame that a patient was in the clinic. The *Edit Tracker* window defaults to highlight *Waiting Room* as the location choice. The front office user will simply click [Done] when this window opens to add the selected patient into the *Patient Tracker* in a timely fashion.

If a patient is not on the schedule, the user will click on the *Patient Tracker* title bar and select a patient by typing the last name in the *Choose Patient* window. This is useful when clinics allow walk-in patients because their name would not appear in the schedule. However, the patient would need to be set up as a new patient first.

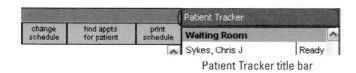

Patient Tracker title bar

In certain areas on the clinic, users may find it more beneficial to display either the *Patient Tracker* or the *Messages List* as the main large window. When changing the main view, the *Appointment List* switches positions with the selected feature and appears as a smaller window on the edge of the screen. To change the main view the users will simply select *Actions* from the main menu, select *Change View* and choose the desired view as seen in Figure 4.7.

A newly created tracker item will appear on the *Patient Tracker* list of every user's screen currently logged onto SpringCharts. The time that the patient is entered into the *Tracker* is recorded. To edit a tracker item and select other defining features, the user will click on any patient in the *Patient Tracker* List. The *Edit Tracker* dialog appears, seen here in Figure 4.8.

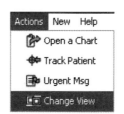

Figure 4.7 Change main view through actions menu.

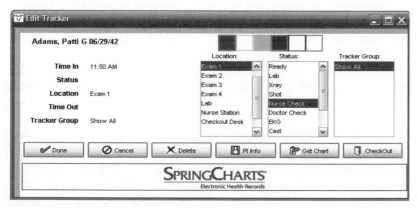

Figure 4.8 Edit tracker window.

From this dialog box, several selection windows and buttons are available:

1. *Color Code:* Enables the patient to be assigned a color status or several color statuses.
2. *Location:* Presents a dialog to change the patient's location in the office.
3. *Status:* Presents a dialog to change the patient's status.
4. *Tracker Group:* Enables the assignment of a particular tracker group to the patient.
5. *Done:* Records the modified information and closes the dialog box.
6. *Cancel:* Cancels the current dialog.
7. *Delete:* Removes this patient from the tracker.
8. *Pt Info:* Shows this patient's demographic information and allows for modification.
9. *Get Chart:* Opens this patient's chart.
10. *CheckOut:* Moves the patient to the lower part of the list, changes the status to "Done," and records the check-out time.

> Note: Setup and modification of *Locations, Statuses,* and *Tracker Groups* is done in the administration panel of SpringCharts Server.

Color Coding

The six-color option used to flag a patient in the *Patient Tracker* is defined by each clinic. It does not interface with any color flagging feature in any PMS software with which SpringCharts may be interoperated. The color flag will remain associated with the patients as they are moved from one location to another and as various status indicators are used. Several colors can be associated with each patient. Some possible applications of the color-flagging are as follows:

1. In a multiprovider clinic the colors could be used to indicate which physician the patient needs to see.
2. In a single-provider environment the colors may be used to indicate which nurse or other clinician would be assigned to the patient.
3. The colors could be used to indicate financial- or insurance-related information: self-pay, workers comp, Medicaid patients, and so on.

Location and Status

The *Location* and *Status* allocations enable the clinic to know exactly where each patient is located in the facility and the status of each patient. These two items are some of the many customizable features of the SpringCharts program. During the time of initial setup, the clinic's various locations and the statuses are entered into SpringCharts Server. They then can be viewed in the *Edit Tracker* window across the network.

Patient Status
Allows the clinical staff to know in general terms what is currently happening with the patient or what needs to be done next. The *Status* is chosen from a drop-down list that is customized by the clinic.

Some examples of a **patient status** could be ready, nurse check, doctor ready, doctor check, nurse orders, facial, lab work, and so on. The *Status* allows the clinical staff to know in general terms what is currently happening with the patient or what needs to be done next. The *Status* in SpringCharts takes the place of the physical flagging system that is often seen outside exam rooms in clinics. For example, if a patient is in the waiting room and all paper work has been processed and insurance verified, the patient would be seen in the *Patient Tracker* showing the time he or she entered the clinic, the *Location* would be "waiting room," the *Status* would be "ready," and the color bar would indicate which nurse needs to call the patient back to the clinic area. The physician and staff will need to be

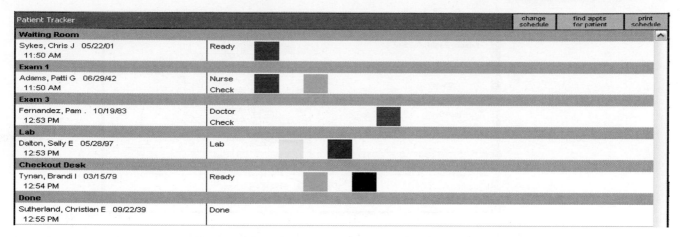

Figure 4.9 Patient tracker window as the main view.

attentive to the changing locations and status of the patients in the *Patient Tracker* in order to know the next activity assigned for each patient. For this reason many clinical staff will want to set their screens to show the *Patient Tracker* as the main screen—seen in Figure 4.9. (Outlined in the previous Patient Tracker section). When a nurse escorts a patient back to an exam room, he/she will change both the location and the status for that patient in the *Patient Tracker*. For example, the nurse may change the *Location* to "exam room 1" and the *Status* to "nurse check." If there are no patients in a specific area listed in the *Location* list, that heading will not be displayed in the *Patient Tracker* screen.

Tracker Group

Clinics that have offices in more than one location usually operate from the same SpringCharts database across the Internet. This enables complete patient medical information to be seen from the various locations. In order to track the patients separately at each location, various *Tracker Groups* can be set up within SpringCharts Server (e.g., Northside Clinic, Southside Clinic). If a clinic is operating with multiple locations, the specific tracker group is also assigned to the patient along with the location and status item in the *Edit Tracker* window. In the *User Preferences* window of the *File* menu each SpringCharts user will choose the default *Tracker Group* that he or she wants to see on the main screen. If *Show All* is selected the user will see the list of patients who are presently in the *Patient Tracker* grid of all the clinics. Setting up distinct tracker groups may also be useful for the single clinic with two waiting areas (e.g., a pediatrician's office that has separate sick and well child waiting rooms).

Patient Info

The patient demographic information can be viewed, printed, and edited from this window. In a linked PMS environment, this information is often imported automatically into SpringCharts from the PMS. If this is the case, changes to the patient's demographics will be done in the PMS program and the modifications will be automatically updated in SpringCharts.

CheckOut

When the patient is finally checked out of the facility the receptionist selects [CheckOut] in the *Edit Tracker* window (seen in Figure 4.10) and the patient's name is moved under a category heading of "done," the status changes to

Focal Point

The tracker group option can be set up for clinics with separate locations that share the same database or for a single medical office with more than one waiting room.

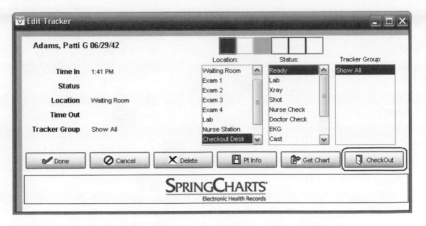

Figure 4.10 CheckOut feature in the edit tracker window.

Patient Tracker		change schedule	find appts for patient	print schedule
Waiting Room				
Sykes, Chris J 05/22/01 2:51 PM	Ready			
Exam 1				
Adams, Patti G 06/29/42 2:51 PM	Nurse Check			
Exam 2				
Dalton, Sally E 05/28/97 2:52 PM	Doctor Check			
Checkout Desk				
Swenson, Christian C 01/24/48 2:53 PM	Ready			
Done				
Dean, Russel J 12/13/35 3:00 PM √ Routing Slip	Done			

Figure 4.11 Checked routing slip stamp in patient tracker window.

"done" and the color flag(s) for the patient are removed, seen in Figure 4.11. The system then logs the checkout time for the patient. The recorded checkout time can be viewed in the *Edit Tracker* window of the "done" patients.

In the *Patient Tracker* window SpringCharts will also display a notification when a routing slip has been generated for the patient after a billed encounter. (A routing slip, discussed in Chapter 6, is synonymous with a charge ticket or superbill and contains the codes and description relevant to the visit.) When a routing slip is created at the completion of a billable office visit, the tracker shows a pink checked *Routing Slip* stamp in the patient tracker, illustrated in Figure 4.11. This routing slip stamp is also displayed in the *Tracker Archive* where records can be searched for non-billed office visits. The routing slips for billable encounters are located under *Edit>Routing Slip* where they can be printed out and manually entered into the PMS program for billing. In an interoperative linked environment with a PMS, the billing transactions may be sent automatically into the PMS software.

Tracker Archive

A record of patients tracked through the *Patient Tracker* is kept in the **Tracker Archive**. The user will select *Tracker Archive* from the *Edit* menu on the main screen. The *Edit Tracker Archive* window is displayed, as seen in Figure 4.12. In

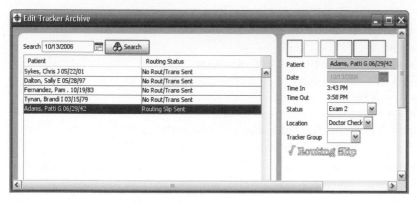

Figure 4.12 Edit tracker archive window.

the *Search* field the user will type the desired date or select from the calendar window and all patients tracked for that date will appear in the window along with such details as time logged in and out of the tracker and whether or not a routing slip was created.

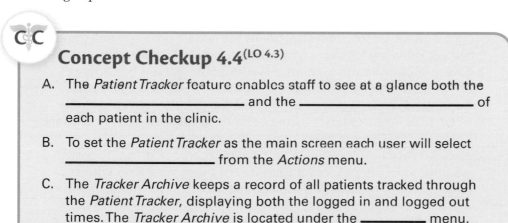

Concept Checkup 4.4(LO 4.3)

A. The *Patient Tracker* feature enables staff to see at a glance both the _____ and the _____ of each patient in the clinic.

B. To set the *Patient Tracker* as the main screen each user will select _____ from the *Actions* menu.

C. The *Tracker Archive* keeps a record of all patients tracked through the *Patient Tracker*, displaying both the logged in and logged out times. The *Tracker Archive* is located under the _____ menu.

Exercise 4.2 Working the Patient Tracker(LO 4.3)

Note: If you complete this exercise on a different day than Exercise 4.1, you will need to add Sally Dalton, Robert Underhagen, and yourself to the schedule before you begin.

1. Click on the patient Chris Sykes in the patient tracker. Change the *Status* in the *Edit Tracker* window to *Ready*. Click the [Done] button.
2. Upgrade the status of Patti Adams in the patient tracker to *Nurse Check*. Click the [Done] button.
3. Using the data that you set up in Exercise 4.1, add Sally Dalton to the patient tracker by clicking one time on the patient's name in the office schedule and selecting the [Track Pt] button. You will notice the program automatically selects *Waiting Room* as the default location. Immediately click [Done]. You will also notice the program stamps the time that Sally Dalton was entered into the patient tracker.

4. Let us assume we are working for a clinic that has allocated color flags as follows:
   a. Blue—A patient visit for Dr. Finchman
   b. Yellow—A patient visit for a nurse check only
   c. Green—A self-pay patient
   d. Red—A patient visit for lab work only
   e. Black—A patient visit for a specific office procedure
   f. Fuchsia—A Medicaid patient

   Click on Sally Dalton's name in the patient tracker and use the color flags along the top of the *Edit Tracker* window to indicate that the patient is coming in for a nurse check and has Medicaid as her primary insurance. Assign her a *Ready* status.

5. Click on Chris Sykes in the waiting room and move him to exam room 2. Give him a status of *Nurse Check* and save him back into the patient tracker.

6. Let us assume the nurse assigned to Patti Adams in exam room 1 is now finished with recording the chief complaints and taking the vitals. Update the patient tracker by changing the status of the patient to *Doctor Check*. Dr. Finchman will notice the update on his patient tracker and will know the location of the patient who now requires his attention.

7. Select Robert Underhagen from the schedule. Robert has arrived and is going straight to the clinic's lab room. Select the [Track Pt] button and place Robert directly in the lab location with the status of lab technician. Indicate by the color flags that this is a nurse check only and for lab work only.

8. Assume your employment is in the clinical area of office. You will want to make the patient tracker into the main screen on your computer. Do this by accessing the *Actions Menu* on the main screen.

9. A walk-in patient has arrived at the clinic. The patient is not on the schedule. This is an established patient. Click one time on the patient tracker header bar and type the last name *Zigman* in the window. Select the patient and click [Done] in the *Edit Tracker* window.

10. The doctor is now finished with the office visit in exam room 1. He or she will click on Patti Adams' name, change the location to *Checkout Desk*, change the status to *Ready*, and click [Done]. Exam room 1 is now available for another patient.

11. Change the status of Chris Sykes to *Doctor Check* and move Sally Dalton into exam room 1 with a *Nurse Check* status.

12. When Patti Adams has been processed at the front desk by setting another appointment and paying her co-pay, the checkout desk personnel will now click on the final [CheckOut] button in the *Edit Tracker* window. You will notice the program changes the location to *Done* and the status to *Done* and removes the color flags from the patient.

13. Add yourself to the waiting room in the patient tracker.

14. Go to the *Tracker Archive* window in the *Edit* menu. The *Edit Tracker Archive* window will display the patients who were processed through the patient tracker today. Click on Patti Adams and notice the *Time In* and *Time Out* stamp on the right-side panel.

15. Click on the [Export] button and export the **list** of names to *Open in Word Processor*.

16. Print out the list of patients, circle your name, and submit to your instructor. Close the *Edit Patient Tracker* window.

LO 4.4 ToDos AND REMINDERS

The *ToDo List* is located just below the calendar on the left of the practice view screen. A ToDo item is set by clicking once on the *ToDo List* title bar. In the *New ToDo/Reminder* window (illustrated in Figure 4.13) one may, 1) notate the ToDo item, 2) send the item to another coworker, 3) link the item to a patient, and/or 4) schedule the ToDo/Reminder for a future date.

In the *New ToDo/Reminder* window the user will type the ToDo/Reminder message in the top text field or select **pop-up text** from the list in the right window. To add to this list of pop-up text for current and future use, the user simply clicks on the *Edit* icon. The link opens the *Edit PopUp Text* feature that enables the user to add, delete, or modify text in many different categories that are used in the system. To modify the text the user will select the *ToDo-Reminders* category on the left side and make necessary adjustments to the text. Lines of text can be moved up or down by clicking on the up and down arrows to the far left. The arrow adjacent to the text will need to be selected to move the text up or down to the next line. Any of the categories of text can be printed out by selecting the [Print] button and highlighting the category. For printing multiple categories you can use the [Shift] and [Ctrl] keys to highlight specific categories or groups of categories.

When a user sends a ToDo/Reminder item to him/herself it is stored in the *ToDo List*, illustrated in Figure 4.14, until the reminder item is completed.

When ToDo/Reminder items are set they will have one of three color indicators, as shown below.

1. A ToDo with a green bar on the right is active and will stay on this user's list until it is selected. Selecting the item will change an active ToDo to a completed ToDo, indicated by a red checked box; selecting it again will reactivate the ToDo back to the original color bar.
2. A ToDo with a blue bar on the right indicates the item is linked to a patient. When this ToDo is selected, the patient's chart will open automatically and the ToDo will be checked as completed. The item may be checked to reactivate again.
3. A ToDo with an orange bar indicates communication between a user and an administrator regarding requested changes to the time clock feature.
4. A ToDo with the red check is a completed item. The next time this user logs on, these items will not be on the list. Clicking on a red check box will activate the ToDo item again. All items without a red check box will continue to roll over to the next day until completed.

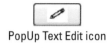

PopUp Text Edit icon

Pop-Up Text

Large groups of text in SpringCharts provides rapid selection of predefined text to complete office visits, letters, reports, and messages. It consists of 34 static categories and 20 categories that can be customized to suit the need of each user. Each category has the capacity to hold 60 lines of customized type.

Focal Point

The ToDo/Reminder feature is a user-defined item that replaces the need for reminder notes.

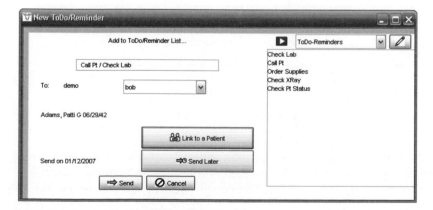

Figure 4.13 New ToDo/Reminder window.

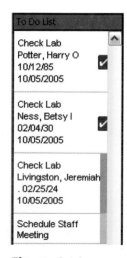

Figure 4.14 Items set in ToDo list.

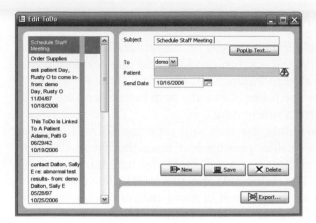

Figure 4.15 Edit ToDo window.

ToDo/Reminders can be linked to a patient, a future date selected, and then sent to another recipient. The ToDo/Reminder will appear on that colleague's *ToDo List* on the selected date, indicating from whom the ToDo/Reminder came. It will be marked with a blue color bar and will open the patient's chart when the recipient accesses the note.

My ToDo List

Current ToDo/Reminders and those that have been scheduled for a future date for the user can be accessed by selecting *Edit>My ToDo List* on the main menu. In the *Edit ToDo* window the various items can be reassigned to different users, reset to a different due date, pop-up text can be edited, and non-linked items can be linked to a patient. Once modifications have been made, the user will click the [Save] button and the corresponding item in the *ToDo List* will be updated. New *ToDoReminder* items can be created from the *Edit ToDo* window as seen in Figure 4.15; the program will automatically add the newly created item to the user's *ToDo List* on the main screen.

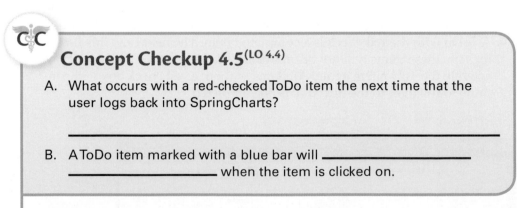

Concept Checkup 4.5(LO 4.4)

A. What occurs with a red-checked ToDo item the next time that the user logs back into SpringCharts?

_____

B. A ToDo item marked with a blue bar will _____
_____ when the item is clicked on.

Exercise 4.3 Working the ToDo List(LO 4.4)

1. You will now function as an office manager. Click on the *ToDo List* header bar. In the *New ToDo/Reminder* window, type *Schedule Staff Meeting* in the empty item field. Click on the [Send] button. You will notice the new ToDo item added to your *ToDo List* with a green bar. Sometime throughout the day you will work on this task. Click the *Schedule Staff Meeting* ToDo item. The program adds a checked box to the item. The next time you log onto SpringCharts this item will have been removed.

2. Again, click on the *ToDo List* header bar. In the *New ToDo/Reminder* window select *Call Pt* and *Check Lab* from the popup text panel. Click the [Link to a Patient] button. In the *Choose Patient* window, type in "*under*" and conduct a search. Highlight Robert Underhagen and select the [Send] button. You will notice the new ToDo item added to your list of tasks. This item will have a blue color bar indicating it is linked to a patient. At some point during the day you will process this task. Click on the Robert Underhagen item. You will notice that Robert's chart opens, enabling you to access the patient's phone number and other important information. Close the patient's chart and notice the red checked box added to this ToDo item.

3. Open a *New ToDo/Reminder* window. From the pop-up text select *Order Supplies*. In the ToDo field also type "*bandages*." In the *To* drop-down list, select *Jan*. Select the [Send Later] button and choose any date next month. Click the [Send] button. This ToDo item will appear in Jan's *ToDo List* on that specific date.

4. Create a new ToDo/Reminder for yourself. Type or select pop-up text. Link it to the patient Rusty Day. Send it to yourself in the future. Go to the main *Edit* menu and select *My ToDo List*. Find the item that you scheduled for yourself in the future. Click on the Red X in the upper right corner to exit this window.

LO 4.5 INTERNAL MESSAGES

The message center is located in the lower right quadrant of the main screen. (see Figure 4.16.) The SpringCharts message system is an intra- and inter-office mail function that enables you to send and receive messages to and from SpringCharts users on the network and e-mail messages over the Internet.

To view a message, the user will click on the message in the *Messages* list. Messages are ordered with the most recent at the top. The display shows from whom the message was received, the date and time it was sent, and the subject line.

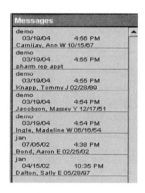

Figure 4.16 Message list window.

Non-Patient Messages

To create a new message, the user clicks on the *Messages* title bar or chooses *New Message* from the *New* menu on the main window. A dialog will appear, asking if this message concerns a patient. If the message does not concern a patient and [No] is selected, a blank message window (Figure 4.17) will appear:

The user will choose the recipient in the *To:* box from the pull-down list of users at the top of the message window.

The user then completes the subject line and types the message body into the text area in the middle of the message and/or pop-up text is selected in the window to the right. One can electronically time- and initial-stamp the message by using the appropriate buttons below the pop-up text window. To add to this pop-up text list for current and future use, the user simply clicks on the

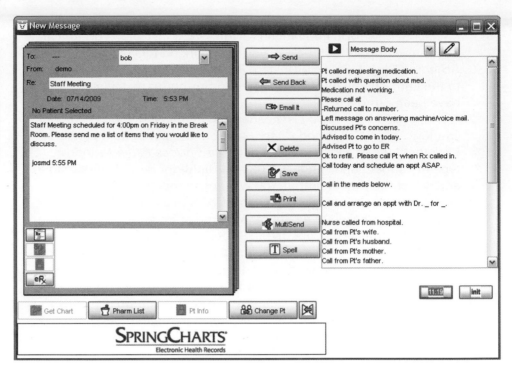

Figure 4.17 New (non-patient) message window.

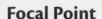

Pop-Up Text Edit icon

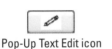

Figure 4.18 Refreshing the pop-up text category.

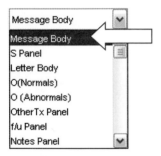

Figure 4.19 E-mail option window.

Edit icon. The link opens the *Edit PopUp Text* feature that enables the user to add, delete, or modify text in many different categories that are used in the system. The appropriate category on the left side (in this case: *Message Body*) is selected and necessary adjustments to the text are made. Lines of text can be moved up or down by clicking on the arrows to the far left of the text that needs to be moved. If the *New Message* window was open before accessing the *Edit PopUp Text* window, any modified text will not immediately appear in the *New Message* window. To see the modified text the user will need to refresh the pop-up text view. Simply click on the category header down arrow and select the category again as seen in Figure 4.18.

The sender will click the [Send] button to send the message in-office, or use the [Email It] button to send the message as an e-mail. When e-mailing a message, the user has access to all of the address book entries that have been made; one can also type in an e-mail address or select the patient's e-mail address if the message has been linked to a patient, illustrated in Figure 4.19.

The user can use the [Send Back] button to send the answered message back to the original sender as an in-office message. If the sender wishes to send the message to more than one user, the [MultiSend] button can be used. To see a list of all of the pharmacies entered into the SpringCharts' address book, the user will click the [Pharm List] button. This button searches the address book for all entries labeled as "Pharmacy." Selecting a pharmacy from the list will add the pharmacy name and work phone number to the body of the message. The [Spell] button accesses a spell checker, seen in Figure 4.20, that enables the user to add new words to an in-program dictionary.

If the message does not concern a patient, the recipient can use the [Save] button to save the message to his/her own private **message archive.** Archived messages can be viewed from the *Edit* menu by selecting *Message Archive.* The

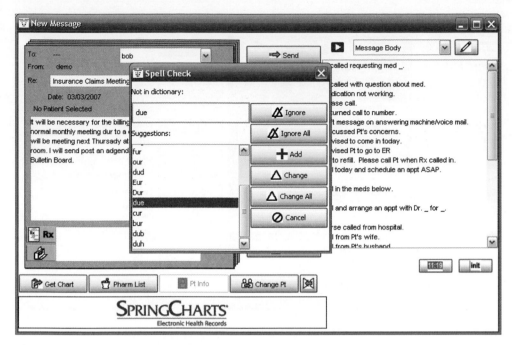

Figure 4.20 Spell check feature in new message window.

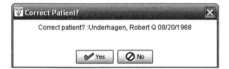

Figure 4.21 Use recent patient prompt window.

message can be re-activated into the Message center from the *Message Archive* window; also, new messages can be created from the *Message Archive* window.

Messages Concerning Patients

If the creator of the message has chosen to link the message to a patient, the message window (Figure 4.21) will appear. SpringCharts remembers the last patient's chart that was accessed during the logged on session and will provide a quick way to select the same patient.

Another way of linking the message to a patient is by selecting the [Change Pt] button in the original *New Message* window that was not linked to a patient. Although the patient demographics are not included with the message, the patient's name will appear as the subject and the [Get Chart] and [Pt Info] buttons will be activated.

By connecting the message to a patient, the recipient will have access to the patient's chart [Get Chart] and the patient's demographics [Pt Info]—seen in Figure 4.22. All the previous options are available: *Send, Send Back, Email It, Print, MultiSend,* and *Spell.* The Rx button gives you access to the patient's routine medications and previous prescriptions as illustrated in Figure 4.23. The user can also select additional medications from the program's database. Once the medication(s) is selected, the user will click on the [Save] button and the medication(s) is added to the bottom section of the *New Message* window.

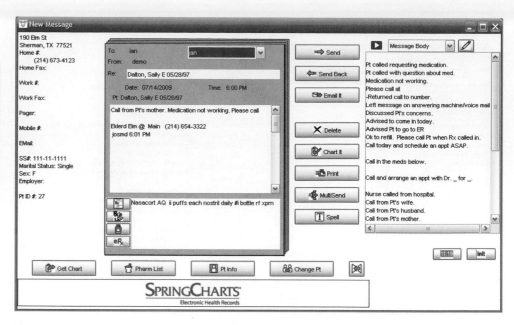

Figure 4.22 New (patient-related) message window.

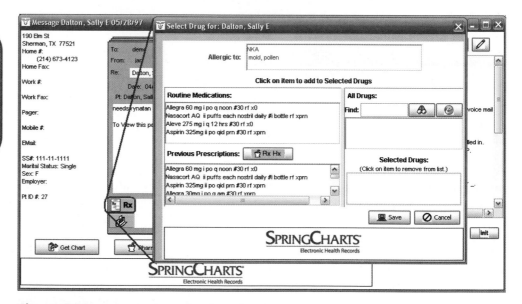

Figure 4.23 Access to the patient's medications.

By clicking on the selected medication in the *New Message* window, the user has the ability to edit that specific medication, illustrated in Figure 4.24. Any changes will only effect the medication information in the message. It does not effect the original medication selected from the patient's chart. The prescription can now be printed out by using the printer icon in the bottom left corner of the message. If *InterFax*™ has been activated on the SpringCharts Server, the prescription can be faxed directly to the pharmacy.

(See Appendix A—*Sample Documents*; Document 1. *Prescription Forms*).

When the message is answered and no longer needed, the recipient will click the [Chart It] button to automatically place the message into the patient's chart. An information window (Figure 4.25) will appear notifying the user that the message has been charted in the patient's chart.

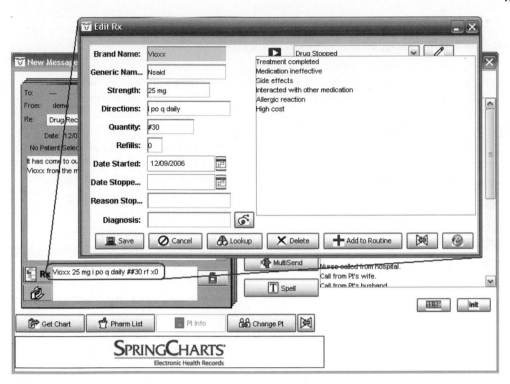

Figure 4.24 Edit prescription window.

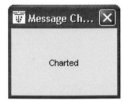

Figure 4.25 Message charted notification.

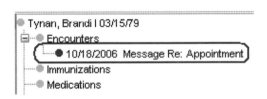

Figure 4.26 Message saved in chart's care tree.

The message will be saved under the *Encounter* tab by default or any other custom-designed tab in the patient's care tree selected by the user. To read or print the saved message at a later date the user will access the message under the chart tab to which it was saved (see Figure 4.26).

Concept Checkup 4.6(LO 4.5)

A. The two methods of sending out a message are:

1. _____

2. _____

B. By connecting the message to a patient, the recipient will have access to the _____ and the _____.

C. To save a message that has been linked to a patient, the recipient must click on the _____ to automatically place the message into the patient's chart.

Exercise 4.4a Working the Messages Center (L.O. 4.5)

1. Once again you will function in the role of the office manager. Click one time in the *Message* header in the lower right quadrant. Click [No] to the question: *Does this message concern a Patient?* In the subject line (RE:), type the subject: *Staff Meeting.* In the body of the message invite the staff to the meeting, giving the time and location. Click in the [MultiSend] button in the middle of the *New Message* window. Check all the staff except the doctor. (Don't select 'scfmd.') Click on the [Send] button. You will notice the new message appears in your own message center at the top of the list displaying the subject, date, and time that the message was sent. This is because you are logged onto the program as *Demo.*

2. As the office manager, you would like to save this message so you can send it out again next month. Click on the staff meeting message in your message center. Click on the [Save] button in the middle panel of the *Message* window. The program will remove the message from the message center and indicate that the message has been archived. In the main *Edit* menu select the *Message Archive* option. The *Message Archive* window will display any archived message. Next month you will want to click on the *Staff Meeting* message then select the [Re-Activate Message] button to send the message back into your message center, from where it can be sent out again to coworkers. Close the *Message Archives* window by clicking on the 'X' in the upper right corner.

Exercise 4.4b Working the Messages Center (L.O. 4.5)

1. Once again, click one time in the *Message* header. Click [Yes] to the question: *Does this message concern a Patient?* In the *Choose Patient* window type the last name *Adams* and conduct a search. Select the patient, *Patti Adams.* You will notice the program adds the patient's demographics to the left side of the *New Message* window and the patient's name in the subject field. Let us now assume you are employed in the doctor's office as a front desk receptionist. You have received a phone call from Patti Adams asking for a prescription refill of Lipitor. No clinic staff workers are available so you will need to send the doctor a message. You will notice that there is no pop-up text in the right panel regarding a patient calling for a refill. You want to add it so you don't have to type this item each time.

Edit PopUp
Text icon

2. Click on the pop-up text edit icon. (See margin illustration.) In the *Edit Pop-Up Text* window, type: *Patient called requesting refill.* on an empty line. Click the [Done] button to save the new pop-up text item. You will now see the line of text that you added into the *Edit PopUp Text* window. Click in that new pop-up text and it will be placed in the body of the new message.

3. Now you will need to select the medication that Mrs. Adams is requesting as a refill. Click on the *Rx* icon in the lower section of the message pad. (See margin illustration.) This will open a window displaying the patient's routine medications and the patient's previous prescriptions that have been prescribed by the clinic. Select Lipitor from the routine medication list, then click the [Save] button. The program adds the medication in question to the message note. Mrs. Adams has asked that her prescription be sent to the *Walshop Pharmacy.*

Click on the [Pharm List] button and select the appropriate pharmacy. The program will ask you if you want to update the patient's chart to reflect this as the patient's default pharmacy. Click on "No." The selected pharmacy is added to the body of the message note.

You would normally send this message to the doctor. However, since we are in a classroom network environment, send the message to yourself. Drop down the list of names in the top portion of the note and select *Demo*. Now click on the [Send] button.

Exercise 4.4c Working the Messages Center (L.O. 4.5)

1. Let us now assume you are the doctor. You will notice the recently received message regarding Patti Adams in the *Messages* center. Click on the message. The doctor will most likely want to check the patient's chart and review lab results and medication history. Click on the [Get Chart] button. In the *Prescription Hx* panel of the face sheet note the occurrences of Lipitor. Close the patient's chart. The doctor wants to refill the prescription without authorizing any more refills and would like to set up an appointment with the patient to conduct another lipid panel. Click on the medication in the lower portion of the *Message* window. Change the *Refills* field to 0 (zero) and click the [Save] button. Click on the Edit pencil icon and edit the doctor's pop-up text and add the following sentences on three separate lines: *OK to refill. Call patient when prescription is called in. Schedule an appointment with patient ASAP to conduct further tests.* Click the [Done] button. In the *Message* window the updated text will be refreshed in the window. Click in the body of the message and hit your enter key to start a new paragraph. Select the three new sentences just added to your pop-up text. Again, hit your enter key to start a new line of text. Click once on the time and initial stamp buttons in the lower right corner of the *Message* window. Send the message back to *Demo*.
2. Open the message sent to you from the doctor. Once you have completed the assigned task you will want to print out the prescription and save this message into the patient's chart. Click on the printer icon located just below the *Rx* button on the message pad. Let's add the doctor's license and DEA number to the script.
Click the [Print Rxs] button to print a copy of the prescription. Write your name on the sheet and turn in to your instructor.
3. Start a new line of text in the message body. Select the following pop-up text: *Called in the meds below. Called and arranged an appt with Dr._____ for_____.* Complete the sentence. Using the time and initial buttons, stamp your initials and the time below your selected sentences.
4. Select the [Chart It] button in the middle of the *Message* window. You will be presented with an option to save the message as an encounter or place the note in another area of the chart. Save it as an encounter. Click the [Save] button.
5. Open Patti Adams' chart by clicking on her name either in the office calendar or in the patient tracker. Click on the [Get Chart] button. Click the "+" sign in the care tree in the upper right panel of the chart. Click on the message that you recently saved. The details of the message can be seen in the lower right corner of the patient's chart. Close Patti Adams' chart.

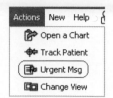

Figure 4.27 Assessing urgent message in actions menu.

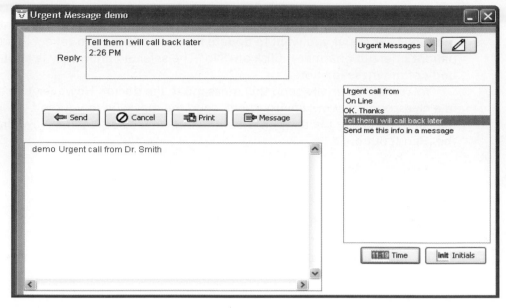

Figure 4.28 Urgent message window.

Urgent Message
The means by which an instant message can be sent to another coworker on the network. The urgent message is not stored with the other messages in the system, rather it is displayed as a pop-up window in SpringCharts.

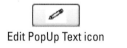

Edit PopUp Text icon

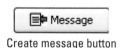

Create message button

LO 4.6 URGENT MESSAGES

To send an **urgent message** to a coworker, the user will simply click on the Actions menu and select *Urgent Msg* as seen in Figure 4.27.

The message is typed or selected from available pop-up text, and then the recipient(s) is selected. As with all pop-up text functions, the *Edit* icon will enable the user to add, delete, or modify text that can be used in this section. Once [Sent], the message will instantly appear on the forefront of the receiving user's screen, as illustrated in Figure 4.28. This eliminates the need to locate a staff member and allows communication with discretion. The urgent messages function like instant messaging; once the user selects [Cancel] the information is *not* saved in the program; however, the urgent message can be printed out.

By clicking on the [Message] button the urgent message is turned into a regular message and can be sent or saved into the message list. This may be necessary if the recipient of the urgent message needs to follow up on the message at a later time.

LO 4.7 E-MAILS

E-mails in SpringCharts function similar to a mail sorting room. All e-mails come to a central location from where they can be sent to specific SpringCharts users. Because of security and electronic virus concerns SpringCharts does not send or receive e-mail attachments—they need to be placed in the body of the e-mail before they are sent out or received. The e-mail service provider is required to have a POP and SMTP address in order for the e-mails to be automatically downloaded into SpringCharts. One e-mail account is set up for the medical office on SpringCharts Server.

A specific user or users will be assigned the security function to receive incoming e-mails. On SpringCharts Server the user(s) who will be responsible for receiving the company e-mails are given security clearance as seen in Figure 4.29.

Focal Point
Urgent messages function like instant messages and are not stored in the program.

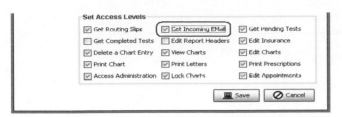

Figure 4.29 User security access window.

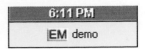

Figure 4.30 E-mail icon in login window.

When e-mail is received into SpringCharts an icon appears alongside the specific user's name who has been assigned the appropriate access level to receive company e-mail. The icon will appear in the yellow login bar—illustrated in Figure 4.30.

When the user's e-mail access level is set, the program opens up the e-mail function for that user located in the *Edit* menu of the main screen. The e-mail submenu is seen in Figure 4.31.

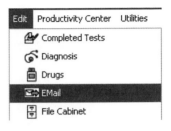

Figure 4.31 Accessing e-mail in the edit menu.

All incoming e-mails will be listed in this window, displaying the senders e-mail address, date and time, and subject heading. SpringCharts e-mail is integrated with the *Message* center and the patients' demographics. When an e-mail item is selected within this window the program opens a *Message* window, placing the body of the e-mail in the message body window and the subject line in the subject field. If the e-mail address from the recipient is set up in SpringCharts' patient database, the program recognizes the e-mail address and attaches all the relevant patient demographic information to the *Message* window as illustrated in Figure 4.32. The e-mail administrator then determines who would be best suited to respond to the e-mail and forwards the e-mail message to the appropriate SpringCharts' user. The message is sent to that user's *Message* center. The e-mail message has all the functionality of a regular SpringCharts message, including access to the patient's chart, pop-up text, messages concerning patients are charted, and so on. The user can e-mail back a response to the sender from this window.

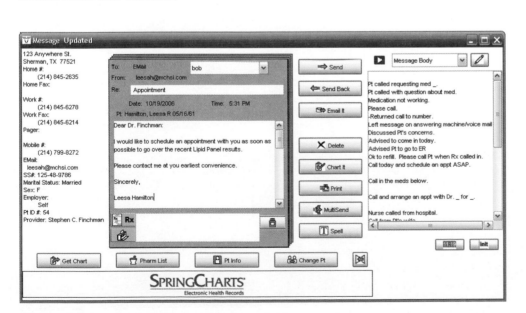

Figure 4.32 Incoming e-mail as new message.

Concept Checkup 4.7 (LO 4.6, 4.7)

A. When an urgent message is sent instantly where does it appear?

_____

_____ .

B. E-mails in SpringCharts function similar to a mail sorting room because

_____

_____

C. If the e-mail address from the e-mail recipient is set up in Spring-Charts' patient database the program will recognize the e-mail address and will

_____

_____ .

Name _____ Instructor _____ Class _____

USING TERMINOLOGY

Match the terms on the left with the definitions on the right.

_____ **1.** Practice view

_____ **2.** Doctor ready

_____ **3.** Tracker group

_____ **4.** CheckOut

_____ **5.** Pop-up text

_____ **6.** Toolbar

_____ **7.** Message archive

_____ **8.** Demographics

A. Logs the recorded checkout time for the patient.(LO 4.3)

B. A sent or received message not regarding a patient will be saved here and can be reactivated.(LO 4.5)

C. A repository of text in SpringCharts enabling clinic staff rapid selection of predefined text.(LO 4.4)

D. A lineup of icons that gives the user shortcut access to the most commonly used functions of the program.(LO 4.1)

E. Clinics that have offices in more than one location will use this feature to track the patients separately at each location.(LO 4.3)

F. A patient's personal statistical data such as name, address, birthday, and so on.(LO 4.2)

G. The first screen displayed upon successful logon.(LO 4.1)

H. An example of a patient status.(LO 4.3)

CHECKING YOUR UNDERSTANDING

Write "T" or "F" in the blank to indicate whether you think the statement is true or false.

_____ **9.** The Tap&Go™ feature utilized on a Tablet PC enables the user to tap once with the stylus pen on a desired item and move to the next one. (LO 4.1)

_____ **10.** SpringCharts gives the clinic the ability to chart a "no show" for patients who miss their appointments.(LO 4.2)

_____ **11.** It is not necessary to add patients to the patient tracker when they arrive in the clinic if they are not on the schedule.(LO 4.3)

_____ **12.** The color-coding feature has six standard colors that have been predetermined to represent different applications.(LO 4.3)

_____ **13.** When the receptionist selects CheckOut in the *Edit Tracker* window, the patient's name is moved to a category heading of "Done."(LO 4.3)

_____ **14.** "Internal messages" is a feature that enables you to record your thoughts, feelings, and hunger cycle.(LO 4.5)

Answer the question below in the space provided.

15. What are the four functions that can be performed in the *New ToDo/Reminder* window?[(LO 4.4)]

a) _____

b) _____

c) _____

d) _____

Choose the best answer and circle the corresponding letter.

16. The e-mail service provider is required to have:[(LO 4.6)]
   a) A POP and JAZZ address
   b) A POP and SMTP address
   c) A SMTP and RSVP address

17. To send an urgent message to a coworker:[(LO 4.8)]
   a) Click on the *Actions* menu and select *Urgent Msg*
   b) Yell with all your might in the coworker's general direction
   c) Create a message and click the [Send Now] button

18. A tracker group is best described as:[(LO 4.3)]
   a) A group of people who follow the patients around in the clinic to keep up with their whereabouts
   b) A small microchip that is inserted into the patient's index finger upon check-in
   c) A classification that is assigned to a patient along with the location and status, in clinics with multiple locations

19. A color-coder flag can indicate certain things, such as:[(LO 4.3)]
   a) Which physician a patient is seeing
   b) Which insurance carrier a patient has
   c) Both a and b

20. By using the appointment calendar the user can:[(LO 4.2)]
   a) Keep up with personal nail and hair appointments
   b) Navigate to prior or future appointments
   c) Get the patient's pending tests

5

The Patient's Chart

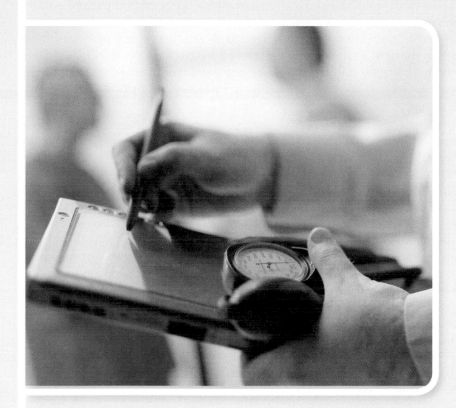

What You Need to Know

To understand Chapter 5 you will need to know how to:

- Start SpringCharts EHR
- Enter new patient demographics
- Create your own electronic patient chart
- Create and edit electronic pop-up text
- Create and edit electronic category preferences

Key Terms

Terms you will encounter in Chapter 5:

Care Tree
Category Preferences
Continuity of Care Record (CCR)
Chart Alert
Electronic Chart
Encounters
Export Chart
Face Sheet
Family Medical History (FMHX)
Imaging Tests
Pending Tests
Past Medical History (PMHX)
Routine Meds

Learning Outcomes

After completing Chapter 5, you will be able to:

LO 5.1 Understand the concept of an electronic chart

LO 5.2 Explain the concept of the chart's face sheet

LO 5.3 Demonstrate how to edit the patient's face sheet

LO 5.4 Explain the concept of a chart's care tree

LO 5.5 Navigate the chart's file menu

LO 5.6 Utilize the chart's edit menu

LO 5.7 Operate the chart's actions menu

LO 5.8 Navigate the chart's new menu

LO 5.1 OVERVIEW

Electronic Chart
The repository for patient medical data created through computer automation in the medical office/clinic. Similar to the traditional paper chart, it holds such static information as the patient's medical history and medical problems, as well as the dynamic information, including office visit notes, tests, letters, and reports concerning the patient.

Open a Chart icon

Face Sheet
Contains more constant patient information such as allergies, problem list, past medical history (PMHX), etc.

Care Tree
The patient's electronic chart lists categories that hold encounters (progress notes), tests, excuse notes, letters, reports, and other current records.

Encounters
A tab in the electronic care tree that stores many of the documents that are created from encounters with the patient.

The **electronic chart** is the repository for patient medical data created through computer automation in the medical office/clinic. Similar to the traditional paper chart, it holds such static information as the patient's demographics, allergies, medical history, and medical problems, as well as the dynamic information, including office visit notes, tests, letters, and reports concerning the patient. In SpringCharts the electronic chart can be accessed from many different places in the *Practice View* screen: by clicking on the patient's name in the *Scheduler*, the patient's name in the *Patient Tracker*, or by selecting a *ToDo* or *Message* associated with a patient. If the patient is not in any of these places, a new patient's chart can be retrieved by clicking on the *Open a Chart* icon on the main menu bar. It can also be accessed from the *Actions* menu and then selecting *Open a Chart*. Figure 5.1 illustrates several options to accessing a patient's chart.

The *Recent Charts* menu provides a drop-down window, as seen in Figure 5.2, that allows the user to access charts that have been opened during the current logon session.

The patient chart is composed of a series of panels on the left for displaying and editing the comprehensive **face sheet.** It contains more constant patient information such as allergies, problem list, past medical history (PMHX), and so on. The dynamic **care tree** on the right side lists **encounters** (progress notes), tests, and other current records and documents.

SpringCharts EHR provides practitioners with a unique view of the entire chart at a glance, as illustrated in Figure 5.3. It's just like having a paper chart open in front of you. The user does not have to navigate to other areas of the program to view various elements of the chart. A patient's chart can be opened by all users in SpringCharts at the same time. In fact, all users can be editing the chart at the same time. However, because of data protection, the same *specific area* of the chart cannot be edited simultaneously by different users. Many different patient electronic charts can be opened simultaneously by the same user.

Concept Checkup 5.1(LO 5.1)

A. The electronic chart is the repository for _____ created through computer automation in the medical office/clinic.

B. The *Recent Charts* menu contains a list of patient charts that have been _____.

C. In SpringCharts a patient's chart can be opened by _____ and all users can _____ the same chart at the same time.

The toolbar in the patient's chart window displays icons for the most commonly used features, seen in Figure 5.4. These features can also be accessed from the main menu bar.

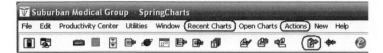

Figure 5.1 Main menu displaying option for opening a chart.

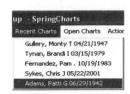

Figure 5.2 Recent charts opened during current logon session.

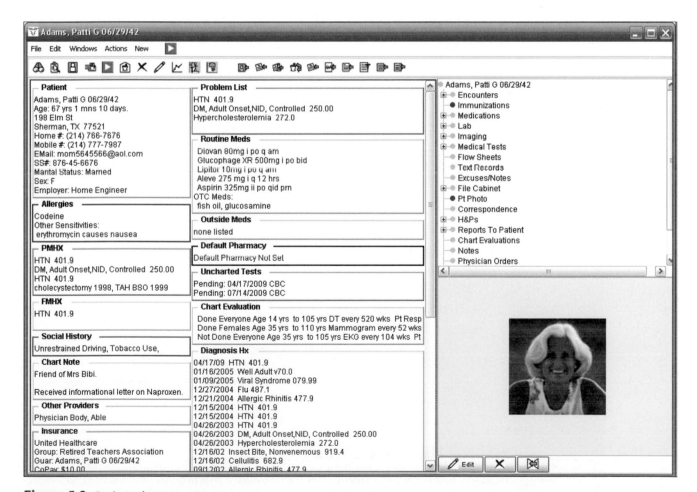

Figure 5.3 Patient chart screen.

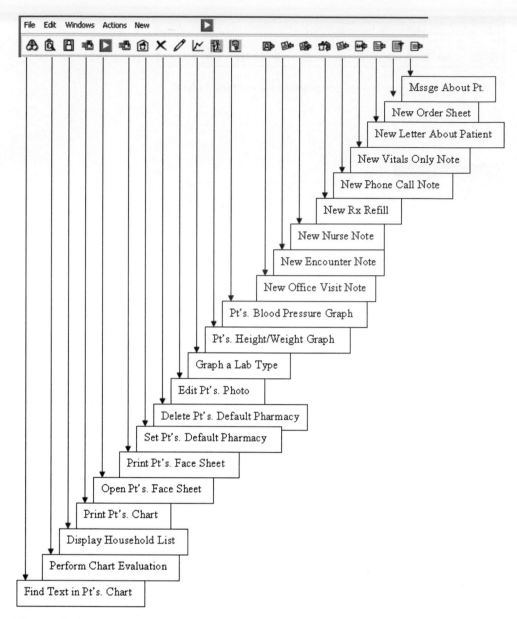

Figure 5.4 Toolbar with icon description.

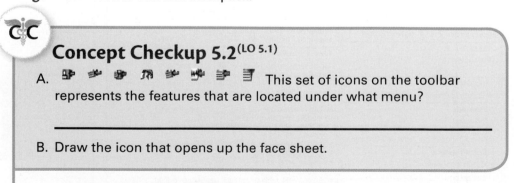

Concept Checkup 5.2^(LO 5.1)

A. This set of icons on the toolbar represents the features that are located under what menu?

_____

B. Draw the icon that opens up the face sheet.

LO 5.2 THE FACE SHEET

In many interfaced environments with practice management system (PMS) software programs, the patient demographics can be imported either in a one-time "data dump" and/or dynamically imported into SpringCharts in "real time"

Open Face Sheet icon

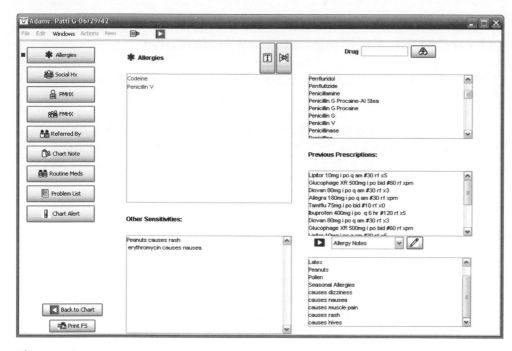

Figure 5.5 Face sheet edit window.

when the patient information is entered into the PMS. The face sheet categories can be edited by simply clicking on the *Open Face Sheet* icon on the chart menu bar. The *Face Sheet Edit* window, shown in Figure 5.5, allows speedy data entry of medical information by the clerical staff. Most subdivisions of the face sheet have a search function to add diagnosis, medicines, and so on, and a pop-up text area for additional clarification. Once the face sheet is opened, the user can select any of the navigation buttons on the left side of the window to edit that particular section.

The social history, past medical and family medical history sections contain medical history items that are set up in the **category preferences** table on the SpringCharts Server (see Figure 5.6). The category preferences table enables the clinic administrator to create predetermined customized lists of medical data. The lists are displayed in SpringCharts on each computer and enable rapid selection of items from these checklists to build the face sheet.

These Server medical lists can be easily customized for each clinic, displaying the items in which the medical office has specific interest. In the initial setup on the Server, the administrator can add up to 30 items in each of these categories.

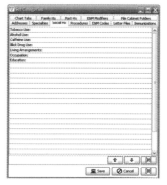

Figure 5.6 Customized lists in category preferences.

Category Preferences
Table on SpringCharts Server enables the clinic administrator to create customized predetermined lists of medical data. The lists are displayed in SpringCharts on each computer and enable the rapid selection of items from these checklists to build the face sheet.

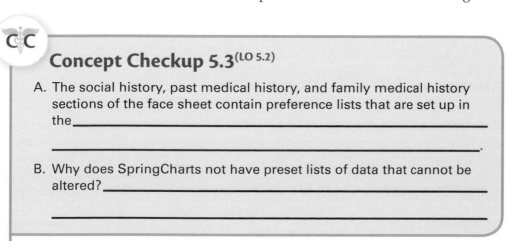

Concept Checkup 5.3(LO 5.2)

A. The social history, past medical history, and family medical history sections of the face sheet contain preference lists that are set up in the _____

_____.

B. Why does SpringCharts not have preset lists of data that cannot be altered?_____

_____

Exercise 5.1   Building Category Preferences(LO 5.2)

1. Close any face sheet and patient's chart that you may have open. On the main menu of SpringCharts select *Administration*. From the drop-down list, select *Category Preferences*.
2. Locate the list for *Social History*. Select each item in the list, backspace to remove the data, and replace the data with the new item. Modify the existing list to the following category preferences: Tobacco Use, Alcohol Use, Caffeine Use, Marital Status, Living Arrangements, and Occupation. Because the list will appear as category headings in the *Face Sheet* window you need to place a colon (:) after each group heading.
3. Locate the *Family History* list. Delete the existing list and create the following categories: Arthritis, Asthma, Cancer, Chemical Dependency, Diabetes, Heart Disease, High Blood Pressure, Kidney Disease, Tuberculosis, Father died at age, Mother died at age, Brothers died at age, Sisters died at age, and Cause of death. There is no need to place a colon after the items in the next sections.
4. Locate the *Past History* list. Delete the existing list and create the following categories: Asthma, Bronchitis, Cancer, Diabetes, Gout, Heart Disease, Hernia, High Cholesterol, HIV Positive, Kidney Disease, Liver Disease, Migraine Headaches, Miscarriage, Mononucleosis, Pacemaker, Pneumonia, Prostate Problems, Stroke, Thyroid Problems, Tonsillitis, Ulcers, and Vaginal Infections.
5. In the *Chart Tabs* list add the following category: Insurance Card.
6. Locate the *File Cabinet Folders* list. Add two categories: Office Forms and Patient Forms.
7. Press [Save] to save the amended categories.

LO 5.3 EDITING THE FACE SHEET

Information to complete the electronic face sheet is taken from the paper intake forms that the patient fills out regarding past medical history, routine medications, current medical problems, and so on. This is typically filled out by new patients in the waiting room while they wait to be processed. Many times, with the implementation of SpringCharts into the doctor's office the paper intake forms will be redesigned to cover the same categories and data flow that appears in the SpringCharts face sheet.

(See Appendix B. *Source Documents—Document 3. Patient Intake Sheet.*)

Allergies

This area allows the adding/editing of drug allergies and other sensitivities. Drug and non-drug allergies can be added by locating them through the *Search* window. For established patients with a prescription history, drugs can also be pulled from the *Previous Prescriptions* display window. A link is available under both the *Allergies* and *Routine Med* categories for direct access to the *Epocrates* website. This popular website provides the user with a current web-based drug interaction and formulary references, thus allowing the provider to make clinical decisions more quickly and confidently. This optional SpringCharts feature

Epocrates link icon

is accessed by pressing the Epocrates link button located in various screens throughout the program.

Other Sensitivities is a text field in the lower half of the *Allergies* window. The information displayed here is shown as a separate category on the face sheet portion of the patient's chart. Pop-up text is available to choose the sensitivity or add descriptive text to the sensitivity, such as specific adverse reactions. Both the allergy and the sensitivities can be removed from the patient's face sheet by highlighting and deleting the entry. If no allergies are entered into the patient's face sheet, the program will automatically enter NKA (no known allergies) into the *Allergies* section of the face sheet.

Social History

Social History allows the adding/editing of the patient's social history. A checklist is provided for rapid entry. The *Preferences* checklist is defined under *Category Preferences* on SpringCharts Server or under the *Administration* menu on a single-user version. Additional defining text can be added to the chosen preference categories by selecting text from the upper *PopUp Text* window, as seen in Figure 5.7.

Past Medical History (PMHX) and Family Medical History (FMHX)

These two areas allow the adding/editing of **past medical history (PMHX)** and **family medical history (FMHX)**. A diagnosis (Dx) may be chosen in a system coded form by ICD code or description in the upper portion of the screen if the desired diagnosis is not located in the *Preferences* list. Again a *Preferences* checklist is provided for rapid entry. The checklist is defined on SpringCharts Server under the *Category Preferences* section. Items from the *Preferences* are added to the *Other PMHX* or *Other FMHX* windows once selected. It is stored in a free text format. This window will also hold free-typed text for further clarification. Whether the patient history has been added from the *Dx* field or the *Preferences* window, selected items can be deleted by highlighting the entry and deleting from within the *Edit Face Sheet* window.

Past Medical History (PMHX)

This category is for recording past medical history in the patient's face sheet.

Family Medical History (FMHX)

This category is for recording family medical history in the patient's face sheet.

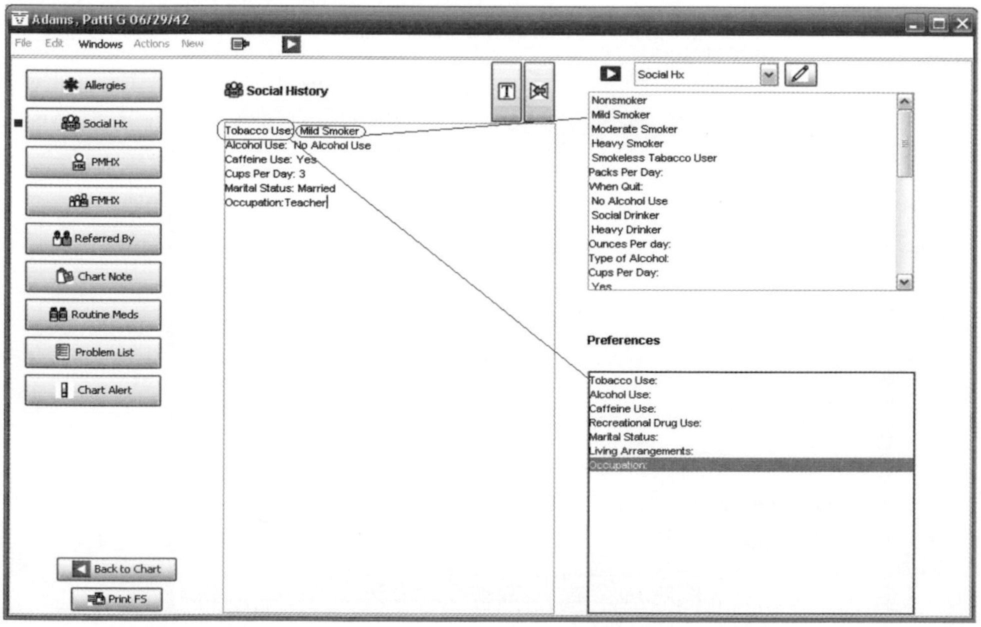

Figure 5.7 Social history setup in edit face sheet window.

Other Providers

This section allows the selection of the referring doctor. Referring physicians must be first set up in the address book in order to be chosen in the face sheet. The user simply types in the physician's last name and conducts a search. The appropriate physician is selected from the list and the name is added to the face sheet.

Chart Note

The chart note section is a location for entering important information about a patient that needs to be seen when opening a patient's chart. Pop-up text is provided in this window to rapidly add predefined text. Many times this section of the chart note will be used by the clinic to record specific medical history based on the specialty of the clinic. For example, an obstetrics and gynecology medical office may use the area to document menstrual history, menopausal history, births, types of deliveries, and miscarriages. A psychologist may use the chart note to record previous psychiatric treatment, substance abuse treatment, history of harmful mood and behavior, and so on.

Routine Meds

Routine Meds
An abbreviation for the patient's current routine medications. They are listed in the patient's electronic chart.

Routine medication allows the entering and editing of the patient's current routine medications and over-the-counter (OTC) meds. Routine medication is chosen by doing a search for the desired medication. Again a direct link is available to the *Epocrates* website to check on drug interactions and formulary references. Pop-up text is presented for **Routine Meds** that will allow easy listing of common medications for the clinic and OTC non-drugs. Medications can be edited by clicking once on the prescription in the *Routine Medication* window and adjusting any of the specifications in the *Edit Rx* window, illustrated in Figure 5.8.

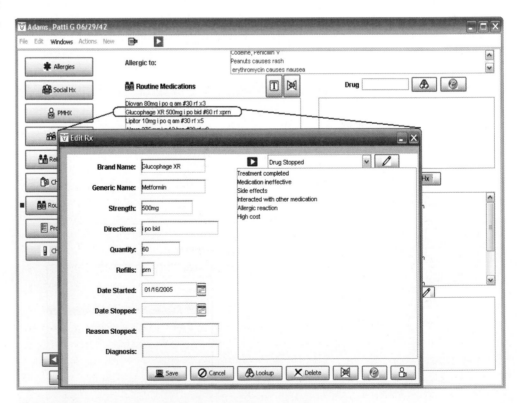

Figure 5.8 Editing drugs in routine medication window.

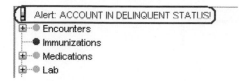

Figure 5.9 Chart alert in patient's chart.

The changes affect only the patient whose chart is open, not the entire database. Displayed in red are the *Allergies* and *Other Sensitivities* in the upper window. The patient's allergies and other sensitivities are displayed each time routine medications are accessed in SpringCharts. The *Outside Meds* section of the face sheet will automatically populate drug data prescribed from other providers when the SpringCharts program sends e-prescriptions across the Internet to the clearinghouse.

Problem List

The problem list allows the adding/editing of the patient's chronic medical problems. Entries can be either diagnosis or text. When a Dx is chosen in the office visit screen it may be also added to the *Problem List* at that time. For established patients who have been previously assigned a diagnosis in a SpringCharts' office visit note, the Dx code and description are available to choose when building the *Problem List* in the face sheet. Again, pop-up text is available to select items from predefined *Problem List* text. SpringCharts automatically stamps the user ID and date at the bottom of the problem list when exiting the *Edit Face Sheet* window. Whenever the problem list is updated, the program will update the user ID and date.

Chart Alert

The **Chart Alert** allows for the inclusion of important text that will appear in red above the *Encounters* category on the charts' care tree as seen in Figure 5.9. The text can be typed in the *Chart Alert* window or selected from predefined text in the *Chart Alert* pop-up text list.

All new and modified face sheet information is saved back into the left-hand side of the chart when the [Back to Chart] button is selected. In many cases it is the clerical staff rather than the clinical staff who build the electronic face sheet from the paper intake sheets after the new patient has filled them out. The newly completed face sheet can then be printed out for new patients to review. This allows the patients another opportunity to revise their medical information. Printing the face sheet is done by selecting the print face sheet button. All information in the *Edit Face Sheet* window is printed except the *Chart Alert*. Thus the *Chart Alert* information is not seen by the patient. The patient's demographics and primary insurance details are also printed on the face sheet form.

(See Appendix A—*Sample Documents*; Document 2. *Patient's Face Sheet*.)

Diagnosis, Prescription, and Procedure History

Three additional windows in the face sheet portion of the chart provide for the automatic recording of diagnoses, prescriptions, and procedures. This information is extracted from the patient's various encounters. As various diagnoses, prescriptions, and procedures are chosen in the office visit screen, they will appear on these lists with the most recent item at the top. These lists can be opened for printing by accessing the *Actions* menu within the patient's chart

Focal Point

The patient's allergies and other medical sensitivities are displayed in SpringCharts any time the user accesses the patient's routine medication or writes a prescription.

Chart Alert

Allows for the inclusion of important text that will appear in red above the *Encounters* category on the chart's care tree.

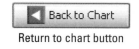

Return to chart button

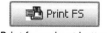

Print face sheet button

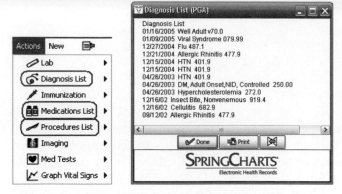

Figure 5.10 Diagnosis list display in patient's chart.

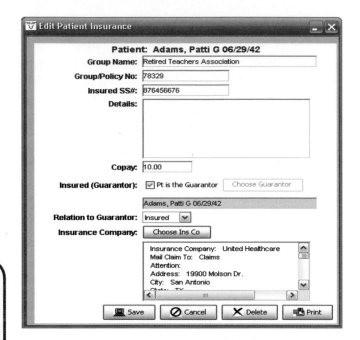

Figure 5.11 Edit Patient Insurance window.

Focal Point

The patient's primary insurance is displayed in the face sheet and is printed out on the face sheet form and routing slip. It can also be added to the physician's order form.

and selecting the appropriate heading, seen in Figure 5.10. A speedier way to open these windows is by clicking on the specific category header in the face sheet of the patient's chart.

Primary Insurance

The primary insurance is added to the patient's face sheet by clicking on the *Insurance* header on the bottom left side of the patient's chart. The *Edit Patient Insurance* window, illustrated in Figure 5.11, allows the user to record such information as policy number, group number, social security number, co-pay amount, and guarantor. The [Choose Ins Co] button within this window is selected to add the patient's primary insurance company from the database list set up in SpringCharts. Insurance companies are set up by accessing the *Edit* menu on the main screen and choosing *Insurance* (see Chapter 3 for details.) The patient's primary insurance information is displayed in the face sheet and printed on the face sheet form and the office visit routing slip. It also may be added to the physician's order form.

Insurance header bar

Choose Ins Co

Add patient's primary insurance button

Concept Checkup 5.4^(LO 5.3)

A. Information to complete the patient's past medical history, routine medications, current medical problems, and so on in the electronic face sheet is taken from _____.

B. What section of the face sheet is not printed out on the face sheet form? _____.

C. The patient's primary insurance information displayed in the face sheet can be printed onto what three different forms?

  1. _____

  2. _____

  3. _____

Exercise 5.2 Building a Patient's Face Sheet^(LO 5.3)

1. If your SpringCharts program was not shut down and rebooted since completing exercise 5.1, you may do so now. This will refresh the program to the new items added in the *Category Preferences* window of the *Administration* menu.
2. Open your own chart by selecting the *Open a Chart* icon on the main menu. Type in the first few letters of your last name in the window. Select your name. Your chart will be empty except for your demographic information.
3. Within your chart, click on the "*Show chart/face sheet*" icon to open your face sheet edit window.
4. The window opens to the *Allergies* section. In the *Allergy* field, type "Peni" and press the search button. Select "Penicillins" from the list. The program adds this drug to your allergy list. Repeat the activity by adding the drug "Codeine" and "Peanut Containing Prod." *Remember that you only need to type the first few letters of the word and then conduct a search. The more letters you type, the more likely you are to make a mistake and then the system will not be able to locate the term.* In the *Other Sensitivities* window type the medication "erythromycin" then select "causes nausea" from the *Allergy Notes* pop-up text.
5. Click on the *Social Hx* navigation button. In the *Preferences* window select the "Tobacco Use" category. (This list is being pulled from the *Administration Category Preferences* setup window.)

Note: If you do not see the list of items that you added under the *Social Hx* portion of the *Category Preferences* window, you will need to close SpringCharts and restart the program.

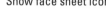
Open a chart icon

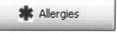
Show face sheet icon

Allergies button

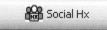
Social history button

Now select the appropriate pop-up text from the *Social Hx* category in the upper window, for example, **Tobacco Use: Non-Smoker.** Also select *Alcohol Use* and *Living Arrangements* categories and add the necessary pop-up text to further define the category.

> Note: You will need to place your cursor after the *Preferences* category item that you selected and then click on the pop-up text item. The placement of the curser determines where the pop-up text is inserted.

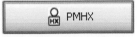

Past medical history button

6. Select the next navigation button—*PMHX.* (Once again you will notice the *Preferences* window displaying up to 30 past medical items that were set up in the *Category Preferences* window of the *Administration* menu.) Select several items from the *Preferences* list. If a patient indicates a medical condition that is not in the rapid-select list, search for the diagnosis by code or description in the *Dx* field in the upper right. Type "HTN" for hypertension, hit the search icon and select the diagnosis.

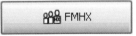

Family medical history button

7. Select the *FMHX* navigation button. Choose several medical conditions that may be appropriate for family medical history. Select "Father Died At Age:," place your curser at the end of this phrase in the *Other FMHX* window and then type an age. Press your [Enter] key to place your cursor on the next line. Select "Cause of Death:" in the *Preferences* list; place your cursor at the end of this phrase and select a medical condition from the list. Repeat this activity with other family members.

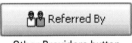

Other Providers button

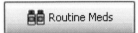

Chart Note button

8. In the *Other Providers* section type "Hart" in the *Address* field. Click the search button and select Dr. Harry Hart as the referring physician.
9. The *Chart Note* contains data about the patient that the medical staff do not want buried in various encounters. Select "Prefers Hospital" and "Religion" then place your cursor at the end of these selections and type in the completed information.

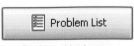

Routine medication button

10. Select the *Routine Meds* navigation button. In the upper right *Drug* quadrant, search and select the following *Routine Meds:* Diovan, Glucophage, and Lipitor. In the *Routine Medications* window, edit Diovan and Glucophage by clicking on each of the medications and removing the strength, directions, quantity, and refills. (Many times a new patient will not know these details, therefore it is important not to have this information in the face sheet if the patient has not supplied these details.) Save the edited medications. Click 'Yes' to the alert question: *Are you sure you want to leave the Strength blank?* Select several OTC (over-the-counter) items from the *Routine Meds* pop-up text in the lower-right quadrant.

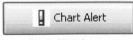

Problem List button

11. The *Problem List* contains all the current medical conditions of the patient. It may be different from the PMHX list because some of the past medical history may no longer be current problems. Select several ailments from the *Problem List* pop-up text. Remember all pop-up text in SpringCharts can be customized for each user.
12. Place your [Caps Lock] on and type "DELINQUENT ACCOUNT" in the *Chart Alert* window. Additional text can be chosen from the *Chart Alert* pop-up text.
13. Click on the [Back to Chart] button. You will notice that all the data selected is now positioned in the various face sheet categories within your chart.

Chart Alert button

14. Click on the Insurance category section in the face sheet of your chart. Enter your group name, policy number, and other details. Select an insurance company from the provided list. Save the information. Your face sheet is now complete. Close the patient's chart and then reopen it so that all the new information is refreshed.

15. Once again, click on the *"Show chart/face sheet"* icon (see open face sheet icon in margin reference) to open your face sheet edit window. Click on the [Print FS] button in the bottom left portion of the screen. This will print out your patient's face sheet report. **Submit your face sheet report to your instructor.**

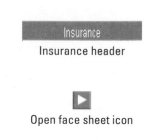

Insurance header

Open face sheet icon

LO 5.4 THE CARE TREE

To edit an item on the right-side care tree diagram, the user will click on the "+" symbol to the left of the category to expand the list and then select the specific item; the particular "branch" item will be displayed in the bottom right window. (On a MacIntosh computer the + sign appears as an arrow.) To edit an item in the care tree the user will click the [Edit] button at the bottom of the screen; SpringCharts will judge the screen size and display as much information as possible to the user.

There are preset categories in the care tree that cannot be altered or edited. When certain documents and tests are saved they are automatically positioned in these appropriate care tree categories. The preset list includes all categories from *Encounters* through *Pt Photo* as seen in Figure 5.12.

However, an additional 30 categories can be added to the care tree list. This provides all users the opportunity to store created documents and imported files under these added categories. Figure 5.12 shows an additional five categories that have been added to the care tree.

Many of the newly created documents will provide the user with an option to choose a care tree category before saving the document. Users may find it more convenient to store certain documents in customized categories rather than under the default *Encounters* tab. Because many of the created forms are initiated from encounters with the patient, the *Encounters* tab is displayed as the default place to save these documents. However, with additional categories added to the care tree the user has other options under which to store documents.

Additional customized categories are added through the setup function of SpringCharts Server in the *Category Preferences* seen in Figure 5.13. Once new items are added to SpringCharts Server, the program will need to be refreshed by shutting down and rebooting in order for the changes to be seen.

After the documents have been saved into the care tree, the category of choice can still be changed by selecting the [Edit] button in the bottom window. Once the window is reopened, the user will choose the [Change Tab] button, illustrated in Figure 5.14, and select another category. The program will move the document from the former category to the newly selected one.

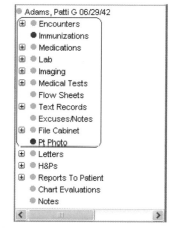

Figure 5.12 Permanent categories in the care tree.

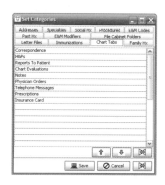

Figure 5.13 Customized chart tab categories in category preference window.

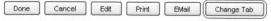

Figure 5.14 Change tab button in document edit window.

Focal Point

An additional 30 categories can be added to the preset categories in the care tree list. Additional categories are set up on the Server.

Concept Checkup 5.5 (LO 5.4)

A. *Encounters* through *Pt Photo* make up preset categories in the patient's care tree that cannot _____.

B. How many additional categories can be added to the patient's care tree? _____

LO 5.5 FILE MENU

The *Find Text* feature in the *File* menu of the patient's chart allows for the searching of specified text in portions of or within the entire chart. The program will display a window showing the text in the appropriate section of the chart and circle the item in red as seen in Figure 5.15. The [Find Again] button opens up other occurrences of the same text.

The *Evaluate Chart* feature will analyze the chart to determine if the patient is up to date with preset tests, screenings, and procedures. A window will display past due items if the patient's record does not indicate that these tests, screenings, and procedures have been done (see Figure 5.16). This function will be discussed in more detail in Chapter 7.

Export Chart
Enables the user to export any portion of the chart as a text file by selecting items from a list of chart entries. Among other things, the text file can be e-mailed and opened in a Word program by the recipient.

Export Chart enables the user to export any portion of the chart as a text file. The *Export Chart* window seen in Figure 5.17 opens with all the items from the patient's chart checked. The list can be unchecked by selecting the [Clear List] button. The user is presented with several export options, including saving the selected material as a text file that can then be emailed to a recipient, copying the material to a clipboard from where is can be pasted into another program, opening the chosen material in the computer's default word processing program, or exporting the material to a PDA or iPod.

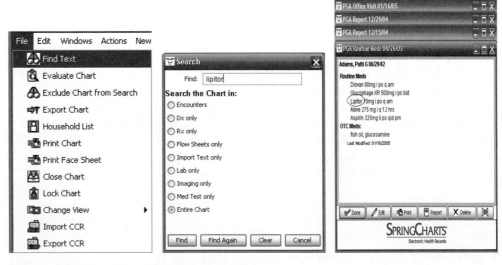

Figure 5.15 Finding text in the patient's chart.

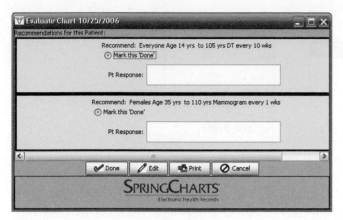

Figure 5.16 Chart evaluation window.

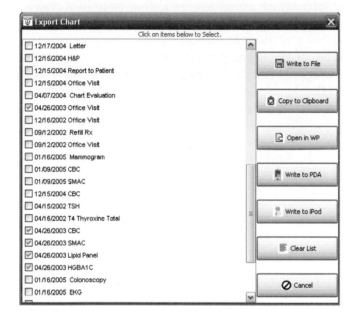

Figure 5.17 Export chart selection list window.

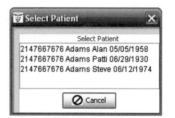

Figure 5.18 Household list window.

The *Household List,* illustrated in Figure 5.18, displays all patients who share the same home phone number. When setting up family members as patients in SpringCharts, users will input the same home number in the patients' demographics to tie them together in the *Household List*.

Similar to the *Export Chart* feature, the **Print Chart** feature enables the user to print the entire chart or selected portions of the charts. If a fax server program has been set up on the network, then the selected portions of the patient's chart can be faxed directly to the recipient from within the program.

(See Appendix A—*Sample Documents*; Document 2. *Selected Items from Patient's Chart*.)

Print Face Sheet takes the user directly to the print window to select the printer where the entire face sheet can be printed out. Patients can peruse and update this information when necessary. Medical clinics are encouraged to print the face sheet for patients who are returning to the clinic after 6 or 12 months. This provides the patient with the opportunity to update their medical records if necessary.

(See Appendix A—*Sample Documents*; Document 3. *Patient's Face Sheet*.)

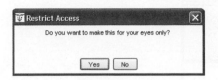

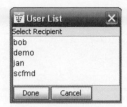

Figure 5.19 Lock chart security window.

Figure 5.20 Selecting records by provider window.

Focal Point

The face sheet, which contains past medical history, family medical history, routine medicines, and so on, can be printed for the patient with each visit and updated.

Close Chart provides an optional way to close the opened chart.

Lock Chart is functional if a user has been set up with the security clearance to lock a chart. The selection of this feature will allow the chart to be modified only by this user. By default, physicians are given the authority to lock charts; however, this authorization can be turned off for specific doctors. A warning box appears before the feature is activated, as seen in Figure 5.19.

Change View affects how the care tree is displayed. *Brief List* will organize the care tree to display only the category headings. *Abbreviated* opens the care tree to display a summary of each of the items under the categories. This view is useful when searching for summary data in the care tree; the items do not have to be opened individually. *Full Details* displays the full details of all the items in the care tree. Again, this is a useful view of the care tree when searching for specific information, because each item does not need to be opened to view the contents. *Sort by Provider* will organize all the attachments in the care tree by the provider whose name is assigned to the attachments.

In a multiple-doctor environment, several doctors may have material in the same patient's chart. *Records of One Provider* will display only the records of the selected provider. In order to refresh the care tree to the original list, the user will select the *Sort by Provider* option again. The *Records of One Provider* may now be chosen again and a different doctor selected from the displayed list as seen in Figure 5.20.

Continuity of Care Record (CCR): Import CCR and *Export CCR* is a standard for transferring patient medical data from one provider's EHR program to another. In practice, the SpringCharts' user can export a pre-defined core set of medical data from a patient's chart, including demographics and the most relevant and timely facts about a patient's medical information, and write it to a patient's USB flash drive, CD, iPod, or PDA. The patient can then carry this CCR to a medical specialist or travel to another state or country and have the CCR imported to a SpringCharts program or any other EHR program.

Continuity of Care Record (CCR)

Developed in response to the need to organize and make transportable a set of basic information about a patient's health care that is accessible to clinicians and patients.

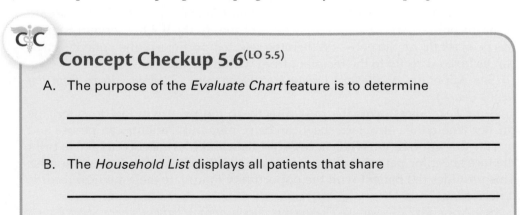

Concept Checkup 5.6(LO 5.5)

A. The purpose of the *Evaluate Chart* feature is to determine

_____

_____

B. The *Household List* displays all patients that share

_____

C. Why are medical clinics encouraged to print the face sheet for patients who are returning to the clinic after 6 or 12 months?

_____

_____

D. What is a CCR?

_____

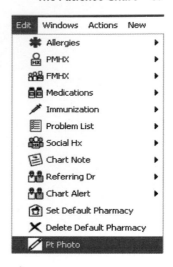

Figure 5.21 Edit menu in patient's chart screen.

LO 5.6 **EDIT MENU**

The *Edit* menu in the patient's chart seen in Figure 5.21 provides another way to access the panels in the comprehensive face sheet of the chart. By selecting the category from the *Edit* menu the face sheet will open to that specific area. The *Edit* menu also contains a couple of items that cannot be edited from the face sheet: *Set/Delete Default Pharmacy* and *Edit Pt Photo*.

When setting up a patient's chart the default pharmacy for the patient can be chosen from a list of pharmacies that have been previously set up in the address book. The default pharmacy along with the phone number is stored in its own category of the face sheet, seen in Figure 5.22. It provides for quick reference when the clinic needs to call in a prescription for the patient. If a user chooses a different pharmacy for the patient when writing a message, the user will be asked if he/she wants to change the default pharmacy for the patient.

Edit Pt Photo allows inclusion of the patient's photograph into the chart. A photo should be taken with a digital camera in the lowest resolution, for example, 150 × 150 pixels. There are two options for importing the patient's photo. First, the image can be retrieved from the digital camera and stored on the computer. By selecting the [Edit] button in the *Photo* window, shown in Figure 5.23, the user can locate and select the stored image to import into SpringCharts. The patient's photo will automatically save itself into the appropriate place in the care tree (*Pt Photo*) and be seen in the lower right window of the patient's chart.

The second option for importing a patient's photo is through the TWAIN/SANE device interface. In this case the user would select the [Scan] button, also seen in Figure 5.23. This technology enables communication between image-capturing devices such as scanners, cameras, webcams, and computer programs. After selecting the [Scan] button, the user will choose the appropriate interface devise.

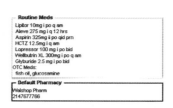

Figure 5.22 Default pharmacy displayed in the face sheet.

Focal Point

A pharmacy must first be set up as an address before it can be placed in the patient's chart as a default pharmacy.

Note: TWAIN technology has been incorporated into equipment manufactured since 2000 and functions in Windows™ and Macintosh OS™ environments. SANE technology, developed more recently, works in other computer environments such as Linux, UNIX, and so on.

The *Source Selector* window seen in Figure 5.24 locates the TWAIN/SANE technology equipment connected to the computer. The user selects the desired piece of equipment and the appropriate graphic user interface (GUI) dialog will open. (The GUI screen will look different for each of the devices that the computer connects to.) From this window the user will be able to extract the image directly

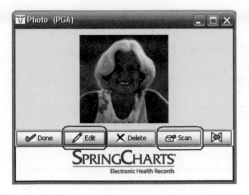

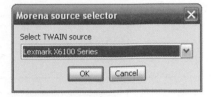

Figure 5.23 Editing or scanning in the patient's photo.

Figure 5.24 Locating a scanning device.

from the appliance without having to save the image to the computer first. The patient's photo will be saved into the appropriate place in the care tree (*Pt Photo*) and be seen in the lower-right window of the patient's chart.

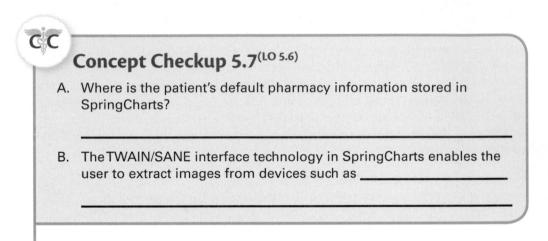

Concept Checkup 5.7(LO 5.6)

A. Where is the patient's default pharmacy information stored in SpringCharts?

_____

B. The TWAIN/SANE interface technology in SpringCharts enables the user to extract images from devices such as _____

_____

LO 5.7 ACTIONS MENU

The *Actions* menu shown in Figure 5.25 contains activities that can be launched within the chart. Various types of tests are ordered for the patient from within the *Actions* menu. Once the tests have been ordered they are stored in the system and await the entry of the test results. When the physician has "viewed" the test results they are then sent to the patient's care tree and filed under the appropriate category. The ordering of labs, imaging tests, and medical tests from within the patient's chart are not recorded on the routing slip or transmitted to a third-party PMS program for billing purposes. Ordering tests from this location would be appropriate when the tests are conducted and billed at another testing facility since the medical office will not need to bill for the activity. Tests can also be ordered within the *Office Visit* screen (discussed in Chapter 6).

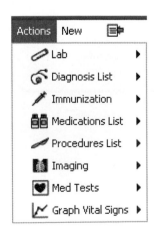

Figure 5.25 Actions menu in patient's chart.

Lab-Graph Type: This option, seen in Figure 5.26, enables the practitioner to view multiple occurrences of the same lab type within a patient's chart to analyze trends over time (Figure 5.27). The most recent test results will appear in the first column.

Order New Lab, Imaging, and Medical Tests: (Creating and modifying tests will be discussed in detail in Chapter 9.) Tests include laboratory tests, imaging tests, and medical tests, identified in Figure 5.28. **Imaging tests** consist of x-rays, CT scans, MRIs, and so on. Medical tests consist of EKGs, stress tests, Doppler flow studies, and so on. Tests are ordered by searching by description (either full name or a portion of it) in the *Order Test* window.

A matching list will appear in the top section. The clinician will select the tests needed to order. Repeated searches can be made for as many tests as the user wishes to order. The bottom section of the window will contain the accumulative list of tests that are being ordered (see Figure 5.29). The test name in the lower window can be clicked on to remove it from your orders. By selecting the [Done] button, the tests are ordered.

Managing and Charting Tests: Once a test (lab, imaging, or other medical test) is ordered, it moves into the **Pending Tests** list located under the main *Edit* menu. When the tests come back from the testing facility, the results will be manually entered into the pending test. Lab results can be automatically entered via SpringLabs *Reference Lab* interface option. After results are entered, the test moves into the *Completed Tests* list. The test is then viewed by the physician and is stored in the patient's chart under the heading for one of these three types of tests in the care tree diagram. For more discussion on the processing of Pending and Completed tests, see Chapter 9.

Diagnosis List, Medications List, and Procedure List: These lists show all diagnoses, medication, and procedures that have been assigned within the patient's office visit note, with the most recent at the top. This data is NOT manually entered into this section, rather the program automatically records the information once it is selected in the office visit screen. This is the same list that is seen in the chart's face sheet. However, by accessing these windows from the *Actions* menu the lists can be printed. In addition to recording the patient's routine medications and previous prescriptions, the program maintains a list of the patient's current medications and stopped medications. A medication is automatically added to the current list when it is initially prescribed; it is automatically removed from the current list when a "date stopped" is manually entered by the prescriber in the *Edit Rx* window or when the assigned dosage amount has expired.

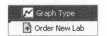

Figure 5.26 Graph lab type window.

Imaging Tests
These tests include x-rays, CT Scans, MRIs, and so on.

Pending Tests
Window displays all the ordered tests (lab, imaging, and medical tests) that are awaiting incoming results.

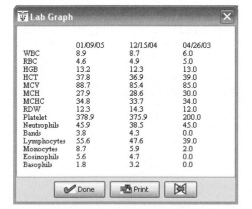

Figure 5.27 Trend graph for lab type.

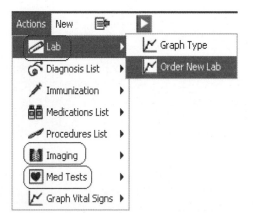

Figure 5.28 Ordering tests under actions menu.

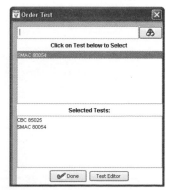

Figure 5.29 Order lab test window.

Immunization: This feature allows the entry of patients' past immunizations and the viewing of the immunization record. Immunizations are also
automatically added to this list when ordered in the office visit screen.
When recording a past immunization entry, the date needs to be entered
manually in the mm/dd/yyyy format or selected from the calendar icon.
The immunization record can be printed for or faxed to the patient or other
entities.

(See Appendix A—*Sample Documents*; Document 4. *Printed Immunization
Record*.)

Graph Vital Signs: Allows the viewing of blood pressure (BP), height/
weight data, body mass index (BMI), and body fat percentage for adults.
Head circumference is graphed for infants. For children aged 2 to 18 years,
data is viewed as a standard growth chart for either "Boy" or "Girl," showing a comparison of the child's vitals against the national percentile, illustrated in Figure 5.30. Infants younger than 36 months of age are graphed
against a backdrop showing the appropriate national percentiles. The graph
type will be adjusted automatically by the program based upon the age of
the patient (infant, child, or adult) and the patient's gender.

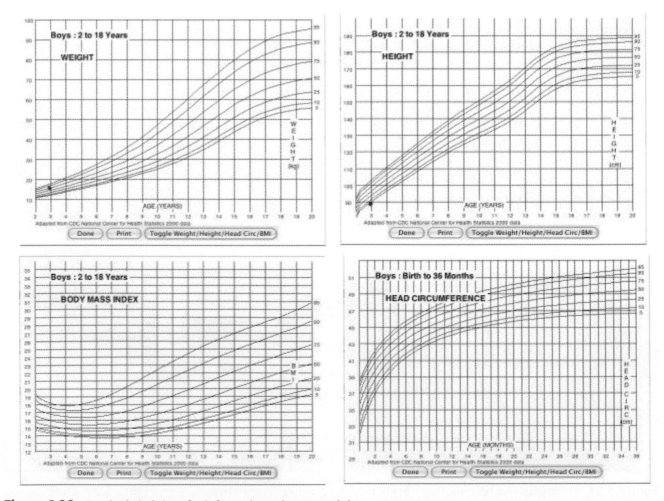

Figure 5.30 Graphed vital signs for infants through young adults.

Concept Checkup 5.8(LO 5.7)

A. The three types of tests that can be ordered in SpringCharts are:

1. _____

2. _____

3. _____

B. A completed test does not get charted into the patient's chart until

_____

C. The graph type of the patient's vital signs is adjusted _____ by the program based upon the _____ of the patient.

Exercise 5.3 Ordering an Imaging Test(LO 5.7)

1. Open the patient chart for Robert Underhagen. Dr. Finchman has recommended a magnetic resonance imaging of Robert's head.
2. Under the *Actions* tab select the *Imaging* submenu. Order Robert an *Imaging Test,* an MRI of the Brain – With & Without contrast. Click the [Done] button.

LO 5.8 NEW MENU

The New menu in the patient's chart presents the user with a large number of documents and reports that can be created and stored in the patient's chart, as seen in Figure 5.31.

New OV creates a new office visit. Office visits are filed in the care tree under "Encounters." The OV will be discussed in detail in Chapter 6.

New Note creates a blank note that enables the user to store any note in the patient's care tree. Pop-up text is available in this screen utilizing the *Notes Panel* category of pop-up text. Pop-up text may be modified from this window. In the lower right panel the user can view comments recorded from previous notes. This material can be copied into the existing note by highlighting the text and selecting the *Copy Note* icon. The New Note window is an ideal place to record information that is not related to a typical office visit or nurse note. Some providers may use it to house hospital consultation notes; medical billers may use it to record information provided by insurance companies. The *New Note* window is equipped with a spell checker. If the user is free-typing the note then the [Spell] button can be selected to spell check the notation. New words identified from the text can be added to the user's dictionary.

The user can time-stamp and/or initial-stamp the note by selecting the *Insert Time/Initial* icons .

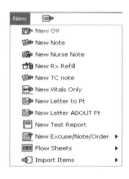

Figure 5.31 New menu in patient's chart.

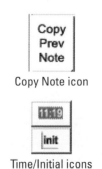

Copy Note icon

Time/Initial icons

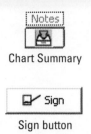

Chart Summary

Sign button

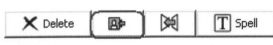

Convert to OV Note button

Also, the user has access to the patient's face sheet information in this window by selecting the *Chart Summary* navigation button on the right side of the screen. The face sheet information can be modified from this screen by right clicking on any face sheet category and selecting *Edit*. Upon doing so, the face sheet window opens enabling revisions to be made.

Before saving the note, the user has the option of initialing or signing and permanently locking the note. This is done by choosing the [Sign] button. When the *Sign* window is displayed, the *Initial Only* option will stamp the user's initials and time at the end of the note; the *Permanently Sign and Lock* option places the user's full name along with the date and time at the bottom of the note, then locks the note. After this point no modifications can be made to the note.

When the *note* is saved into the care tree, the user will be given the option to create a billable routing slip for this encounter or save it into the patient's care tree without creating a billing form.

The *New Note* can be transposed into a regular office visit note by selecting the [Convert Note] button at the bottom of the screen. This action will change the note into an office visit note and place all the selected verbiage in the *Objective* portion of the SOAP note. This now gives the provider a wide range of other pop-up text to add to the note, like diagnoses, procedures, and so on. Once changed to an office visit note, the original *new Note* cannot be filed separately.

New Nurse Note creates an encounter note for a nurse visit. This is similar to the new *OV* note but not as extensive. It does not have note panels for *Review of Systems* and *Exam*. Nurse Notes are filed in the care tree under "Encounters." A nurse note will be discussed in further detail in Chapter 6.

New Rx Refill creates a new medication refill form and a new prescription form. The *New Rx Refill* window seen in Figure 5.32 displays the patient's *Routine Medications* and *Previous Prescriptions*. Medication can be chosen

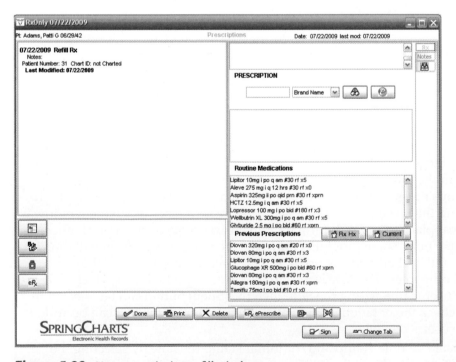

Figure 5.32 New prescription refill window.

from either of these windows. Also, the [Rx Hx] button is available to view all the previous prescriptions by date; the [Current] medication button produces a window that displays the patient's current medications. (All prescribed medications remain on the current list until an expiration date is added in the *Edit Rx* window or the number of days to use the prescribed quantity expires.) It is important in any EHR program that an accurate current medication list is kept in order for the system to perform a drug interaction check against new prescriptions. The allergy information from the chart's face sheet can be seen in red in the upper window.

If the drug is not listed in the *Routine Medications* or the *Previous Prescriptions* areas, the clinician will type the first portion of the name in the "Prescription" field and click on the *Search* icon. The user may search for a medication by either the brand or the generic name. The appropriate drug is then selected from the displayed material. Once selected, the drug may be modified by clicking once on the chosen medication, which opens the *Edit Rx* window. In this window the strength, directions, quantity, and number of refills, among other things, can be altered for this specific prescription. If the practice subscribes to the *Epocrates* Internet service and has the SpringCharts interface, an *Epocrates* icon will be displayed in the *Rx Only* and the *Edit Rx* window.

The *New Rx Refill* window allows for the addition of notes when documenting the new prescription(s). The *Notes* tab is located in the upper right navigation panel and displays pop-up text from the *Notes* category, enabling the clinician to record pertinent information regarding dialogue with the patient. The window also displays documented notes from previous prescription encounters with the patient. These prior notes can be copied into the current encounter by highlighting the preferred note and selecting the *copy note* icon. The user is also able to utilize the *time* and *initial* stamps in the *Notes* window.

As with the *New Note* feature mentioned previously, the *Rx Only* window also enables the user to transpose the prescription encounter into a regular office visit note. This may be used when a nurse practitioner determines that a patient may need to be seen by the physician while in the process of documenting a prescription. In this case the *Convert Note* icon is selected and the prescription note is placed in the *Objective* portion of the SOAP note while the prescription is placed as part of the *Plan*. The physician can now open the saved office visit note and continue to document. When the *New Rx Refill* note is transposed to an office visit note, there is no longer any record of the *New Rx Refill* note filed separately.

The clinician is also able to view the patient's face sheet information by selecting the *Chart Summary* icon in the navigation panel. Items in the face sheet window can be modified or added to by right-clicking on the desired category and selecting the *Edit* option.

SpringCharts provides allergy checking and drug-to-drug interaction checking through an optional feature called Pharmacy Web Services. This feature checks new prescriptions or refills for potentially dangerous interactions with the patient's existing medications and allergies. Allergy-drug and drug-drug interaction checking can be done anywhere a drug is prescribed: *New Rx Refill* in the patient's chart, *Rx* in an Office Visit, Nurse Note, New TC Note and a Message concerning a patient. The *Drug/Allergy Interaction Checking* icon button is shown under the Print Prescription icon. Selecting this button produces the Internet *Drug-Allergy and Drug-Drug Interaction* results from the Pharmacy Web Service. This results window shows the details of the prescribed

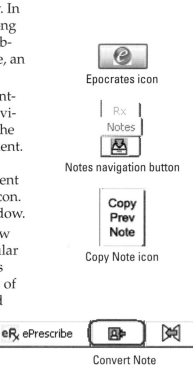

Epocrates icon

Notes navigation button

Copy Note icon

Convert Note

Chart Summary

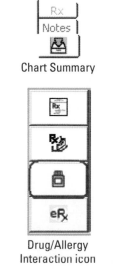

Drug/Allergy
Interaction icon

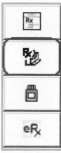

Printer icon

drug(s) checked against the patient's list of the Routine Medications, Current Medications, and Allergies cataloged in the chart. The severity level of any interactions and ensuing discussion are displayed. The results window is for viewing purposes only and cannot be printed out.

The *printer* icon enables the medical personnel to print the script in the office or fax it directly to a pharmacy using the integrated InterFax™ interface. Selecting the *printer* icon produces a *Prescription Printing Options* window, shown in Figure 5.33 , from which all medication or selected medication may be chosen for printing as scripts. Each medication will be printed as a separate script note.

The choice to have the doctor's signature print on the bottom of the script(s) is only available if the user is logged on as a physician and the doctor's digital signature has been added in the *Set User Preferences* window mentioned (discussed in Chapter 4). If no digital signature has been added to the program and the *Use Digital Signature* option has been selected in the *Prescription Printing Options* window, the phrase "Electronic Signature Verified" will appear above the physician's printed name at the bottom of the script. If the *Use Digital Signature* option is **not** selected the script forms will print a line above the physician's name on the script upon which the physician may manually sign. Also available in the *Prescription Printing Options* window is the choice to have the provider's license, Drug Enforcement Administration (DEA), and National Provider Identification (NPI) numbers printed on the script(s). These various choices can be set as defaults by selecting the [Save Rx Prefs] button before the scripts are printed.

Focal Point

In the *Rx Only* window a medication refill can be chosen from the routine medications panel, from the previous prescriptions panel, or from the database.

> SpringCharts EHR has the ability to recognize the state in the practice's address and format the prescription form layout according to state requirements.

If a fax server program is available on the network or if the clinic has subscribed to SpringCharts' Internet faxing option, then the script(s) can be faxed directly to the pharmacy without the need of printing the document in the office.

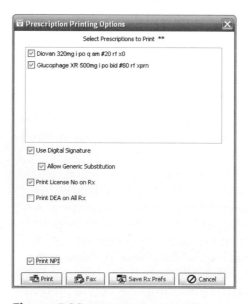

Figure 5.33 Prescription printing options window.

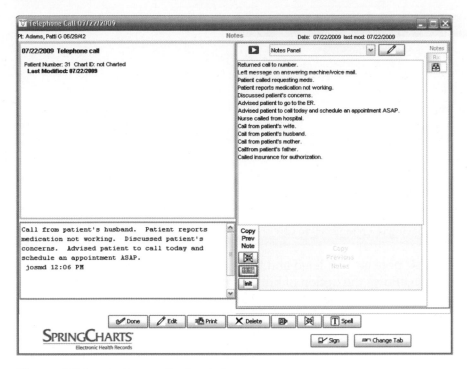

Figure 5.34 Telephone call edit window.

(See Appendix A—*Sample Documents;* Document 1. *Prescription Forms.*)

The [Sign] button gives the clinician the opportunity to *Initial Only* or *Permanent Sign & Lock* the *New Rx Refill* note. Once the note is locked, it cannot be unlocked or edited, even by the user who permanently locked it. When the user "permanently signs" the Rx refill, the clinician's full name, date, and time are stamped at the end of the note.

> *New TC note* creates a new telephone call encounter form. Text can be chosen from predefined pop-up text in the displayed window (see Figure 5.34). Text from previous telephone call notes appears in the lower right quadrant. This prior text can be highlighted and copied into the existing note by the use of the *Copy Note* icon. The date stamp and initial stamp is also available in this window enabling the user to initial their note.

> The [Rx] navigation button also appears in this window displaying the patient's *Routine Medications* and a list of *Previous Prescriptions*. If medication needs to be prescribed as a result of the conversation, the provider is able to document and print the patient's prescription by selecting from these lists or adding the medication after searching the database. (For an enhanced discussion of the Rx window features, see previous topic in the *New Rx Refill* section above.)

> As with the *New Rx Refill* window, the *Chart Summary* panel is available to display the entire patient's face sheet information.

> Also available in this window is the ability to convert a telephone call note into an office visit note. Once the *convert note* icon has been selected, text from the TC note will appear on the *Objective* portion of the office visit note and any prescribed medication will appear in the Plan section on the SOAP note.

> The [Sign] button in the telephone call note screen provides the same functionality as discussed earlier in the *New Rx Refill* screen.

Focal Point

Only those logged into SpringCharts as providers have the ability to add an electronic signature to prescriptions.

Copy Prev Note

Copy Note

Focal Point

In the *Telephone Call* window, prescriptions can be created as well.

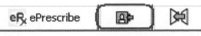

Convert Note icon

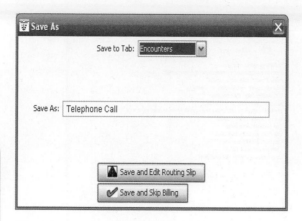

Focal Point

SpringCharts will automatically calculate the BMI from the height and weight of the patient.

Figure 5.35 Saving telephone call to care tree.

When the TC note is completed and the user selects the [Done] button, the program allows the option of billing for the phone consultation (see Figure 5.35). In several states patient telephone consultations are a billable encounter.

When the TC notes are completed and the user selects [Done] the program allows the option of billing for the phone consultation, seen in Figure 5.35. In several states telephone consultations with the patient are a billable encounter.

New Vitals Only creates a new vitals form. Vitals forms are filed in the care tree under "Encounters." This feature in SpringCharts is only used when patients come to the medical clinic for the sole purpose of having their vitals taken. The vitals may also be taken within the office visit encounter which will be discussed in the next chapter. The *Vitals* window contains security settings that warn the user if the vitals are out of line with the accepted minimum and maximum values, illustrated in Figure 5.36. The HC box is where the head circumference is recorded for infants. The body mass index is grayed out; the program will calculate this item from the patient's height and weight. The clinician has the option of right-clicking in any vitals' box and selecting a vital from the displayed drop-down lists. This feature is

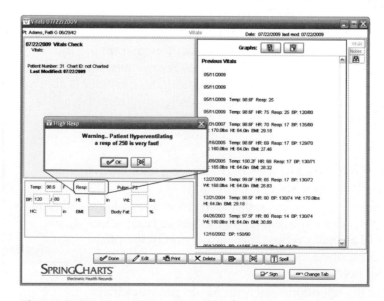

Figure 5.36 New vitals only window.

particularly useful when medical personnel are using a PC Tablet or other portable computer without a keyboard.

A *Notes* navigation button is available in this window providing pop-up text to record any clarification to the vitals. A *previous notes* section is displayed in the lower right quadrant from where notes recorded in prior visits can be viewed and copied as current notes. A time and initial stamp in the *Notes* panel enables the user to record when the vitals were taken.

Three additional customized fields can be created within the *Vitals* window to record other medical details. These additional fields are added in *Administration* panel under the *Vitals* section. In the *Custom Vitals Editor* the label, units, and minimum and maximum values are added. Once "enabled," the newly created vital will be displayed in the *Vitals* window as an additional field. SpringCharts Client programs will need to be shut down and rebooted to see any additional items added to SpringCharts Server.

The vital signs and notes can be transposed into a regular office visit note by selecting the [Convert Note] button at the bottom of the screen. This action will change the recorded information into an office visit note and place the vitals and note in the *Objective* portion of the SOAP note. This now gives the provider a wide range of other pop-up text to add to the note, such as diagnoses, procedures, and so on. Once changed to an office visit note, the original *New Vital Only* note cannot be filed separately. A nurse or medical assistant may change the vitals and note into an office visit note if he or she realizes that the patient should be seen by the physician in the same encounter. The ability to convert any kind of patient encounter note into an office visit note reduces documentation time and increases efficiency.

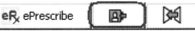

Convert to OV Note

Before saving the vitals note, the user has the option of initialing or signing and permanently locking the note. This is done by choosing the [Sign] button. When the *Sign* window is displayed, the *Initial Only* option will stamp the user's initials and time at the end of the note; the *Permanently Sign and Lock* option places the user's full name along with the date and time at the bottom of the note and then locks the note. After this point no modifications can be made to the vitals or note.

Sign button

New Letter to Pt creates a new letter addressed to the patient. The program automatically defaults in the patient's name, address, greeting, and salutation. The user has only to complete the body of the letter. This can be done by typing in the text field or by choosing appropriate pop-up text. (See Appendix A—*Sample Documents*; Document 5. *Letter to a Patient*.)

New Letter ABOUT Pt creates a new letter concerning the patient, illustrated in Figure 5.37. Recipient and address information can be easily retrieved from the [Get Address Book] button in the right-hand panel. Pop-up text is available in the displayed *Letter Body* category. As with all pop-up windows, text may be modified and added by selecting the *edit pen* icon. If multiple practices and/or physicians have been set up in the program, alternate letterhead and doctor's signature name can be chosen by selecting the appropriate navigation buttons to the right. A pre-typed letter can be selected by accessing the [Get from File] button in the right-hand panel. These previously created letters can be added to the body of the letter. All entries in the patient's care tree are also available to add into the body of the letter by selecting the [Add Chart Notes] button. This is useful when sending office visit notes to a referring physician, such as test results, encounter notes, or information from the face sheet. The [Chart It] button will save a copy of

Focal Point

Letters to or about the patient can be quickly created by using drop-in addresses and pop-up text and adding chart notes.

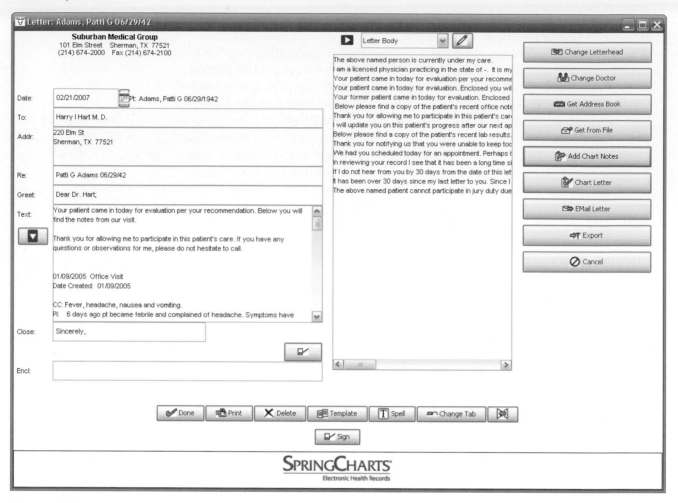

Figure 5.37 New letter about patient window.

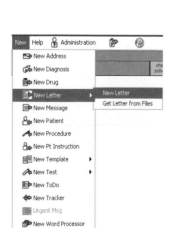

Signature icon button

Figure 5.38 New Letter
option on main menu.

the letter to the care tree, although this will automatically happen when clicking on [Done]. To activate a spell checker for the letter content, the user will click on the [Spell] button. The letter can be printed out or e-mailed to a recipient. The [Export] button enables the user to export the letter to another word processing program where it can be reformatted in greater details, if necessary. The signature icon (see marginal reference) located at the bottom of the letter enables the user to choose which signature will be placed on the letter. The options are the user's name or the default doctor's name that was chosen in the *User Preferences* window during setup. If a user wants to permanently lock a letter so that no changes can be made to it after it is sent, then the [Sign] button needs to be accessed and the [Permanently Sign and Lock] button activated. Once a letter has been signed and locked and saved, it can be viewed but not edited, even by the author.

(See Appendix A—*Sample Documents*; Document 6. *Letter About a Patient*.)

Users can also produce correspondence in SpringCharts that may not be related to specific patients. Letters may be created for attorneys, hospitals, accountants, and so on. Letter categories are set up in the *Administration* menu under the *Category Preferences* window. Non-patient letters are created in SpringCharts Client under *New>New Letter* on the main menu bar, illustrated in Figure 5.38.

These letters can be written by selecting pop-up text, typing in the specific fields, handwriting on a PC Tablet, or through voice recognition software. The template layout looks similar to the one used when creating *New Letter to Pt* and *New Letter ABOUT Pt* in the patient's chart, except for the addition of the [File it] button. These letters cannot be charted. Once the letter is created the user will select [File it] and choose a category file where the letter will be saved. Letters are retrieved by selecting *New>New Letter>Get Letter from Files*. A filed letter can also be incorporated into a letter to or about a patient by selecting the [Get from File] button in the New Letter window in the patient's chart.

New Form enables a clinic to create an electronic form of questions and possible answers that can be used to interview the patient or guardian. After completed, the form is stored in the Care Tree and can be printed. (See Chapter 10, Productivity Center and Utilities, for creating and using forms.)

New Test Report creates a blank test reporting form. Completed tests for this patient can be added to the report from the selection list (see Figure 5.39). The program comes with a layman's explanation for many of the tests. Identified *problem* areas and *recommendations* can be added from the pop-up list. The user chooses the appropriate pop-up text categories to access this text. The completed test report can be either printed out or e-mailed to the recipient. Test descriptions for these reports are created and edited by selecting *Edit>Tests Explanations* from the main screen. When the specific test is selected from the patient's *Select Test* list, the report explanation will automatically be added.

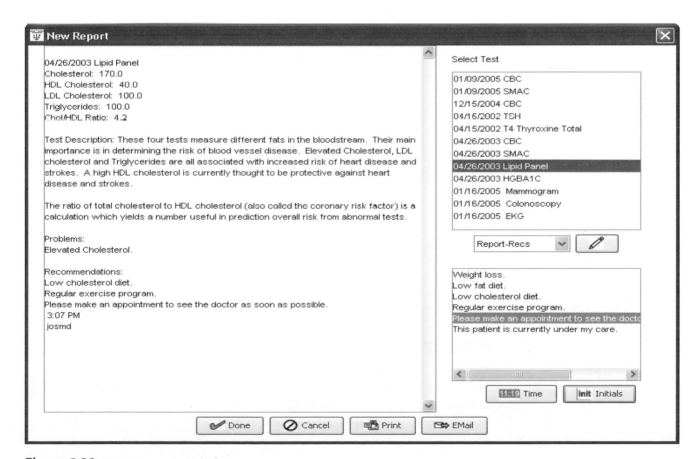

Figure 5.39 New test report window.

(See Appendix A—*Sample Documents*; Document 7. *Test Report to Patient*.)

New Excuse/Note/Order provides the creation of printable forms for work or school excuses, notes, and orders. Again, pop-up text is available to avoid typing a note each time. Excuse notes are automatically saved under the *Excuses/Notes* category of the care tree. When completing an order form the user will be given the option to chart the order in the patient's care tree. Order forms are used to record the ordering of lab, imaging, and medical tests that typically will be conducted at a third party facility. Within the order window the user will be able to select a diagnosis(es) from the patient's *Previous Dx* window thus associating a relevant diagnosis with the ordered test(s). The program automatically prints the ordering provider's name on the order form. The user will be given the option to have the order form signed electronically by adding the phrase "Electronic Signature Verified" to the form.

(See Appendix A—*Sample Documents*; Document 8. *Patient's Excuse Note*.)

Flow Sheets provide two types of flow sheets allowing for the creation of simple documents for repeated use. They are commonly used for tracking changes and results of a patient's response to medication and/or treatments. Once a flow sheet is created, it is automatically saved in the care tree under the *Flow Sheets* category and can be opened routinely and modified.

The first flow sheet option provides a text writer format.

The second flow sheet/table functions as a spreadsheet, seen in Figure 5.40, and sets tabs when the user presses the [Tab] key. This enables the user to add columns and/or row headings under which to record ongoing information. The flow sheets can be printed out.

Should a wide data entry be made in the spreadsheet, the column width will be reset when the flow sheet is re-opened. The table flow sheets are arranged in a spreadsheet layout with invisible grids; the user simply clicks in an area to add data.

Import Items allows the import of a text file (.txt) or an image (.jpg or .gif) into the patient's chart. *Import New Text File* is commonly used to import

Focal Point

Tests reports are created for patients. They contain the test result and a test description. The provider can also add text identifying problem areas and recommendations.

Focal Point

Excuse notes are created for work or school absentees and are automatically saved under the Excuses/Notes category in the patient's care tree.

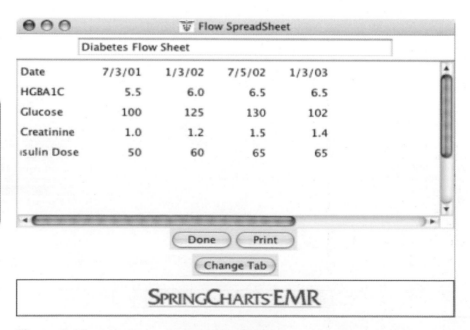

Figure 5.40 Flow sheet—spreadsheet window.

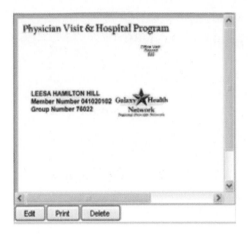

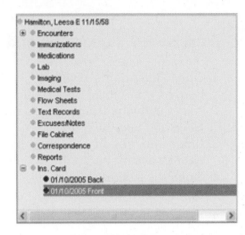

Figure 5.41 Imported image into care tree.

Figure 5.42 Care tree showing new category window.

previous records. The imported document needs to have been saved in a .txt format before it can be imported. Once imported, the document can be edited before being saved to the care tree. After the .txt document has been saved, it cannot be edited. *Import Picture* enables the import of a .jpg or .gif file. Graphics are saved in their original resolution and can be resized or printed once imported. To resize an image the user will click on the [Edit] button and choose the appropriate percentage from the *Resize* list. The newly imported image is visible in the lower window when the item is highlighted in the care tree (see Figure 5.41). A new category in the care tree can be created under which to store these imports, as shown in Figure 5.42.

Additional categories for the care tree are added in the *Category Preference* window on SpringCharts Server.

Importing unlimited types of files in the patient chart will be discussed as clinical tools in Chapter 7.

Focal Point

Importing text documents, images, and scans into SpringCharts is an ideal way to store additional items in the patient's charts.

Concept Checkup 5.9(LO 5.8)

A. *New TC note* creates a new

_____.

B. The *New Vitals Only* feature in SpringCharts is only used when

_____.

C. What navigation button is used in the *New Letter ABOUT Pt* window to include test results, encounter notes, or information from the face sheet when writing to a referring physician?

_____

D. The *Import Picture* feature enables the import of what types of files?

_____

Exercise 5.4 Recording and Viewing Vitals(LO 5.8)

1. Open Patti Adams' chart. Under the *New* menu select *New Vitals Only*.
2. Record your vitals. Click on the *Notes* tab in the upper right and select verbiage from the pop-up text. Click the [Done] button and *Save and Skip Billing*.
3. Close and reopen your chart by selecting your name from the *Recent Charts* menu on the Main menu bar.
4. Open the *Actions* menu within the patient's chart. Select *Graph Vital Signs* and view the various graphed vitals.
5. Open the Body Mass Index graph and print a copy. Write your name on the sheet and submit to your instructor.

Exercise 5.5 Creating a Letter About a Patient(LO 5.8)

1. Open Patti Adams' chart. Under the *New* menu select *New Letter ABOUT Pt.*
2. Select the referring physician, Dr. Harry Hart, from the [Get Address Book] button.
3. Choose the pop-up text that begins with: "Thank you for allowing me to participate . . ."
4. Click on the *Edit PopUp Text* icon.
5. Add the following sentence on an empty line: *Below please find a copy of the patient's recent lab results.* Click on the [Done] button.
6. Place the cursor in the letter body on a new line and select the newly added pop-up text sentence. Also, click on the sentence: *I will update you on this patient's progress after our next appointment.*
7. Click on the [Add Chart Notes] button and select the lipid panel results from the *Chart Entry* window. The lab test results will be added to the body of the letter. Select the Signature icon and select a signature (see marginal reference).
8. Print the letter on your letterhead and submit to your instructor.
9. Click on the [Done] button and select *Letters* as the category where the letter will be stored in the patient's care tree.
10. In your chart, click on the "+" expand symbol beside the *Letter* category in the care tree to see the saved copy of the letter.

Edit PopUp Text icon

Signature icon button

Exercise 5.6 Creating a Test Report for a Patient(LO 5.8)

1. Open Patti Adams' chart. Under the *New* menu select *New Test Report to Pt.*
2. Highlight the lipid panel in the *Select Text* window. You will notice that the program automatically adds the test description to the bottom of the test results.
3. Place your cursor in the body of the report under the section heading *Problems.* Select *Elevated Cholesterol* from the pop-up text in the lower right panel.
4. Click on the down arrow in the pop-up text category window to reveal the list of pop-up text categories. Select *Report-Recs.* Place your cursor under the section heading *Recommendations.* Now select the following pop-up text line items: *Low cholesterol diet. Regular exercise program. Please make an appointment to see the doctor as soon as possible.*
5. Print the test report and submit to your instructor.
6. Click on the [Done] button and store a copy of the report under the *Reports to Patient* category in the care tree. You will notice a "+" expand symbol has been placed beside the *Reports to Patients* header in the care tree. Click the "+" symbol to see the saved report.

Name _____ Instructor _____ Class _____

USING TERMINOLOGY

Match the terms on the left with the definitions on the right.

_____ 1. Care tree

_____ 2. Category preferences

_____ 3. Chart alert

_____ 4. Electronic chart

_____ 5. Encounters

_____ 6. Export chart

_____ 7. Face sheet

_____ 8. FMHX

_____ 9. Imaging

_____ 10. Pending tests

_____ 11. PMHX

_____ 12. Routine meds

A. The patient's past medical history.(LO 5.3)

B. Enables you to export any portion of the chart as a text file.(LO 5.5)

C. Tests that include x-rays, CT scans, MRIs, and so on.(LO 5.7)

D. The family medical history records.(LO 5.3)

E. The patient's routine medications and over-the-counter (OTC) meds.(LO 5.3)

F. The portions of a patient's chart that displays the patient demographics, medical history, and medical information. (LO 5.2)

G. After new lab, imaging, and/or medical tests have been ordered they are sent to this area.(LO 5.7)

H. Located on the right side of the patient's chart, it lists encounters (progress notes), tests, and other records.(LO 5.4)

I. This window on SpringCharts Server enables the clinic administrator to create predetermined customized lists of medical data.(LO 5.3)

J. Allows for the inclusion of important text that will appear in red above the *Encounters* category on the chart's care tree.(LO 5.3)

K. A category in the care tree that stores many of the documents that are created from encounters with the patient.(LO 5.4)

L. The equivalent to a patient's paper chart containing face sheet information and ongoing medical encounter documentation.(LO 5.1)

CHECKING YOUR UNDERSTANDING

Write "T" or "F" in the blank to indicate whether you think the statement is true or false.

_____ 13. SpringCharts EHR provides practitioners a unique electronic view of the patient's chart similar to a paper chart.(LO 5.1)

_____ 14. All of the preset categories in the care tree can be altered or edited.(LO 5.4)

_____ 15. *Edit patient photo* allows you to manipulate the picture, such as add a moustache, gray the hair, or age the face of a patient's photograph in the chart.(LO 5.6)

_____ **16.** The *Evaluate Chart* feature will analyze the chart to determine if the patient is up to date with preset tests, screenings, and procedures.(LO 5.5)

_____ **17.** The *Category Preferences* window enables the clinic administrator to create a collections module for 30 to 60 days, 60 to 90 days, or 90+ past due accounts.(LO 5.2)

_____ **18.** Information to complete the electronic face sheet is taken from the intake forms that the patient fills out regarding their PMHX, routine meds, and current medical problems.(LO 5.3)

Answer the question below in the space provided. (3 points)

19. List four advantages of having electronic patient charts rather than using a paper chart system.(LO 5.1)

1. _____

2. _____

3. _____

4. _____

Choose the best answer and circle the corresponding letter.

20. Graphing vital signs allows the viewing of:(LO 5.7)
   a) Blood pressure, height/weight data, body mass index
   b) An infant's head circumference with a comparison against the national percentile
   c) Both a and b

21. Under the *New* menu option, a new Rx refill creates a new medication refill form that can be:(LO 5.8)
   a) Printed or faxed in the physician's office
   b) E-mailed directly to the patient
   c) Both a or b

22. A flow sheet can be used to:(LO 5.8)
   a) Track a woman's menstrual cycles
   b) Track the amount of time a patient waited in the waiting and exam rooms
   c) Track changes and results of a patients response to meds and/or treatments

23. In the *Prescription Printing Options* window the feature is available to use electronic signature. This is accessible for:(LO 5.8)
   a) Only the physician
   b) All users of SpringCharts
   c) The pharmacist who acknowledges the receipt of the prescription(LO 5.3)

6

The Office Visit

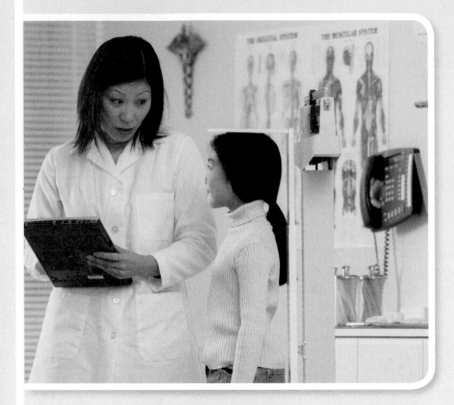

Learning Outcomes

After completing Chapter 6, you will be able to:

LO 6.1   Understand the concept of an office visit note

LO 6.2   Create a new office visit record

LO 6.3   Demonstrate how to activate a new diagnosis code

LO 6.4   Demonstrate how to activate a new drug/medication

LO 6.5   Explain how to discontinue medications for patients

LO 6.6   Describe how to edit pop-up text in an office visit note

LO 6.7   Create various office visit reports

LO 6.8   Utilize features of the Edit menu

LO 6.9   Understand features of the Actions menu

LO 6.10 Understand features of the Tools menu

LO 6.11 Create a routing slip

LO 6.12 Edit an office visit note by adding an addendum

LO 6.1 OVERVIEW

The most common encounter with the patient is the **office visit.** A new office visit encounter is created by selecting the *New* menu within the patient's chart and clicking *New OV*. Depending on the user preferences chosen, one of two different formats will appear. Figure 6.1 shows the "Large Screen" view.

> Note: If your SpringCharts office visit screen does not look like Figure 6.1, then you need to adjust your User Preferences setting. Refer to Figure 3.1 in chapter 3 to select the 'large screen' view of the office visit note.

An *OV* window is in three main sections. Typically the left side panel displays the patient's chart overview. This panel allows the practitioner to view the face sheet items without having to exit the Office Visit display. Any of these face sheet categories can be added into the office visit note to document that the provider discussed these issues with the patient. The middle panel is the portion where the notes will be stored. It is in the **SOAP** format, containing the subjective, objectives, assessment, and plan areas. All of the text items selected in the Office Visit pop-up text categories or manually added to the text fields will automatically save into one of these areas. Below the OV note section is the work area where the text can be created and modified. The right side of the *OV* screen is the pop-up text window along with the Navigation Panel tabs that access different information that will be selected for the Office Visit note.

The left and right panels in the Office Visit can be reversed. Left-handed users typically like to have the Navigation Buttons on the left side of the screen so that their hand is not covering the OV note when selecting the *PopUp Text* icon. This is especially true when using a PC Tablet. You will remember that the office visit orientation is determined by selecting either the right or left options under *Preference 2* tab in the *Set User Preferences* window.

Office Visit
Defined in SpringCharts as an encounter with a medical provider in which the patient's chief complaints, body systems, vitals, physical exam, diagnoses, and medications, among other things, are reviewed and documented.

SOAP
An acronym for SUBJECTIVE, OBJECTIVE, ASSESSMENT, and PLAN. The SOAP note is a convenient way for healthcare providers to layout the documentation of an office visit exam and to improve communication among medical staff members.

Office Visit Orientation: Right ▾

✔ Save

OV Orientation button in User Preferences

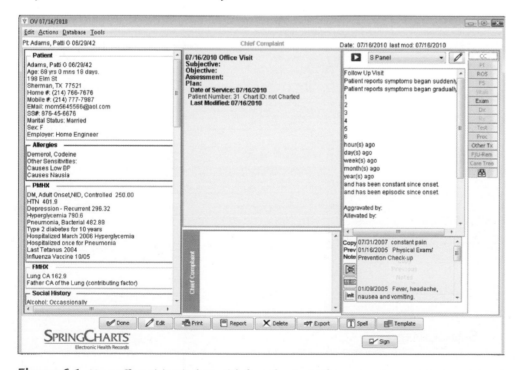

Figure 6.1 New office visit window with face sheet panel.

The SOAP format

The *Subjective* component consists of the patient's current medical condition from the patient's point of view. It generally includes the symptoms, the history of the present illness, and a review of the patient's body systems.

The *Objective* component is a continuation of the narrative from the practitioner's perspective and will generally include the vital signs and findings from the physical exam.

The *Assessment* component details the diagnosis(es) based on the exam. Possible diagnoses are usually listed in order of the most likely to the least likely.

The *Plan* component is what the health-care provider will do to test and treat the patient's symptoms. It may include prescribed medications, tests that need to be run, any counseling and advice given to the patient, as well as the setting of a time for follow-up or future review.

Concept Checkup 6.1 (LO 6.1)

A. The SOAP acronym stands for:

S. _____

O. _____

A. _____

P. _____

B. The _____ panel is seen on the left side of the *Office Visit* screen when first entering the window.

LO 6.2 BUILDING AN OFFICE VISIT

The navigation panel along the right side of the screen, seen in Figure 6.2, enables the provider to proceed through the office visit in a logical flow; however, the various panels may be chosen in any order. Included in the panel are chief complaint *(CC)*, history of present illness *(PI)*, review of systems *(ROS)*, face sheet *(FS)*, vitals, exam, diagnosis *(Dx)*, prescriptions *(Rx)*, tests, procedures *(Proc)*, other treatment *(Other Tx)*, and follow-up and reminders *(F/U-Rem)*.

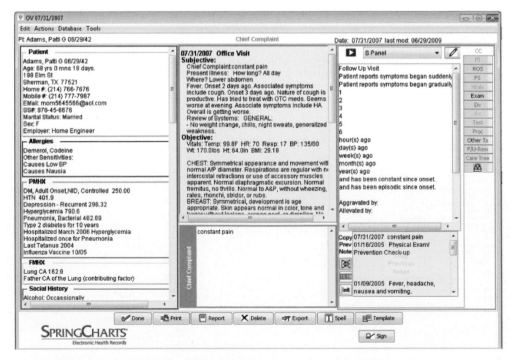

Figure 6.2 Office visit screen with pop-up text.

Once a panel tab has been selected, a list of pop-up text relevant to that tab of the navigation panel will appear in the third panel of the screen, also seen in Figure 6.2. Data can be entered by: 1) tapping with a stylus tool (as with a Tablet PC), 2) clicking on pop-up text items with a mouse, 3) typing directly into the text box, or 4) through a third-party voice recognition program the user can dictate and have the text automatically entered into the text field. Also, on a Tablet PC with handwriting recognition software, hand script will be recognized and automatically typed into the text box. However, it is recommended that pop-up text be utilized rather than these other methods of data entry. The use of pop-up text is the most rapid way of building documentation for an office visit note.

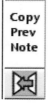

Figure 6.3 Copy previous note function.

The *Chief Complaint, Present Illness, Review of Systems, Examination, Procedure, Other Treatment,* and *Follow-up/Reminder* areas have the addition of notes from previous encounters in the bottom right window. A clinician can highlight any previous note text and copy it to the present note by clicking on the *Copy Note* icon, displayed in Figure 6.3. These previous notes are dated and organized by most recent first. Past encounter notes enable the clinicians to refresh their memory with past visits and copy any similar note quickly into the current office visit if necessary. The previous note panel will only display that portion of previous office visit documentation specific to the area selected on the navigation panel.

To the left of the previous note panel is a time and initial button that enables the clinician to time- and initial-stamp that portion of the office visit note. This feature allows various medical providers to be involved in the same patient encounter. For example, a medical assistant may record the illness when first admitting the patient to the exam room. The identification and time can be recorded in the *chief complaint* portion of the OV note. Similarly, a nurse may administer an injection after the physician has completed the examination and initial- and time-stamp that procedure. Thus, the one OV note can document the actions of other authenticated users along with the primary physician.

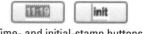

Time- and initial-stamp buttons

You will notice that the *Present Illness* panel navigation button accesses the same *S Panel* pop-up text as the *Chief Complaint* panel button, seen in Figure 6.4. This is because both sections of text will be housed in the subjective area of the SOAP format. However, they are broken out as separate categories on a **History & Physical report**.

Although the program will default to the appropriate pop-up text category when a specific navigation button is selected, additional lists of pop-up text are located by category in the pop-up text header field, seen in Figure 6.5. By accessing this list, the practitioner has multiple categories of text to choose from. Any selected text from other categories besides the default category will be added to existing text in the panel section that the user has currently opened. For example, a practitioner may create a new category of text specific to a certain procedure that he or she performs or a unique review of systems, or the practitioner may want a category specifically for chief complaints. Regardless of what category of pop-up text the text is chosen from, it will always go into the appropriate *SOAP* format based upon the navigation panel that is open at the time of text selection. The program offers an additional 20 user-defined categories that can be added to the pop-up text feature. (Customizing pop-up text is discussed in detail in Chapter 8.)

To add the chosen text into the body of the *SOAP* format, the user simply clicks the *In Box* or selects any other navigation panel tab. By clicking on the *In Box*, the user can view the entire OV note in the upper middle section. The

History & Physical Report
Often referred to as an **H & P.** It is the documentation of the patient's medical history combined with the physical exam. The H & P is the initial clinical evaluation and exam of the patient.

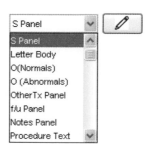

Figure 6.4 S panel category in pop-up text window.

Inbox

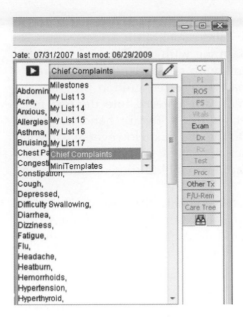

Figure 6.5 Pop-up text category list showing chief complaints.

Chief Complaint, Present Illness (History), *Review of Systems, Examination, Other Treatment*, and *Follow-Up/Reminder* all operate in similar manner with the appropriate pop-up text appearing on the right side.

The *FS* navigation tab allows the provider to add part or all of the face sheet to the encounter documentation by simply clicking on one or more of the category icons. The face sheet items selected will be placed in the *Subjective* area of the OV note. If the provider wants to add the entire face sheet to the office visit documentation he or she will click on the icon at the top of the screen beside *"Face Sheet—Add All to this Note."*

> Note: To change information in the face sheet, the user must edit the face sheet itself. Changes made to the information in the Office Visit note that was supplied from the FS tab will not modify the information in the patient's face sheet.

Along with all typical nine basic vitals, three additional custom vitals can be added to the program, such as peak flow rate, oxygen saturation of the blood, and so on. These are added to SpringCharts Server and will appear in the *Vitals* section of the *Office Visit* screen and in the *New Vitals Only* window of the patient's chart. The BMI (body mass index) is automatically calculated for the user based upon the patient's height and weight. See Table 6.1 for a manual calculation of BMI and Table 6.2 to see how disease risk is affected by BMI.

SpringCharts will display all four vital charts (height, weight, blood pressure, and **Body Mass Index [BMI]**) by accessing the *Growth Chart* icons at the top right in the *Vitals* panel. Growth charts backgrounds differ by the age and gender of the patient for the purpose of showing appropriate national percentiles for children. Figure 6.6 displays vitals for a boy between the age of 3 and 18 years.

The diagnosis (*Dx*), prescription (*Rx*), (*Test*), and procedure (*Proc*) navigation tabs operate differently by offering a search feature of the database rather than using pop-up text. The diagnosis, prescription, and procedure panels also offer the user a choice from items logged from previous patient chart entries. Selecting the *Dx* navigation tab produces a dialog widow enabling the user to choose diagnoses from the *PMHX + Problem List* window or the

Graphs: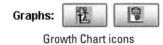

Growth Chart icons

Body Mass Index (BMI)

The measurement of choice for studying obesity. BMI is calculated by a mathematical formula that divides a person's weight by their height in meters squared. (BMI = kg/m²).

Table 6.1 BMI Calculation Table

To calculate the body mass index (BMI), locate the appropriate height in the left-hand column and the weight in the same row. The number at the top of the column is the BMI for that height and weight.

BMI (kg/m²)	19	20	21	22	23	24	25	26	27	28	29	30	35	40
Height (in.)							Weight (lb.)							
58	91	96	100	105	110	115	119	124	129	134	138	143	167	191
59	94	99	104	109	114	119	124	128	133	138	143	148	173	198
60	97	102	107	112	118	123	128	133	138	143	148	153	179	204
61	100	106	111	116	122	127	132	137	143	148	153	158	185	211
62	104	109	115	120	126	131	136	142	147	153	158	164	191	218
63	107	113	118	124	130	135	141	146	152	158	163	169	197	225
64	110	116	122	128	134	140	145	151	157	163	169	174	204	232
65	114	120	126	132	138	144	150	156	162	168	174	180	210	240
66	118	124	130	136	142	148	155	161	167	173	179	186	216	247
67	121	127	134	140	146	153	159	166	172	178	185	191	223	255
68	125	131	138	144	151	158	164	171	177	184	190	197	230	262
69	128	135	142	149	155	162	169	176	182	189	196	203	236	270
70	132	139	146	153	160	167	174	181	188	195	202	207	243	278
71	136	143	150	157	165	172	179	186	193	200	208	215	250	286
72	140	147	154	162	169	177	184	191	199	206	213	221	258	294
73	144	151	159	166	174	182	189	197	204	212	219	227	265	302
74	148	155	163	171	179	186	194	202	210	218	225	233	272	311
75	152	160	168	176	184	192	200	208	216	224	232	240	279	319
76	156	164	172	180	189	197	205	213	221	230	238	246	287	328

Previous Diagnoses window, seen in Figure 6.7. The *PMHX – Problem List* displays diagnoses from these areas of the patient's face sheet and the *Previous Diagnoses* window displays all the diagnoses from previous encounters with this patient in the clinic. These features enable for rapid selection of diagnoses, drugs, and procedures within the office visit; many times a practitioner will be choosing diagnoses, medications, and procedures that have been used previously.

Table 6.2	BMI Disease Risk Table

Risk of Associated Disease According to BMI and Waist Size

BMI	Obesity Level	Waist less than or equal to 40 in. (men) or 35 in. (women)	Waist greater than 40 in. (men) or 35 in. (women)
18.5 or less	Underweight	--	N/A
18.5–24.9	Normal	--	N/A
25.0–29.9	Overweight	Increased	High
30.0–34.9	Obese	High	Very high
35.0–39.9	Obese	Very high	Very high
40 or greater	Extremely obese	Extremely high	Extremely high

The prescription (*Rx*) navigation tab allows the user to view information windows from the patient's chart related to *Allergies* and *Other Sensitivities*. Medications can be chosen from *Routine Medications* and *Previous Prescriptions* windows. This provides the clinician with valuable information from which to make informed medical decisions. Medication prescribed during the office visit can be added to *Routine Medications* by clicking on the specific selected medication in the lower center window in the *Office Visit* screen and selecting *Add to Routine*, seen in Figure 6.8.

The strength, dosage, and so on, also seen in Figure 6.8, can be edited for this specific prescription without changing the system's original medication information. In the *Edit Rx* window, displayed when the user highlights the

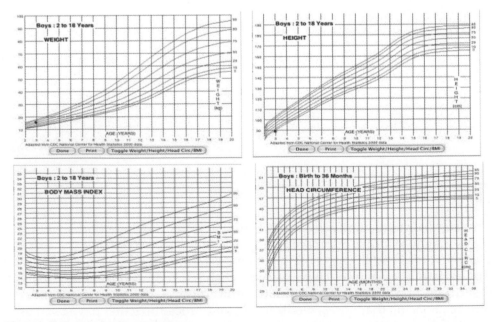

Figure 6.6 Graphs for vitals data.

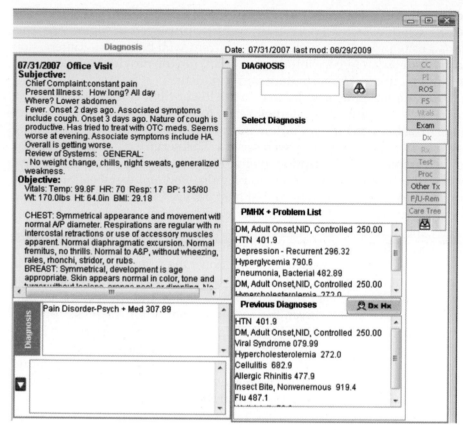

Figure 6.7 Diagnosis panel showing other resources.

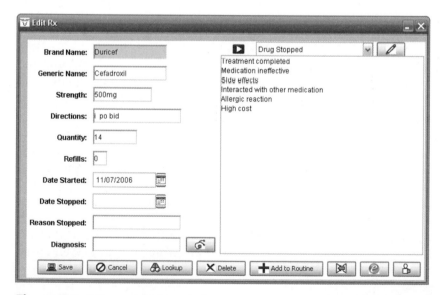

Figure 6.8 Edit prescription window.

prescribed medication, the provider can associate the medication with diagnoses. By accessing the diagnosis search button the user is shown the patient's previous diagnoses window and diagnoses listed in the past medical history and problem list from the patient's face sheet. Diagnoses can be selected from any of these sources and associated with the medication.

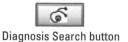

Diagnosis Search button

PRESCRIPTION

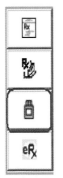

Figure 6.9 Access to the Epocrates website.

Drug Formulary

A database of approved medications in drug therapy categories and includes information on preparation, safety, effectiveness, and cost.

Drug Monographs

Highly detailed and thoroughly documented studies on drugs. They provide such information as the composition, description, method of preparation, dosage, adverse effects, overdose, warnings, and research.

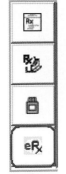

Drug Allergy/Interaction Checking button

SpringScripts button

Once again, a direct link is provided in the main *Prescription* window and the *Edit Rx* window to the Epocrates™ website, displayed in Figure 6.9. This popular website provides the user with a current web-based drug interaction and **drug formulary** reference information, allowing the provider to make clinical decisions more quickly, accurately, and confidently.

The **Drug Monographs** icon located in the lower right corner of the *Edit Rx* window allows the physician Internet access to information necessary to prescribe the drug by searching for automatic matches within the First Data drug monographs from the *NewCrop™* web service. This service gives such information as the composition, description, method of preparation, dosage for drugs, instruction sheets, and so on. Monographs also contain specifications (tests, procedures, and acceptance criteria) that help ensure the strength, quality, and purity of the named items. The practitioner is able to access patient handouts for the specific medication on the NewCrop™ website directly from SpringCharts, seen in Figure 6.10. Patient medication handouts can be printed out.

The printer icon in the lower left panel allows the printing or faxing of the prescription(s) from the *Office Visit* screen. Once the data filter preferences have been made in the *Prescription Printing Options* window and the [Print Rxs] button selected, the user will be given the option to print or fax the prescription(s) directly from SpringCharts, illustrated by Figure 6.11. If the prescription is created by a user who is not set up in SpringCharts as a physician, then the script will need to be printed to receive the physician's signature. Only users set up as providers will have the *Use Digital Signature* option in the *Prescription Printing* option. If a doctor is creating the prescription, the *Use Electronic Signature* check-box option will be available in the *Prescription Printing Options* window. If this is checked the prescription will show *Electronic Signature Verified* above the doctor's name on the script form if the doctor's digital signature was not added to the *User Preferences* window. If the provider has added his/her signature into SpringCharts, the digital signature will be printed onto the prescription(s). This form can now be sent electronically directly to the pharmacy's fax machine from SpringCharts. The *Electronic Signature Verified* phrase informs the pharmacy that the prescription was sent by the doctor. Whether or not the prescription has been electronically signed by the physician, the program still records the provider's name on the script from the *Print Name As* field in the *Doctor Information* setup window on SpringCharts Server.

(See Appendix A—*Sample Documents*; Document 1. *Prescription Forms*.)

Once selected, the *Drug Allergy/Interaction Checking* button in the *Rx* text box will access the Pharmacy Web service and check the selected prescriptions for potentially dangerous interactions with the patient's existing current medications, routine medications, and allergies. This feature will be discussed in more detail in the next chapter.

The SpringScripts icon shown as the last of four buttons in the prescription window allows for the prescription to be sent electronically to a Web-based

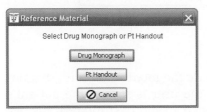

Figure 6.10 Drug monographs access window.

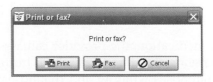

Figure 6.11 Print or fax option for prescription form.

e-prescribing clearing house and then on to the pharmacy. SpringScripts is also discussed in greater detail in the next chapter.

Tests may be ordered within the office visit by accessing the *Test* navigation tab. Once all the tests have been chosen the user must click the [Order Selected Test] button, displayed in Figure 6.12, to send the tests to the lower center information window.

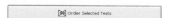

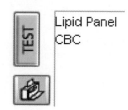

Figure 6.12 Order selected tests button in the test panel.

> Note: For a non-physician user to order tests in the *Office Visit* screen, the user must have first selected a physician in his/her *User Preferences* window (*File>Preferences>User Preferences*). Once set up, the program will allow the user to order tests.

Figure 6.13 Printer icon for test order form.

After selecting the [Order Selected Tests] button, a window will display, listing the doctors who are set up in SpringCharts Server. The user will select the physician for whom the tests are being ordered.

The tests can now be printed out or faxed as a physician order by selecting the printer icon in the lower center quadrant (see Figure 6.13). The order window will automatically add the selected test(s) and the diagnoses from the office visit note. Tests that will be conducted in the clinic can be deleted from the order form. The user has the option of adding selected pop-up text from the *Orders* category or adding a preset orders template by selecting the [Template] button. (See Chapter 8 for further discussion on templates.) The patient's primary insurance information recorded in his or her chart can be added to the order form by selecting the [Add Pt Ins] button, as illustrated in Figure 6.14. The order form for tests conducted at a third-party facility can now be printed and given to the patient.

(See Appendix A—*Sample Documents*; Document 9. *Test Order Form*.)

The order form can also be used to create a referral form. Because the program automatically places the diagnosis codes from the OV note onto the form

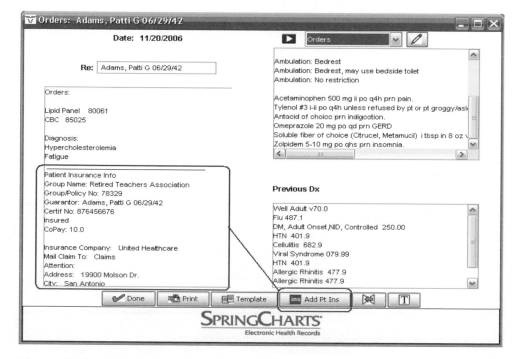

Figure 6.14 Order form showing patient's primary insurance.

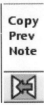

Copy Previous Note button

Create a reminder button

and provides the user with preset pop-up text and templates, a referral form can be created quickly, printed for the patient, and then stored in the patient's chart. The form is printed with the clinic's letterhead and contains the patient's name, address, and date of birth.

Procedures are chosen by first selecting the *Proc* navigation tab then the correct procedure category. Each category displays only the specific CPT codes that have been activated under these categories. Limiting the number of codes to those which the clinic typically uses enables speedier selection. (See Chapter 9 for further discussion on activating new procedure codes.) The user may also select procedures from the *Previous Procedure* window in the lower right corner. These procedures were conducted in prior encounters with the patient. Once a procedure has been selected, additional notes can be added to the procedure to document injection sites, medication strengths, patient education, and so on. (Chapter 9 will discuss notation of procedures further.)

Other Treatment is documented from within the *Office Visit* window. The *Other Tx* navigation tab allows the provider to select text from the default pop-up category for counseling or coordination of care items. Once again, text that was used in previous encounters with the patient relevant to the *Other Tx* section is available in the lower right window for previewing and/or copying into the current visit. If the same "coordination of care" counseling is conducted, the physician simply highlights previous text (not including the date) then selects the [Copy Prev Note] button to add this previous portion of the note to the existing office visit.

The *F/U-Rem* navigation tab allows for the selection of a follow-up period and referral notes. Text may be chosen from the default popup text category or selected from the previous note window containing text used in prior encounters.

In the lower left window the user will find a *"create a reminder"* icon that will enable the provider to send a *ToDo/Reminder* item to another person in the clinic or to him/herself. Clicking on the icon will activate the *New To/Do Reminder* window, seen in Figure 6.15. The dialog box will automatically be linked to this patient. Pop-up text is available for rapid selection of text. The *"create a reminder"* icon is useful for communication to the front desk personnel to

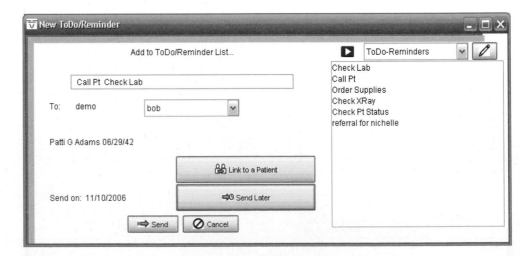

Figure 6.15 New *ToDo/Reminder* window in office visit screen.

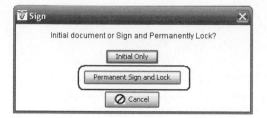

Figure 6.16 The sign window in the office visit.

Date Created: 04/26/2003
Date of Service: 04/28/2003
Patient Number: 31   Chart ID: 12
Last Modified: 11/22/2006

Figure 6.17 Dates automatically recorded in the office visit.

schedule a follow-up appointment or to schedule a follow-up call or procedure with the patient. When the recipient clicks on the item in his/her *ToDo List*, the patient's chart will open, giving the user all necessary information to execute the scheduled activity.

Selecting the [Sign] button in the OV screen provides the practitioner with the opportunity to *Initial Only* or *Permanent Sign & Lock* the office visit, as seen in Figure 6.16. *Initial Only* allows the office visit note to be recalled for further edits made by anyone with chart editing privileges. Portions of the office visit note can be completed and saved into the patient's chart without the entire note being finalized. This enables various health-care providers to take responsibility for segments of the health-care process. For example, a nurse or medical assistant may document the chief complaints and record the vitals in an office visit note, then save the partial note into the patient's chart. A physician may then open the same note, accessed from another computer, and complete the exam, assign diagnoses, prescribe medication, and so on, then create a routing slip for billing purposes. The office visit is placed in the patient's chart by selecting the [Done] button. A provider will not want to lock an office visit note, even if he/she has completed the routing slip, if the medical assistant needs to reopen the OV note and document details about a procedure that was administered after the provider left the exam room.

Once the office visit is locked, by selecting *Permanent Sign & Lock*, it cannot be unlocked or edited, even by the physician who permanently locked it. However, addendums can be amended to the bottom of an office visit note in this case. If an unlocked office visit note is edited at a future date, the *Last Modified* date will be updated, as illustrated in Figure 6.17. The *Date Created, Date of Service*, and *Last Modified* date are recorded automatically at the bottom of office visit note.

The *Date of Service* will automatically default to the date that the office visit note was first created. If a doctor wants to chart an office visit note on another day subsequent to the actual encounter, the *Date of Service* will require changing. On the office visit menu the physician would select *Tools>Date Of Service*. The desired date of service would be chosen in the dialog box. This will cause the office visit to be saved in the care tree *Encounter* category with the appropriate date of service. This date will be transferred to the PMS software for billing or printed on the routing slip regardless of the actual charting date.

Focal Point

Various clinicians can work on the same OV note. An MA may be first to document medical information and then hand off the OV note to be completed by another provider.

Concept Checkup 6.2^(LO 6.2)

A. Once a navigation tab has been selected in the *Office Visit* screen, _____ _____ will appear on the right side of the screen.

B. The *Copy Note* icon in the OV window enables the clinician to _____ _____

C. Along with all nine basic vitals, _____ additional custom vitals can be added to the program.

D. The diagnosis (*Dx*) and prescription (*Rx*) navigation buttons operate differently by offering _____.

E. The strength, dosage, and so on can be edited in the *Edit Rx* window without _____ _____

F. Procedures are chosen by first selecting the correct _____

Each category displays only the specific CPT codes _____ _____

Exercise 6.1 Building an OV Note (Part 1—MA)^(LO 6.2)

1. Open your own patient's chart. On the chart menu select *New>New OV.* In the *Office Visit* screen notice the face sheet information on the left-hand side of the window.
2. Add another past medical history item to your face sheet by right-clicking in the PMHX section of the face sheet panel on the left side and selecting *Edit.* In the face sheet window choose another medical item either from the list of *Preferences* in the lower left or search for a new diagnosis in the upper right. Click the [Back to Chart] button in the lower left.

Note: The OV screen will be positioned behind the patient's chart window. To bring it to the foreground simply click on the top edge of the OV window.

3. Let us assume your patient is visiting the doctor because of a flare-up with seasonal allergies and you are the medical assistant. Click on the [CC] navigation tab on the right side of the *Office Visit* screen. Notice the *S Panel* of pop-up text that appears in the right-hand panel.

You do not have all the appropriate pop-up text that you need to document the chief complaints of seasonal allergies. Click on the edit pencil to the right of the pop-up text category to open the *Edit PopUp Text* window. In the empty space at the bottom, type *Allergies, Runny nose, Itchy eyes* all on separate lines. (Place a comma after each symptom.) Click the [Done] button to return to the *Office Visit* screen. The added words will now appear in your list. In the pop-up text list, select *Allergies, Runny nose, Itchy eyes.* The words will be added to the lower middle work area. Click on the time and initial insert buttons in the lower right section to add the time and your initials to the note.

4. Select the [Vitals] navigation tab on the right. All previously created text is now added to the *SOAP* format. Fill out some vital information on yourself. Remember you do not have an abnormal temperature. *HC* stands for head circumference and is used by pediatricians to record head measurements for developing infants. BMI (body mass index) is grayed out because the program will calculate this item from the height and weight measurements.

5. Click on the [Done] button in the OV screen. Click the [Save and Skip Billing] button. We will come back later, finish the note, and create a routing slip for this office visit. The OV note has been added to the list of encounters in the care tree of your patient's chart. Close the chart.

Exercise 6.2 Building an OV Note (Part 2—Doctor)(LO 6.2)

Note: Now that the medical assistant has completed the initial assessment, the office visit is handed over to the physician. The physician will not start a new office visit note (as the medical assistant did), rather he/she will edit the existing office visit note.

1. Open your chart. Click on the "+" sign beside the *Encounters* heading in the care tree. Select the office visit entry you started in Exercise 6.1. Click on the [Edit] button at the bottom of the window.

Note: In the office visit screen the provider can view the information already collected by the medical assistant. SpringCharts has office visit templates for some of the most common ailments. This enables the provider to quickly select the appropriate template to populate the office visit note. All that remains is tweaking the notes for the specific patient.

2. Click on the [Template] button in the bottom right corner of the office visit screen. From the displayed list select: *Allergic Rhinitis.* Notice the entire note has been built very quickly.

3. The doctor will now complete the note for this patient. Click on the *PI* navigation tab on the right-hand side. The text from the template appears in the lower middle work area. Move the scroll bar to the top of this window and complete the following sentence: *Pt c/o red, itchy eyes, congested, itchy and runny nose (clear fluid), post-nasal drip, sneezing, itchy ears, scratchy throat and occasional cough for the past _ weeks.* Place your curser in front of the word *weeks*, highlight the underscore mark and type *3*.

Note: The physician will continue this way through the entire note making changes and additions where necessary for this specific patient.

4. A diagnosis will need to be added. Click on the *Dx* navigation tab on the right-hand side. Search for *Allergic Rhinitis* in the *Diagnosis* field in the upper right. Select *Allergic Rhinitis 477.9* from this list.
5. Next the physician will prescribe a medication. Click on the *Rx* navigation tab on the right side. In the *Prescription* field search for and select *Allegra 180mg* and *Flonase 50mcg*.
6. The physician may want you to come back into the exam room and administer a subcutaneous allergy shot. He/she will order the injection by choosing the *Proc* navigation tab on the right side. Click on the drop-down arrow beside the *All* category on the upper right side. Select the category *InjectMed.* From the list displayed below, choose *Allergy Injection – 1.*
7. Click on the [Done] button in the OV screen. Click the [Save and Skip Billing] button. The medical assistant will need to re-open this office visit note and document the administration of the allergy injection. The OV note has been added to the list of encounters in the care tree of your patient's chart. Close the chart.

Exercise 6.3 Building an OV Note (Part 3—MA)(LO 6.2)

Note: The physician will now communicate with the medical asistant regarding administrating the allergy shot. This may be done via the *Patient Tracker* by changing the *Tracker Status.*

1. Open your chart. Click on the "+" sign beside the *Encounters* heading in the care tree. Select the office visit entry you amended in Exercise 6.2. Click on the [Edit] button at the bottom of the window.
2. Click on the *Proc* navigation tab on the right side. Click on *Allergy Injection – 1* in the lower center work area.
3. In the *Edit Procedure* window you will need to document the injection administration that you just gave. Choose the pop-up text *Lot#* and type in a lot number. On the next line choose the pop-up text *Site: Left arm.* Click on the [D & T] button and the [Initials] button. Click on the [Save] button.
4. Click on the [Done] button in the OV screen. Click the [Save and Skip Billing] button. The doctor will now complete the routing slip and bill for the encounter. The OV note has been added to the list of encounters in the care tree of your patient's chart. Close the chart.

ICD-9 codes
Stands for the *International Classification of Diseases, Ninth Revision.* The ICD has become the international standard diagnostic classification for all medical data dealing with the incidence and prevalence of disease in large populations and for other health management purposes, for example, "474.00 - Tonsillitis (chronic)."

CPT Codes
Stands for *Current Procedural Terminology.* The CPT five-digit codes were developed by the American Medical Association (AMA) and have been adopted by insurance carriers and managed care companies as the means to identify common medical procedures, for example, "82270 - Fecal occult blood test."

LO 6.3, 6.4 ACTIVATING A NEW DX CODE AND DRUG IN THE OFFICE VISIT

New DX Code

SpringCharts is installed with the complete AMA library of **ICD-9 codes** and **CPT codes.** However, the clinic will need to activate the specific codes it intends to use. This method enables the clinic to have a restricted number of codes to choose from thus speeding the selection time. When SpringCharts is initially

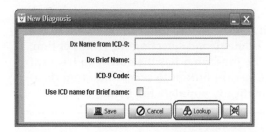

Figure 6.18 Activating a new diagnosis code.

installed a limited set of diagnosis and procedure codes are automatically activated at that time. While in the office visit screen, if the practitioner needs a particular diagnosis that has not been activated, he/she should choose *New Diagnosis* from the *Database* menu within the office visit window. New diagnosis description and code can be manually added directly into the appropriate fields. However, by selecting the [Lookup] button, seen in Figure 6.18, the program will access the ICD-9 database, enabling the user to search for a new diagnosis by either code or description. When the desired diagnosis code has been selected the *Dx Brief Name* field will need to be filled out. Whatever is typed into the *Dx Brief Name* field will determine the text for which the practitioner will search when selecting a diagnosis in the office visit. If the clinic normally uses the same text that appears in the ICD-9 database, the provider will simply check the *Use ICD name for Brief name* field to copy the ICD-9 name into the *Dx Brief Name* field, then click the [Save] button and the diagnosis code and description will be activated to the SpringCharts diagnosis list.

> Note: A new diagnosis can be activated from the *Edit* menu if the user is not in an office visit screen. The same functions as described above are available in this area. New ICD and CPT codes are created or modified by the Center for Medicare and Medicaid Services (CMS) annually. All EHR databases are updated yearly because of changes to these codes.

New Drug

SpringCharts also comes with the **American Medical Association (AMA)** dictionary of drugs/medications. In order to activate another drug during an office visit, the provider can access the database within the office visit screen. From the *Database* menu in the office visit screen he/she will select *New Drug*. The user can fill out the fields directly or search the database by clicking on the [Lookup] button. Once the chosen drug is selected, the program will auto-fill all the appropriate fields, as illustrated in Figure 6.19. The physician can make whatever modifications are necessary.

American Medical Association (AMA) Acronym for the American Medical Association, which was founded in 1847. Its purpose is to promote the art and science of medicine in order to improve professional and public health concerns in America's healthcare system.

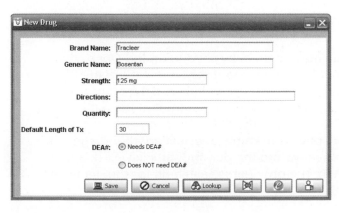

Figure 6.19 New drug setup in the office visit screen.

Note: If the user is not in an office visit screen, a new drug can be added to the drug database by accessing the main *Edit* menu and selecting the *Drugs* option. Once again, in the *New Drug* window, the prescriber has the ability to free-text medication information or select the [Lookup] button to access the drug database and select a drug which will automatically populate the fields.

From the *New Drug* window the provider has access to the Epocrates™ website to check for drug interactions, formulary references, and pill identifiers and access to drug monographs and patient handouts through the NewCrop™. website, also seen in Figure 6.19, thus allowing the provider to make clinical decisions more quickly and confidently.

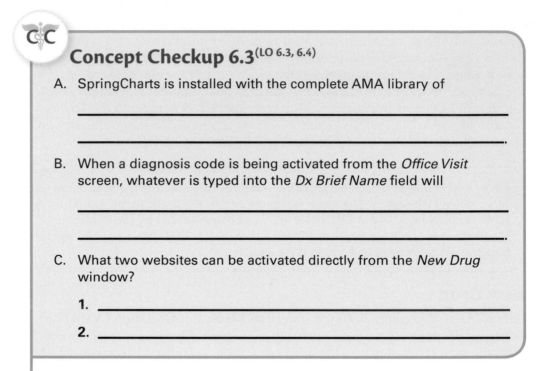

Concept Checkup 6.3(LO 6.3, 6.4)

A. SpringCharts is installed with the complete AMA library of

_____

_____.

B. When a diagnosis code is being activated from the *Office Visit* screen, whatever is typed into the *Dx Brief Name* field will

_____

_____.

C. What two websites can be activated directly from the *New Drug* window?

1. _____

2. _____

Exercise 6.4 Activating a New Diagnosis(LO 6.3)

Open Chart icon

1. Open your chart. This may be done by clicking on the *Open Chart* icon. Select your chart by typing in your last name. Click the "+" sign next to the *Encounters* in the care tree. Highlight the office visit that you recently created. In the lower right quadrant of the patient chart select the [Edit] bottom to open the *Office Visit* screen.
2. Let's assume that the physician wants to select another diagnosis that has not been activated into the SpringCharts list. Click on the [Dx] navigation button. The provider is searching for the diagnosis

Pulmonary congestion. In the diagnosis search field type: *pulm* and click the search icon. Pulmonary congestion is not yet activated.

3. Click on *Database* on the menu bar and select *New Diagnosis*. In the *New Diagnosis* window click on the [Lookup] button. In the search field type: *pulmonary* and search the database for *Pulmonary Congestion And Hypostasis.* Highlight this diagnosis to add it to the *New Diagnosis* window. The physician will use the same description as supplied by the database so check the *Use ICD name for Brief name* box. Save the newly activated code.

4. Back in the *Office Visit* screen, search for the new diagnosis by typing *pulm* in the diagnosis search field. Select the new ICD-9 code 514. It will be added to the patient's diagnosis for this office visit.

Exercise 6.5 Activating a New Medication(LO 6.4)

1. The provider needs to add another medication that is not yet activated to the SpringCharts list. Click on the [Rx] navigation button. In the prescription field type: *deconsal*. It is not in the list. Once again, select *Database* on the OV menu bar, then *New Drug.* The provider has the option to fill out the details of the new drug or click the [Lookup] button and search for Deconsal in the drug database. Click on the [Lookup] button. In the *LookUp Drug* window type: *deconsal* search and select *Deconsal 60 mg – 200 mg Cap.* In the *New Drug* window type: *1-2 cap PO q12h* in the *directions* field and *30* in the *Quantity* field. Put 0 in the *Refills* field. Save the new medication.

2. In the prescription search field of the OV screen search for Deconsal again. Select the newly activated drug.

3. Click the [Done] button in the OV screen and *Save and Skip Billing* of the office visit. Close the patient's chart.

LO 6.5 DISCONTINUED MEDICATION IN THE OFFICE VISIT

When medication needs to be stopped for a patient, an *Encounter* with that patient will need to be created. This would typically be done within an office visit, nurse note, new TC note, and messages or anywhere in SpringCharts where the patient's drug list can be accessed. To discontinue a patient's medication select the specific prescription and highlight it to open the *Edit Rx* window, seen in Figure 6.20. This graphic user interface (GUI) will enable the practitioner to input a *Date Stopped*, a *Reason Stopped*, and link the medication to a *Diagnosis.* The *Reason Stopped* can be selected from preset popup text.

The *Diagnosis Search* icon in the *Edit Rx* window will open up the patient's list of *Previous Diagnoses, PMHX, and Problem List* diagnoses. The provider can rapidly select a diagnosis or several diagnoses to accompany the medication information, thus associating an identifiable medical problem to the assigned medication.

Focal Point

To remove a medication from the patient's routine or current medication list, the provider must place a stopped date in the medication edit window.

Diagnosis Search button

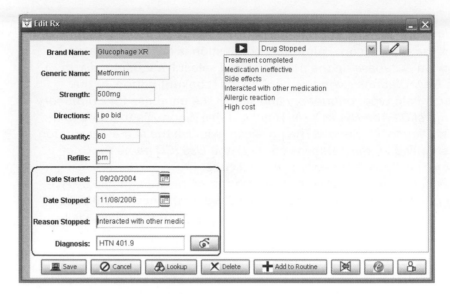

Figure 6.20   Edit prescription window.

Again, the *Edit Rx* window enables access to the Epocrates™ and NewCrop™ interactive websites to retrieve such information as formulary references, pill identifiers, drug monographs, and patient medication handouts.

Concept Checkup 6.4^(LO 6.5)

A. List at least four places in SpringCharts where a provider can open the *Edit Rx* window in order to stop a medication:

1. _____

2. _____

3. _____

4. _____

B. What kinds of information can the clinician retrieve from the Epocrates™ and NewCrop™ websites?

_____

_____

LO 6.6 EDITING POP-UP TEXT IN THE OFFICE VISIT

Additional items can be added to existing pop-up lists or pop-up text line items modified within the office visit by clicking on the edit button to the right of the pop-up text category field, seen in Figure 6.21.

The *Edit PopUp Text* window, illustrated in Figure 6.22, allows for 60 line items to be added to any pop-up text category. In addition to the 34 preset categories headings that are automatically installed the program (that cannot be altered), there are 20 customizable categories in the side menu. (Some may

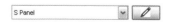

Figure 6.21   Accessing the edit pop-up text window.

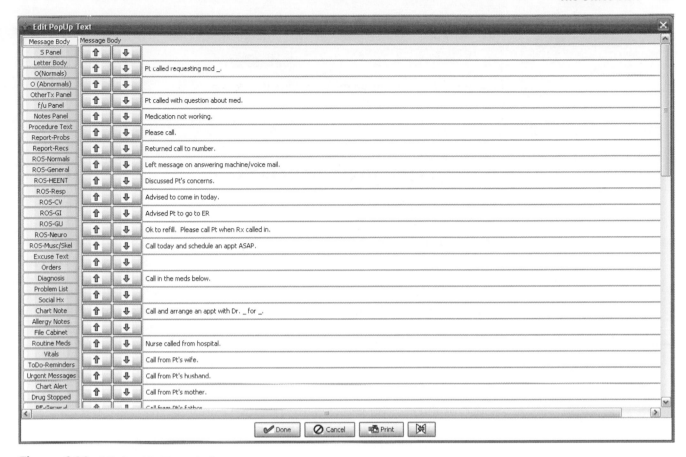

Figure 6.22 Edit PopUp Text window.

already be in use if customized **TemplateWare**™ was installed.) Text can be edited, deleted, or added in the *Edit PopUp Text* window. Added text can be manipulated to other positions by using the up and down arrows to the left of the text. (See Chapter 8 for further details.) Once changes have been made in the *Edit PopUp Text* window, the user will select the [Done] button and the modified text will be seen in the office visit screen, as seen in Figure 6.23.

In the office visit screen work area the selected text can also be edited in the lower center panel by traditional methods for insertions, deletions, and changes. The cursor may be placed in a sentence and additional pop-up text added to that area. (This feature is optional and may be selected on the main menu under *File>Preferences>User Preferences - PopUp Text Insert: Insert at Cursor.*

TemplateWare

SpringCharts add-on feature that provides prebuilt office visits notes, orders, and letters, as well as pop-up text for specific specialists. Installing these powerful templates saves time and facilitates more complete patient documentation with a minimum of effort. Some of the specialty TemplateWare includes family practice, gastroenterology, internal medicine, pediatric, psychiatry, and pulmonary medicine.

Concept Checkup 6.5 (LO 6.6)

A. How many lines of type can be added to each pop-up text category?

_____

B. How many additional categories of pop-up text can be added to SpringCharts?

_____

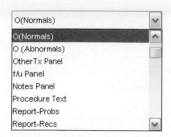

Figure 6.23 Refreshing the pop-up text category.

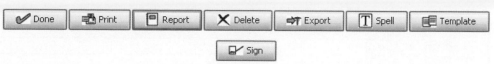

Figure 6.24 Speed button menu in *Office Visit* screen.

LO 6.7 OFFICE VISIT REPORTS

Report to Patient

The [Report] button in the office visit screen, seen in Figure 6.24, enables the printing/faxing/emailing of this specific physical exam *to the patient*. Any test results that have been entered into the pending tests and saved into the patient's chart are printed next to the name of the tests that were ordered in the office visit and the normal range is printed to the right of these results. Ordered tests that have not been added back into the chart will also be listed in this report and will state *Pending* beside the test's name. Identified *Problems* and *Recommendations* are headings located at the end of the report in which the diagnoses and treatment are detailed, respectively. The pop-up text categories of *Report-Probs* and *Report-Recs* are also available to further clarify these areas with additional text. An alternative way to create an exam report for the patient is to click the [Report] button in the lower left quadrant of the patient's chart once the office visit note has been selected in the care tree. This enables the user to create a report without having to open the *Office Visit* screen.

(See Appendix A—*Sample Documents*; Document 10. *Report to Patient*.)

> **Focal Point**
>
> Creating a report of the OV note provides the patient with the provider's notations of the exam along with the diagnoses and treatment plan.

Office Visit Note

The [Print] button within the *Office Visit* screen and the [Print] button located in the patient's chart will allow for the printing/faxing of the office visit note itself. The office visit note does not add tests results or additional information like letterhead and notation to the patient. It will simply detail the note in the *SOAP* format.

(See Appendix A—*Sample Documents*; Document 11. *Office Visit Report*.)

History & Physical Report

The *History & Physical Report* generator, seen in Figure 6.25, is located in the *Tools* menu within the *Office Visit* screen illustrated in Figure 6.26. The H&P is a more elaborate report than the standard reports mentioned above; it pulls information from the patient's chart, such as allergies, current medication, past medical, family medical and social history, as well as aspects of the current physical exam and test results. This report is more suitable for hospitals and referring physicians. The *H&P Report* is stored in the care tree once the [Done] button is activated.

(See Appendix A—*Sample Documents*; Document 12. *History & Physical Report*.)

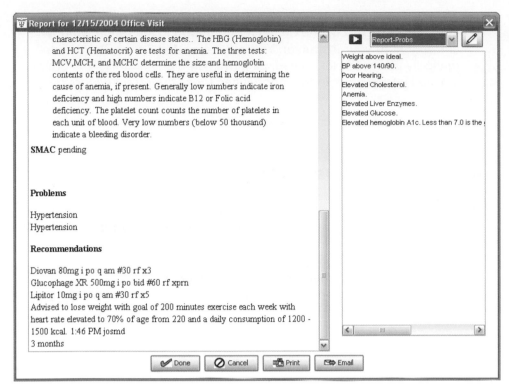

Figure 6.25 Creating an exam report from an office visit.

Figure 6.26 Creating a
History & Physical Report.

Concept Checkup 6.6(LO 6.7)

A. If tests have been ordered in the office visit and the results have been
    entered into the pending tests and then saved into the patient's chart
    the results will appear along with the ordered tests in what two reports?

1. _____

2. _____

B. Along with information from the current exam, the H&P also con-
    tains information from the patient's chart such as:

    _____

    _____

Focal Point

The H&P Report is more
elaborate than the patient
report and the SOAP
note because it includes
a lot of other medical
information from the
patient's chart.

Exercise 6.6 Creating an Exam Report(LO 6.7)

1. Open your patient's chart. Highlight the recent office visit note. Click
    on the [Report] button at the bottom of the patient's chart screen.
    The program will automatically open the OV window and display
    the exam report on the screen.

2. Print the report by clicking on the [Print] button in the report window and submit to your instructor. You will notice that SpringCharts automatically places the letterhead, patient's name and address, the greeting, and introduction in the report letter. Close the report window.

Exercise 6.7 Creating an H&P Report(LO 6.7)

1. In the OV window, click on the *Tools* menu and select *H&P*. The *History & Physical Report* is speedily created. You can see that a H&P contains relevant information from the current physical exam as well as documentation from the patient's face sheet.
2. Print the report and submit to your instructor.
3. Click the [Done] button and save the H&P under the *H&P* category in the care tree.

Exercise 6.8 Creating an OV Note Report(LO 6.7)

Focal Point

The provider has immediate access to the patient's face sheet from the OV screen where modifications can be made.

1. With your office visit window still open, click on the [Print] button and print the entire office visit note. As you will see the OV note is not pre-addressed to any entity and may be used to send to a referring physician or other consultant.
2. Submit the OV note to your instructor. You have already seen that office visit notes, among other things, can be added to the body of a letter and printed, faxed, or e-mailed to the patient or other concerned entities.
3. Close the OV window.
4. In the patient's chart you will notice the *Report to Patient* and the *Office Visit* saved as *Encounters* in the care tree and *H&P* saved under that category in the care tree. Click on the "+" sign beside the *H&P* category and highlight the recently created H&P report. The report will be seen in the lower right quadrant from where it can be edited and printed.
5. Close the patient's chart.

LO 6.8 EDIT MENU

The *Edit* menu in the *Office Visit* screen, seen in Figure 6.27, provides quick access to the face sheet chart categories. By selecting any of these face sheet items the user is taken immediately to that feature of the *Edit face sheet* window of the patient's chart. This enables the practitioner the ability to add additional items to the face sheet during the office visit encounter (e.g., additional past medical or family medical information supplied by the patient at the time). As mentioned

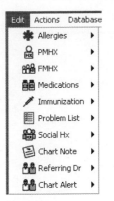

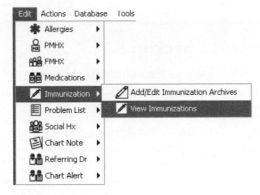

Figure 6.27 Edit menu in *Office Visit* screen.

Figure 6.28 View Immunizations from the edit menu.

earlier, the provider can also access the patient's face sheet by right-clicking on the appropriate section of the face sheet panel in the OV screen and selecting *Edit*.

In addition to the face sheet items in the *Edit* menu, the immunization record can be accessed, viewed, and printed, seen in Figure 6.28. Past immunizations can also be added in this window to bring the vaccination record current. New vaccines administrated in the clinic will not be added here; immunizations are automatically added to the list when selected as a *Procedure* in the office visit. When entering past immunizations the date must be typed in the mm/dd/yyyy format or the *Select Date* calendar used.

LO 6.9 ACTIONS MENU

The *Actions* menu within the *Office Visit* screen, displayed in Figure 6.29, provides some of the same functions as the *Actions* menu inside the patient's chart. However, no test can be ordered from this menu. The *Lab* feature in the *Actions* menu enables the physician to display the patient's previous labs on a table flow sheet for comparisons and trend analysis, as seen in Figure 6.30.

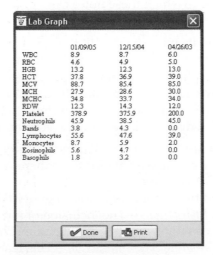

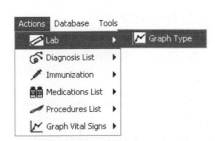

Figure 6.29 Graph lab type from actions window.

Figure 6.30 Comparison lab graph accessed in office visit.

Concept Checkup 6.7(LO 6.9)

A. In addition to the face sheet items in the *Edit* menu of the *Office Visit* screen, the _____ can be accessed, viewed, and printed.

B. The *Lab* feature in the *Actions* menu of the *Office Visit* screen enables the physician to display

_____

_____

_____

LO 6.10 TOOLS MENU

The *Tools* menu in the office visit provides access to:

1. *H&P*—The creation of a History & Physical Report is discussed within the *Office Visit Reports* of this chapter.
2. *Calculators*—There are three types of calculators available in SpringCharts: 1) the conversion calculator, 2) the pregnancy EDD calculator, and 3) the simple calculator. (These are discussed in detail in Chapter 10.)
3. *Care Plan*—A plan of care can be attached to the office visit record by accessing a stored care plan on the computer or copying and pasting a care plan from National Guideline Clearinghouse. (The care plan feature is discussed in more detail in Chapter 7.)
4. *Chart Tab*—The chart tab feature enables the user to save an existing office visit note under a different care tree tab separate from where it was originally saved, illustrated in Figure 6.31. By default the program will save OV notes under the *Encounter* category; other categories can be created in the care tree to which these notes can be saved.
5. *Draw*—the draw program will be discussed in detail in Chapter 7.

The draw item is stored with the office visit note. The *Follow-Up* segment on the note is stamped with the word: *Graphic*, as seen in Figure 6.32. To view the attached graphic from within the patient's chart without opening up the office visit simply click on the specific office visit in the care tree, then click the word: *****Graphic***** in the lower right detail panel of the chart and the *Draw item* window will display along with the accompanying office visit note.

6. *New Excuse/Note/Order*—This note writer feature enables the practitioner to create an excuse note for the patient or create a test order form within the *Office Visit* screen. It has the same functionality as the *New Excuse/Note/Order* in the patient chart screen under the *New* menu.
7. *Patient Instructions*—The inclusion of patient instructions handouts within the office visit is discussed in detail in Chapter 7.
8. *Resend Routing Slip/Transaction*—This feature enables the office visit note to be sent again either as a **routing slip** or the transactions sent to the PMS interface. New information does not need to be added to the OV note for another routing slip to be produced. Once selected this option will display the *Routing Slip* window for editing.

Routing Slip
Form that contains the medical office's most common procedure and diagnosis codes and descriptions. It also contains the patient's name, demographics, and billing information and may or may not include pricing. In a paper environment the physician usually indicates on the routing slip which procedures and diagnoses were used in the office visit. With an EHR only the codes and description that were selected in the office visit will print on the routing slip. Some other names for a routing slip are superbill, encounter form, and fee ticket.

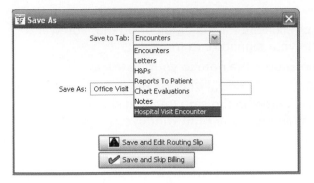

Figure 6.31 Saving office visit note under alternative tab.

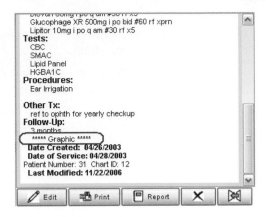

Figure 6.32 Office visit note stamped with graphic label.

9. *Spell Check*—The built-in spell checker will scan the entire office visit note and suggests appropriate spelling corrections. Words can be added to the internal dictionary.

10. *Template*—The various functionalities of SpringCharts' templates, including office visit templates, will be discussed in detail in Chapter 8.

11. *Date of Service*—If the practitioner is documenting the office visit note on a day subsequent to the actual date of service, this feature will need to be accessed and the real date of service selected from the supplied calendar. Unless the *Date of Service* is selected, the program will automatically stamp the system date when the office visit note was first created.

Concept Checkup 6.8(LO 6.10)

A. Office visit notes that were saved under the *Encounter* category in the care tree can be opened and resaved under a different category by selecting _____ in the *Tool* menu of the *Office Visit* screen.

B. If the physician needs to send another routing slip without adding new data to the office visit note, he/she will need to select _____ from the Tools menu in the *Office Visit* screen.

C. How does a physician document the correct office visit date of service if the office visit note is created after the date of service?

_____

_____

Exercise 6.9   Creating an Excuse Note(LO 6.10)

1. Open your patient's chart. Open the recent office visit note. Click on the *Tools* menu and select *New Excuse/Note/Order* then *New Excuse/Note*. In the *Note* window select pop-up text to excuse

the student's absence from college for the time period that you were at the doctor's office. Add your signature to the note.

2. Print the excuse note and submit the note to your instructor.

3. Click the [Done] button in the OV screen. Click on the "+" sign to the left of the *ExcusesNotes* category in the care tree and see the saved note. The note is displayed in the lower right window.

LO 6.11 ROUTING SLIP

A *Routing Slip* is created from the *Office Visit* screen and contains all the billable items from the office visit note. When the provider selects [Done] in the *Office Visit* screen a window is displayed, giving the user the options of *Save and Edit Routing Slip* or *Save and Skip Billing*, seen in Figure 6.33.

The *Routing Slip*, illustrated in Figure 6.34, gives the user access to the **E&M Coder**, which will recommend the appropriate level of office visit code and additional billable codes from the customized *Superbill*. (The superbill will be discussed in further detail in Chapter 7.)

The Evaluation & Management code is calculated from:

1. The patient type (new or established or consulting),
2. The complexity of the presenting problem,
3. The level of history reviewed,
4. The extent of the exam and review of systems, and
5. The level of medical decision making.

E&M Coder

Stands for Evaluation & Management Coder, which is a built-in function of Spring-Charts that recommends the correct evaluation and management code for office visits. The coder looks for keywords used within the review of systems and exam of body areas, organs, and systems in the office visit note. The E&M coder then uses this information along with the number of diagnoses to determine the E&M code level for billing.

Focal Point

The routing slip window provides the practitioner with a recommended E&M code based on documentation in the OV note.

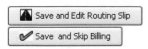

Figure 6.33 Routing slip option when saving OV.

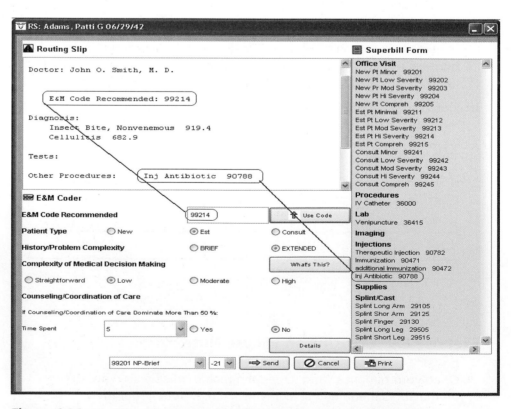

Figure 6.34 The electronic routing slip showing E&M coder and superbill.

Although these areas are selected automatically by the program based upon an intricate formula, the user can overrule the recommendation by clicking on the appropriate radio button for *Patient Type, Problem Complexity*, and *Complexity of Medical Decision Making*. If the time element for coordination of care and counseling is used to determine the E&M code, then all the other criteria listed above have no bearing on the specific code recommended. The code will be based solely on the time indicated, not the level of care.

SpringCharts' *E&M Coder* is an advanced elaborate program that automatically evaluates the review of systems and exam text of the office visit note and recommends the level of care based on terminology used. The words, phrases, and abbreviations used in the OV note give evidence to the number of body areas and systems examined, and the extent of the exam, thus affecting the evaluation and management level. If a low code is recommended the provider may need to review the OV documentation for accuracy. The *Office Visit* screen causes the practitioner to observe the patient's past medical, family medical, and social histories. The *E&M Coder* in turn gives the provider credit for reviewing these areas.

The physician may use the recommended code by selecting the [Use Code] button. The *E&M Coder* will recommend a level of code based upon a new, established, or consult visit to a physician's office. If the exam/encounter was conducted at another facility then a code may be chosen from the drop down window of other E&M codes in the bottom section of the window. The codes in this list are set up in the *Category Preferences* window on SpringCharts Server in the *E&M Codes* sub-window.

The [Details] button is selected to view the *E&M Code Factors* that were used to determine the specific recommended code. If the provider wishes to use the *Time Spent* feature to support the selection on the E&M code, the time in this field needs to be chosen and the *Yes* radio button activated. The *E&M Code Recommended* field will now show the new recommended E&M code based upon the time factor of the coordination of care of the patient encounter. The two different criteria for recommending an E&M code is seen in Figure 6.35.

The user will then click *Send* to send the routing slip to the PMS interface (if available) or to place the routing slip on file within SpringCharts. Stored routing slips can be accessed under the *Edit* menu on the main window from where they can be printed out by the billing personnel or resent to the PMS interface, as seen in the View *Routing Slip* window, illustrated in Figure 6.36.

(See Appendix A—*Sample Documents*; Document 13. *Routing Slip*.)

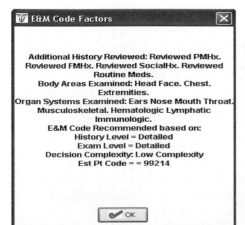
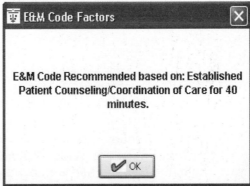

Figure 6.35 E&M code based upon level of care or time factor.

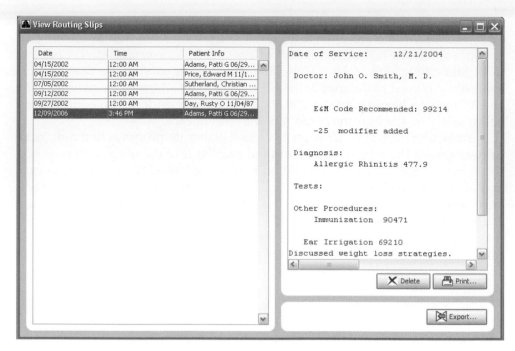

Figure 6.36 Stored routing slips.

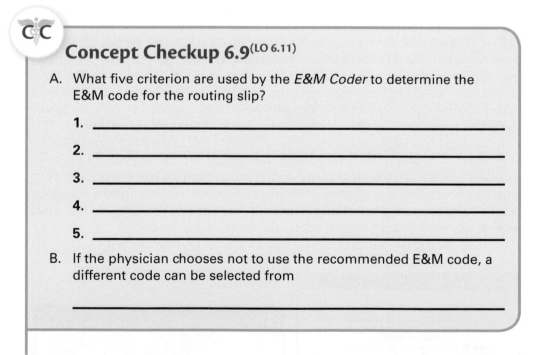

Concept Checkup 6.9^(LO 6.11)

A. What five criterion are used by the *E&M Coder* to determine the E&M code for the routing slip?

1. _____

2. _____

3. _____

4. _____

5. _____

B. If the physician chooses not to use the recommended E&M code, a different code can be selected from

_____

Exercise 6.10   Creating a Routing Slip^(LO 6.11)

1. Open your patient's chart. Open the recent office visit note. Click on the *Tools* menu and select *Resend Routing Slip/Transaction.* You will see in the *Routing Slip* window the diagnoses and follow-up information recorded from the OV note. The *E&M Coder* in the middle

section is recommending the E&M code of 99202. Click on the [Details] button in the bottom area of the *Routing Slip* window and read about the body systems and areas that were reviewed during the office visit. Click [OK] and use the recommended code by clicking on the [Use Code] button.

2. Print the *Routing Slip* by clicking the [Print] button and submit to your instructor.
3. Click on the [Send] button. Close the patient's chart.
4. In the main *Practice View* screen, select the *Edit* menu and choose the *Routing Slips* option. In the *View Routing Slip* window you will see the routing slip you just created. This is where the billing person will come to retrieve the routing slips for each day in order to bill the insurance companies or other responsible parties. In a linked environment to a PMS program, this routing slip code information will have been sent to the PMS interface.

LO 6.12 ADDING ADDENDUMS TO AN OFFICE VISIT

Providers have the ability to lock an office visit note so that no additional material can be entered into the note, even by themselves. Office visit notes are locked by clicking on the [Sign] button ion the OV screen. The user will be given the option to either initial the note or permanently sign or lock the note, as seen in Figure 6.37. Office visit notes that have been *permanently signed and locked* can be amended. In an existing "Signed & Locked" office visit located in

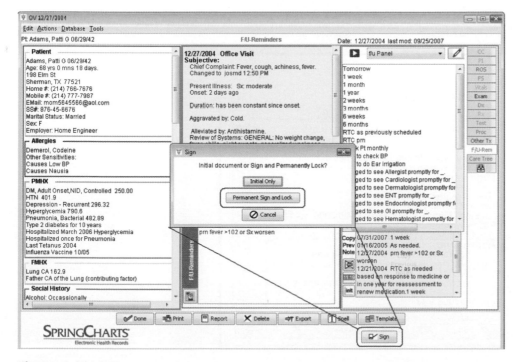

Figure 6.37 Office visit notes can be permanently locked.

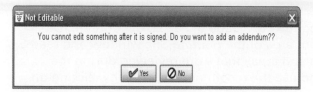

Figure 6.38 Adding an addendum to a locked office visit note.

Addendum
Medical note added subsequent to the original note that will supplement the clinical information.

the care tree, the user will select the [Edit] button in the lower right panel in the patient's chart. The user will be given the option of adding an **addendum** to the office visit note, illustrated by Figure 6.38.

> **Note: This option will not appear if the office visit note was not** *permanently signed and locked*. **In this case the office visit note may be opened and information added or modified in the body on the previous note. The system will update the** *Last Modified* **date at the bottom of the note.**

The added addendum note will be placed at the bottom of the existing office visit note. The program will automatically date, time, and initial-stamp the addendum when it is saved. Additional addendums can be added to the same office visit note, illustrated in Figure 6.39.

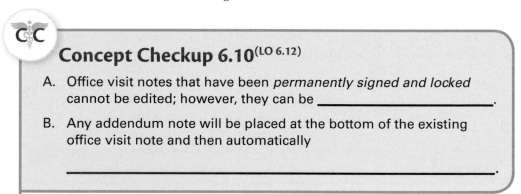

Concept Checkup 6.10 (LO 6.12)

A. Office visit notes that have been *permanently signed and locked* cannot be edited; however, they can be _____.

B. Any addendum note will be placed at the bottom of the existing office visit note and then automatically

_____.

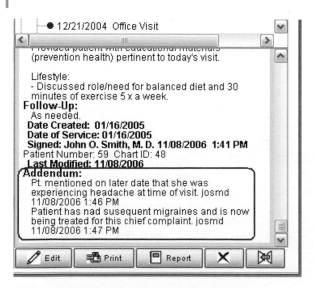

Figure 6.39 Office visit note addendum.

Name _____ Instructor _____ Class _____

USING TERMINOLOGY

Match the terms on the left with the definitions on the right.

_____ 1. SOAP format

_____ 2. BMI

_____ 3. Drug formularies

_____ 4. ICD-9

_____ 5. CPT

_____ 6. E&M coder

_____ 7. Routing slip

_____ 8. Drug monograph

_____ 9. History & Physical

_____ 10. AMA

_____ 11. Addendum

_____ 12. Office visit

A. Definition for the International Classification of Diseases, Ninth Revision. (LO 6.3)

B. This association was founded in 1847 with the purpose of promoting the art and science of medicine. (LO 6.4)

C. A medical note added subsequent to the original note. (LO 6.12)

D. The documentation of the patient's medical history combined with the physical exam. (LO 6.7)

E. An encounter with a medical provider whereby the patient's chief complaints are reviewed. (LO 6.2)

F. A convenient way for health-care providers to lay out the documentation of an office visit exam. (LO 6.1)

G. Current procedural terminology. (LO 6.3)

H. The measurement of choice for studying obesity. (LO 6.2)

I. A sophisticated algorithm that determines the appropriate E&M codes. (LO 6.11)

J. Databases of approved medications in drug therapy. (LO 6.2)

K. A form that contains the medical office's procedures, diagnosis codes, and charges for an office visit. (LO 6.11)

L. Highly detailed and thoroughly documented studies on medications. (LO 6.2)

CHECKING YOUR UNDERSTANDING

Write "T" or "F" in the blank to indicate whether you think the statement is true or false.

_____ 13. The navigation tabs enable the provider to proceed through the office visit and includes the chief complaint (CC). (LO 6.1)

_____ 14. The use of *Build-Your* text is the most rapid way of building documentation in an office visit. (LO 6.6)

_____ 15. SpringCharts is installed with the complete AMA library of ICD-9 and CPT codes. (LO 6.3)

_____ 16. SpringCharts will not allow you to activate any of the ICD-9 or CPT codes that are listed in the AMA library. (LO 6.3)

_____ 17. SpringCharts comes with a large hardbound AMA dictionary of drugs/medications. (LO 6.4)

_____ 18. OV notes that have been permanently signed and locked cannot be amended. (LO 6.12)

Answer the question below in the space provided.

19. What four components make up the SOAP format?(LO 6.1)

_____

_____

_____

_____

Choose the best answer and circle the corresponding letter.

20. The tools menu in the OV provides access to:(LO 6.10)
    a) History and physical report and the care plan
    b) The draw program and stored patient instructions
    c) a and b

21. There are three types of calculators in SpringCharts. They are:(LO 6.10)
    a) Conversion, simple, and metric calculators
    b) Conversion, pregnancy EDD, and simple calculators
    c) Pregnancy EDD, metric, and financial calculators

22. The *Edit* menu in the OV screen provides quick access to the face sheet items including:(LO 6.8)
    a) New diagnosis
    b) H&P Report
    c) None of the above

23. When medication needs to be stopped for a patient, an encounter with that patient will need to be created. Medications can be recorded as stopped in:(LO 6.5)
    a) The OV note and nurse note
    b) New TC note and messages
    c) a and b

24. In the lower left window of the *Office Visit* screen, the user will find a "create a reminder" icon that will enable the provider to send a ToDo/Reminder item to:(LO 6.2)
    a) A patient's home e-mail
    b) Another person in the clinic
    c) An outside lab

25. The abbreviation "ROS" stands for:(LO 6.2)
    a) Routine oral surgery
    b) Registered oncology school
    c) Review of systems

7

Clinical Tools

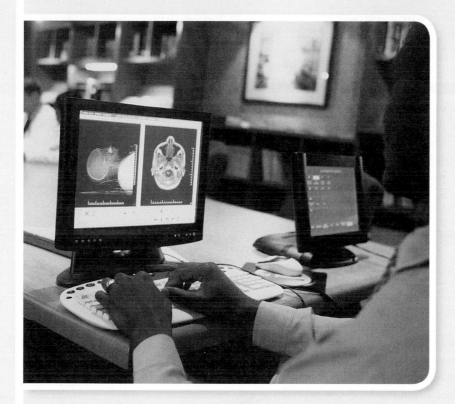

What You Need to Know

To understand Chapter 7 you will need to know how to:

- Open a patient's chart
- Open a new office visit
- Navigate in an *Office Visit* screen
- Add new pop-up text
- Refresh pop-up text
- Create a routine slip

Key Terms

Terms you will encounter in Chapter 7:

Care Plan

Chart Evaluation

Superbill

Wellness Screenings

Learning Outcomes

After completing Chapter 7, you will be able to:

LO 7.1 Create and conduct a chart evaluation item

LO 7.2 Demonstrate how to order a test in the office visit screen

LO 7.3 Understand the function of the E&M coder

LO 7.4 Demonstrate how to add items to a superbill

LO 7.5 Create and administer a patient instruction sheet

LO 7.6 Describe how to add a care plan to an office visit

LO 7.7 Perform a drug allergy check

LO 7.8 Understand the purpose of the draw program

LO 7.9 Demonstrate how to import a document to a patient's chart

LO 7.1 CHART EVALUATION

Chart Evaluation
Used to define criteria to search patient charts for health needs in order to support disease management, routine preventive services, and wellness health-care standards.

SpringCharts' **chart evaluation** feature allows users to define preventive health criteria and then assess patients' charts by these criteria. This enables the physician to be proactive in the **wellness screenings** of patients. In order to set up chart evaluations, the administrator will select *Chart Evaluation* from the *Administration* menu, seen in Figure 7.1. (In a networked environment the *Administrator* panel is accessible on SpringCharts Server.) From this window the user can access the *National Guideline Clearinghouse* (NGC) through the Internet to evaluate medical standards for wellness screenings. This information from NGC can then be set up within SpringCharts to provide ongoing chart evaluations.

Selecting the [New] button presents the *Evaluation Item* window for setting up evaluation criteria, illustrated in Figure 7.2.

In the setup window, users will define criteria specifications by:

Wellness Screenings
Periodic medical checkups to test for or inoculate against significant diseases. Wellness screenings are preventive services given before the onset of chief complaints.

1. *Gender*—Select whether a criterion is specific to male, female, or either one.
2. *Age*—Select the age within which the criteria should be met.
3. *Actions*— Indicate the *Test, Procedure,* or *Encounter* required to meet the criteria.

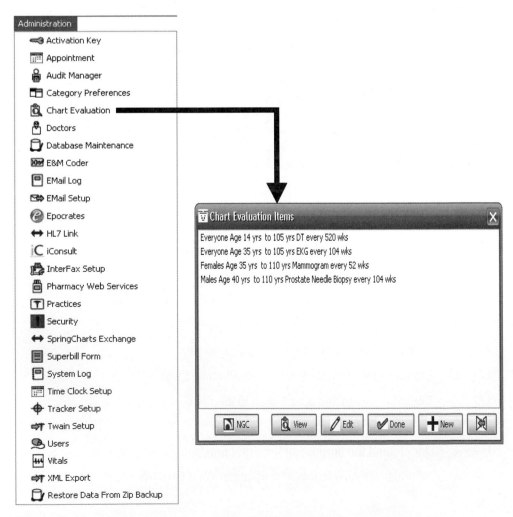

Figure 7.1 Accessing the chart evaluation from the administration menu.

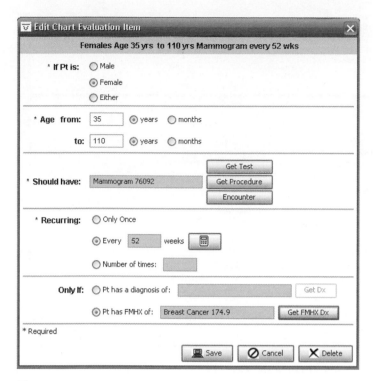

Figure 7.2 Edit *Chart Evaluation* window.

4. *Recurring*—Specify if this is a recurring criterion or one-time event. If recurring, enter the time span in number of weeks or the number of screenings needed in the patient's life time.
5. *Diagnosis(es)*—Specify if this criterion is required only if a patient has specific diagnosis(es) or if it is linked to a family medical history diagnosis(es).

Having the wellness screening item linked to a diagnosis from the patient's chart is optional. These preventive guidelines can be accessed on SpringCharts Server in the future and modified due to updated medical information.

Individual patients can be screened by accessing *File > Evaluate Chart* from within the patient's chart. There is also a speed icon on the patient chart's tool bar that will activate this feature. It is recommended that a chart evaluation be run by clinic personnel with each patient encounter. Each evaluation recommendation, seen in Figure 7.3, that has not been completed in the patient's chart is listed; each recommendation has a field in which to document the patient's response. The recommendation may be made to the patient; however, the patient may decline to have the test, injection, or procedure done on that day. The clinician may also choose to override any automated prompt and not make any recommendation to the patient. If a verbal recommendation is made to the patient, the clinician will check the *"Mark this Done"* radio button. After the main [Done] button is selected, the patient's response and a summary of the evaluation item(s) are then automatically recorded and dated in the chart's care tree under the *Encounter* category.

If the patient is up to date with the evaluations and health management screenings the user will receive a message: *Pt up to date with recommendations* when the *Evaluate Chart* feature is activated in the chart. If the user receives the following message: *No criterion set*, it indicates that no chart evaluations have been set up on SpringCharts Server.

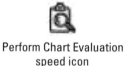

Perform Chart Evaluation
speed icon

Focal Point

Chart evaluation criteria will change from clinic to clinic based on the specialty.

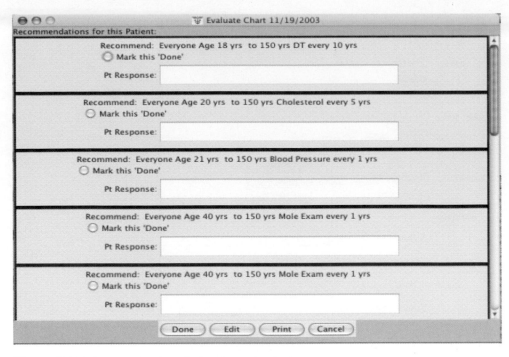

Figure 7.3 *Chart Evaluation* window in patient's chart.

SpringCharts also has the ability to scan the entire patient database and apply the chart evaluation criterion to all patient charts. When this activity is necessary the administrator will click on *Utilities* menu on the main *Practice View* screen and select *Evaluate All Charts*. SpringCharts will list all the patients in the database and display those who have outstanding evaluation screenings. Patients listed as *UTD* indicate that they are "up to date" with the medical screenings, displayed in Figure 7.4.

> Note: Because all charts are evaluated, this process could take some time and should be run after hours.

Focal Point

SpringCharts has the ability to conduct a chart evaluation on specific patients or run an evaluation on the entire patient database.

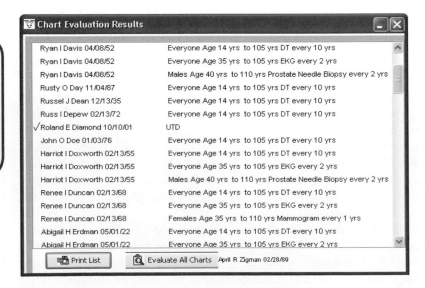

Figure 7.4 Chart evaluation results from database.

Concept Checkup 7.1(LO 7.1)

A. The chart evaluation feature in SpringCharts allows users to define

_____

_____.

B. The message: *No criterion set* indicates

_____

_____.

C. The chart evaluation feature can be run for specific patient charts or

_____.

Exercise 7.1 Creating and Conducting a Chart Evaluation(LO 7.1)

1. Open the *Administration* menu in the main *Practice View* screen. Select *Chart Evaluation*. Highlight the *Chart Evaluation Item* that deals with mammogram screening and click the [Edit] button. Look at the details of this wellness check item. Let's narrow down our screening criteria by linking this item to a family medical history diagnosis. In the lower portion of the window click on the radio button that deals with the FMHX. Select a diagnosis by clicking on the [Get FMHX Dx] button. In the *Rapid Select* window type: *breast* and select *Breast Cancer 174.9*. Click the [Save] button. This chart evaluation item will now only recommend an annual mammogram for female patients between 35 and 110 years if their chart shows a family medical history of breast cancer. Remember, the chart evaluation is activated manually in a patient's chart and will reveal only disease management items that are not up to date.

2. We will now add a new wellness screening item. Let's do some research and find the criteria we need to know in order to create the conditions for a Pap smear. In the opened *Chart Evaluation Items* window click on the [NGC] button. Once on the National Guideline Clearinghouse™ website, type in *pap smear* in the *Search* field and conduct a search. Locate the title for *Cervical screening*. Read through a portion of the article and note down the appropriate age that Pap smears should begin and end, who should get them, and how frequently they should be conducted. Close the web browser and click on the [New] button in the *Chart Evaluation Items* window. Fill out the details in the *Edit Chart Evaluation Item* window with the

information you have gathered. **Note:** A Pap smear will be a test, not a procedure. We will not link a Pap smear to any specific diagnosis. Save the new item and close the *Chart Evaluation window*.

3. Because the *Chart Evaluations* are normally set up on SpringCharts Server in a network environment, you will need to close SpringCharts and reopen it. This will enable you to see the changes that were made on the server. Once the program is rebooted, open your patient's chart. Locate the *Chart Evaluation* icon on the toolbar and conduct a chart evaluation. Let's assume we recommend all the displayed criteria to the patient so we will check the *Mark this Completed* radio buttons. Record the patient's response. Perhaps the patient is declining the DT shot and will schedule on the next visit. If the Pap smear screening is displayed, go ahead and indicate the patient has agreed to have it done today. Click the [Done] button.

4. Click on the "+" sign to the left of the *Encounter* category in the care tree and notice the addition of the chart evaluation screenings. The details will be seen below.

Exercise 7.2 Ordering a Test in an Office Visit(LO 7.2)

1. Let's go ahead and order the Pap smear screening. Open a new office visit in your patient's chart. In the OV screen, select the *Routine Well Visit* pop-up text under the [CC] navigation button.
2. Record some routine well vitals under the [Vitals] navigation button.
3. Select the diagnosis code for a *Well Woman* under the [Dx] Navigation button.
4. Now let's order the Pap smear test. Choose the appropriate navigation panel button for tests and type *pap* in the search field. Selecting the test will place it in the lower window. Click the [Order Selected test] button at the bottom and the test is added to the OV note.
5. To print the order for the test, click on the printer icon *below* the [TEST] button in the lower left text panel. You will notice the diagnosis added to the *Orders* window from the OV note. Add the patient's insurance information to the Order form by clicking the [Add Pt Ins] button.
6. Print the order note, electronically sign it, and submit the printed Order Form to your instructor.
7. Click the [Done] button inside the *Orders* window and chart the order form under the *Encounters* category in the care tree.
8. Record a 3-year follow-up for the patient from the [F/U-Rem] navigation panel. If you do not have *3 years* in your pop-up text then you need to add it by clicking on the edit pencil icon. Remember to choose the appropriate category in the *Edit PopUp Text* window, add the new text, and then move it up to the most suitable position. Return to the OV screen and refresh the pop-up text panel.

9. Send a *New ToDo/Reminder* to the front desk to *Schedule appointment in 3 years*.
10. Close the office visit and create a routing slip. Choose the recommended E&M code in the *Routing Slip* window.
11. Print the *Routing Slip* and submit to your instructor.
12. Click the [Send] button to send the *Routing Slip*. Close the patient's chart.

ToDo/Reminder button

LO 7.3 EVALUATION & MANAGEMENT CODER

SpringCharts *E&M Coder* helps the physician determine the correct evaluation and management code for office visit encounters.

To set up this feature, the administrator will select the *E&M Coder* from the *Administration* menu in the *Practice View* screen.

> Note: SpringCharts Server's administrator menu in a networked environment is accessible on SpringCharts Server. Once selected, the E&M coder setup window will be displayed, seen in Figure 7.5.

In the setup, users may define keywords for review of systems and examination of body areas and organ systems. SpringCharts *E&M Coder* uses these keywords to search an office visit note to determine if a body system or area has been reviewed or examined. It is important that any words or abbreviations that are added to the *E&M Coder* are also set up as text in the pop-up text that will be used in the office visit. When the *E&M Coder* matches these words it will give the practitioner credit for examining that specific body area or system.

The *E&M Coder* comes with a comprehensive list of terms and abbreviations. It is only necessary to add terms for specialties that focus on specific body areas.

Based on: a) the thoroughness of terms and phrases used in the OV note that match key terms in the *E&M Coder*, b) the number of diagnoses used, c) the

Focal Point

Key terms and phrases are set up in the E&M coder on SpringCharts Server. The program analyzes the Review of Systems and the Exam verbiage in the OV note for these terms and then gives the provider credit for reviewing the body areas. The number of body areas examined affects the level of E&M code recommended by the program.

Focal Point

The number of encounters, the number of diagnoses, the extent of the history in the CC and PI portion of the OV note, and the number of body areas reviewed all have bearing on the level of suggested E&M code.

SpringCharts® SetUp

SpringCharts E&M Coder

Review Of Systems keywords

Constitutional Symptoms	Eyes	Ears Nose Mouth Throat	Cardiovascular	
General	Eye	HEENT	CV	
Constitutional	vision	ENT	Cardiovascular	
fever	diplopia	ear	heart	
weight	blurred	nose	hrt	
chill	ophth	mouth	chest	
fatigue	tear	teeth	palpitation	
headache	glaucoma	gum	beat	
ha	cataract	tongue	pnd	
vision		throat	orthopnea	
blurr		neck	angina	

◄ ► Cancel Setup

Figure 7.5 E&M coder setup window.

number of procedures conducted, and d) the history of encounters in the patient's care tree, the routing slip will:

1. Automatically evaluate the type of patient encounter as *new, established,* or *consultation*
2. Automatically suggest the complexity of the present illness/problem
3. Automatically calculate the complexity of medical decision making

From this information the routing slip then recommends the appropriate E&M code.

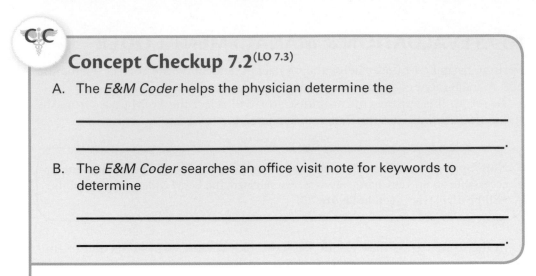

Concept Checkup 7.2(LO 7.3)

A. The *E&M Coder* helps the physician determine the

_____

_____.

B. The *E&M Coder* searches an office visit note for keywords to determine

_____

_____.

LO 7.4 SUPERBILL FORM

Superbill

Typically contains the medical office's most common procedure and diagnosis codes and descriptions for the purposes of recording the physician's selection and billing. However, in SpringCharts the superbill is designed to display codes and items that are often overlooked or not available in the OV exam and can be billed.

SpringCharts provides a customized **superbill** that can be set up to contain all additional and ancillary codes not usually selected from within the *Office Visit* screen. The superbill may display procedures and codes such as venipuncture, administration of injections, administration of immunizations, surgical trays, splints, and other billable items that may not have been addressed during the encounter. The routing slip window provides the practitioner the opportunity of viewing the superbill for additional items that can be added to the routing slip.

Note: The E&M coder is designed to recommend an administrative code (evaluation and management) based upon a visit to the doctor's office. However, if the provider is creating a routing slip based upon an encounter with a patient in another facility, for example, inpatient facility, skilled nursing facility, and so on, appropriate ranges of administrative codes will need to be added to the superbill form so the provider can select them in the routing slip window. Also, the superbill is an ideal place to store wellness screening administrative codes since the recommendation of these codes is beyond the E&M coder's capabilities.

The superbill is set up on SpringCharts Server under the *Administrator* panel or in the *Administration* menu on the single computer version, seen in Figure 7.6. The administrator simply adds the category heading and lists the code and item. The superbill items are then displayed as a gray panel in the *Routing Slip* window. From here items can be clicked on and automatically added to the routing slip.

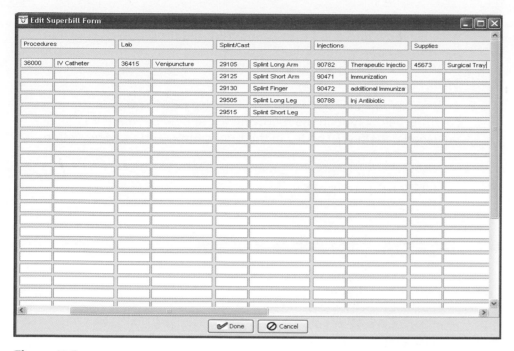

Figure 7.6 Superbill setup window.

Concept Checkup 7.3(LO 7.4)

A. The purpose of the superbill in the SpringCharts routing slip window is to

_____

_____ .

B. What two entries are added to the superbill under each category heading?

1. _____

2. _____

Exercise 7.3 Adding Items to the Superbill(LO 7.4)

1. Open the *Superbill* form in the *Administration* menu. In the left column you will notice a list of E&M codes that will be displayed in the superbill panel within the *Routing Slip* window. Let us assume that our physician performs preventive wellness exams for Medicaid patients. Listing these regular office visit E&M codes here is redundant

because the codes can be accessed from the drop-down list within the *Routing Slip* window. Let's replace these with wellness checkup E&M codes. Highlight and delete all fifteen codes under the *Office Visits* heading.

2. In the *Section Titles* field type: *Preventative E&M Codes*. In the two columns below type in the following list of new patient (NP) and established patient (EP) codes in the first column and the description in the next column.

   99381 NP < 1 yr old
   99382 NP 1–4 yrs old
   99383 NP 5–11 yrs old
   99384 NP 12–17 yrs old
   99385 NP 18–39 yrs old
   99386 NP 40–64 yrs old
   99387 NP 65+ yrs old
   99391 EP < 1 yr old
   99392 EP 1–4 yrs old
   99393 EP 5–11 yrs old
   99394 EP 12–17 yrs old
   99395 EP 18–39 yrs old
   99396 EP 40–64 yrs old
   99397 EP 65 + yrs old

3. Under the *Supplies* heading, type the following codes and descriptions:

   A4550 Surgical Tray
   D5982 Surgical Stent
   D5988 Surgical Splint

4. Click on the *Universal Export* button and copy the material to a clipboard (first option) and paste the material in a word processing document (NotePad, WordPad, or MS Word). Format the document for printing so that the layout looks acceptable.

5. Print the document. Write your name on it and submit it to your instructor.

6. Click the [Done] button in the *Edit Superbill Form* window.

LO 7.5 PATIENT INSTRUCTIONS

Focal Point

Many great patient information sheets can be found on the Internet and imported into SpringCharts.

Patient instructions can be created in SpringCharts or imported into Spring Charts and then accessed in the *Office Visit* screen to print or e-mail for the patient. To create a new patient instruction sheet, the users will first generate a document they wish to use and save the document in RTF (rich text format) on the computer. In a Windows environment, documents created in Word Pad are automatically saved in the RTF format.

Under the *New* menu on the main window the users will select *New Pt Instruction*. The users are then given the option to either import an RTF file or to create their own patient instruction document, seen in Figure 7.7.

If the user chooses the *Write your own* option, a window is displayed in which patient instructions may be typed out or copied and pasted here. Many routine patient instructions can be found on *www.familydoctor.org* or other more specialized websites. The user would simply save the article as a "printer-friendly version" on the website, highlight the desired text, then

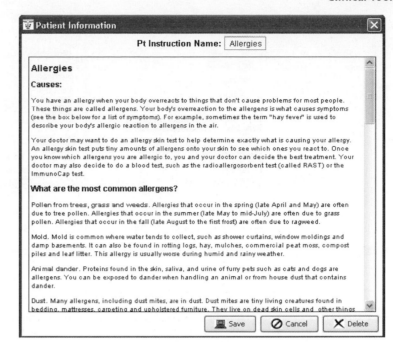

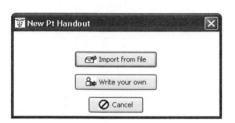

Figure 7.7 Creation option for a patient instruction.

Figure 7.8 Newly imported patient instruction sheet.

copy and paste the article into SpringCharts' *Patient Instruction* window. The article may be further edited before saving in SpringCharts. The new patient instruction sheet must be given a title before saving, illustrated in Figure 7.8.

> Note: Within SpringCharts the mouse right-click button may not support cut/copy/paste; however, the keyboard keys can be used as follows: [Ctrl]+[X] = Cut; [Ctrl]+[C] = Copy; [Ctrl]+[V] = Paste.

If a patient instruction sheet has been previously created and save in an RTF format on the computer the user can import the document by selecting the *Import from file* option. This feature will open a browse window from where the document can be selected.

The *Patient Instruction Manager* is accessed from the main window by selecting *Edit>Patient Instructions*. From here existing patient instructions can be modified as well as new ones created.

To administer a *Patient Instruction*, the provider will open either a new or existing office visit note from a patient's chart. After the OV note has been created and it is necessary to give out an information sheet, the provider will select the *Tools* menu and choose *Patient Instructions*, illustrated in Figure 7.9. A list of all instructions that have been created in SpringCharts are available from which to select. The user will be provided with the options to either print or e-mail the selected patient instruction sheet. Once the OV note has been saved the program will stamp the note recording the administering of the information sheet, as displayed in Figure 7.10.

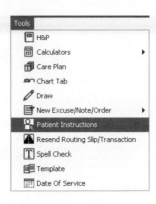

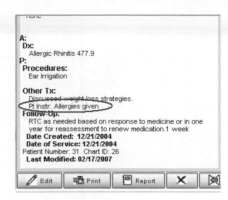

Figure 7.9 Administrating a patient instruction sheet.

Figure 7.10 Record of patient instructions given.

Concept Checkup 7.4(LO 7.5)

A. To import an existing patient instruction document into Spring-Charts, it will need to be in _____ format.

B. The patient instruction sheet is administered in the _____ screen.

Focal Point

Patient instruction sheets are administered in the OV screen. When printed for the patient, the program adds reference to the OV note indicating the information was given.

Exercise 7.4 Creating a New Patient Information Sheet(LO 7.5)

1. Click on the *New* menu in the main *Practice View* screen and select the *New Patient Instruction*. Click [OK] in the information window and select the [Write your own] button.

2. Open your web browser and type in the URL address: www.familydoctor.org. In the *Women* section click on the *More* link. Under the *Reproductive Health* section choose the instruction information of *Pap Smears*. Select *Printer friendly version* in the upper right. To highlight this information, place your cursor at the beginning of Pap Smears, and with your left mouse button depressed, drag the cursor to the end of the instruction page. Right-click on any highlighted area and choose *copy*. Close the web page and return to the SpringCharts program. Click in the *Patient Instruction* window. Using your key pad, press the [Ctrl] + [V] keys. Highlight the bottom section of the instruction that begins with *Reviewed/Updated* and delete this section. Delete the phrase "Return to top" throughout the document. At the bottom of the instruction sheet type: *For more information contact our office at (214) 674–2000.*

3. Change the *Patient Instruction Name* to *Pap Smears* and click the [Save] button.

4. To view all the patient instructions in the program select the *Edit* menu and choose *Patient Instructions*. You will notice your Pap smear instruction sheet listed here. In this window instruction sheets can be modified, exported, and deleted, and new ones can be created. Close the window.

Exercise 7.5 Administering a Patient Instruction Sheet (LO 7.5)

1. Open your patient's chart. Locate the office visit note in the *Encounter* category of the care tree that dealt with the well woman visit. Highlight the OV note and click [Edit] in the lower window.
2. In the OV screen select the *Tools* menu and choose the *Patient Instructions* option. Click on the *Pap Smear* instruction sheet in the *Choose Patient Instruction* window.
3. Print the instruction sheet. Write your name on it and submit it to your instructor. Close the OV note and skip billing.
4. View the bottom on the OV note in lower right window of the patient chart. Notice the phrase: *Pt Instr: Pap Smear given* recorded in the OV note. This now becomes a permanent record in the patient's chart.

LO 7.6 PLAN OF CARE MANAGER

Practitioners may also attach a text document with *Plan of Care* or *Practice Guidelines* to a patient's office visit note. This document then remains a permanent record associated with that office visit. To access a plan of care the provider will select the *Tool* menu from within the office visit screen and choose *Care Plan*, as seen in Figure 7.11. Once selected SpringCharts opens an interface window to enable the user to import a *Plan of Care* document stored on the computer, which may be a site-specific care plan document, or access *The National Guideline Clearinghouse*™ (NGC). The NGC is a comprehensive database of evidence-based clinical practice guidelines and related documents. The NGC website holds numerous medical treatment plans containing objective, detailed clinical information for physicians, nurses, and other health-care professionals. The user simply searches for and highlights the specific document then pastes it into the patient's *Care Plan/Guideline* window using the [Ctrl]+[V] keys. A saved Plan of Care Guideline is displayed in Figure 7.12.

The selected *Care Plan* document will be a permanent record associated with this office visit. The *Care Plan* may be viewed at the bottom of the office visit note when selected in the patient's chart Care Tree, illustrated in Figure 7.13.

Care Plans or **Practice Guidelines**
Specific documents that provide a "road map" to guide all who are involved with a patient's care, outlining the appropriate treatment to ensure the optimal outcome. A caregiver unfamiliar with the patient should be able to find all the information needed to care for this person in the care plan.

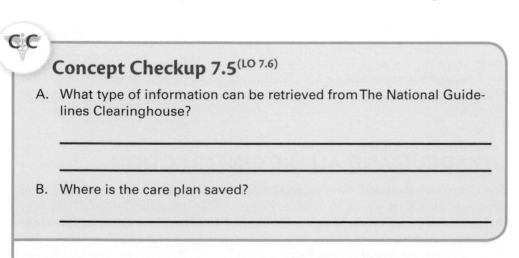

Concept Checkup 7.5 (LO 7.6)

A. What type of information can be retrieved from The National Guidelines Clearinghouse?

_____

_____

B. Where is the care plan saved?

_____

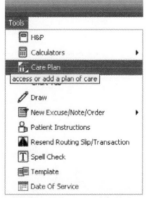

Figure 7.11 Accessing a care plan in the office visit.

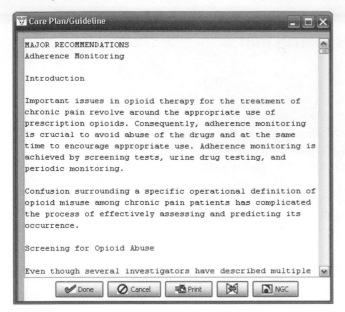

Figure 7.12 Care plan selected either from computer or NGC website.

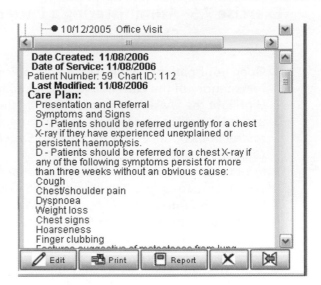

Figure 7.13 Care plan attached to office visit note.

Exercise 7.6 Adding a Patient's Care Plan(LO 7.6)

1. Let's add a care plan to a patient's chart. Open your patient chart. Select the OV note in the care tree that dealt with the allergy symptoms. Edit the OV note.
2. In the OV screen select the *Tools* menu and choose *Care Plan*. In the *Care Plan/Guideline* window click on the [NGC] button. (Care plans can be attached from a location stored on the computer or a computer on the network or downloaded from the *National Guidelines Clearinghouse*.)
3. On the NGC website, enter *seasonal allergies* in the search field and search for the care plan. Locate and open the *Allergic Rhinitis* plan. Highlight the recommendations, copy the information, and close the web browser. Paste the material into the *Care Plan/Guideline* window by using the [Ctrl]+[V] keys. Click the [Done] button, close the OV screen, and skip billing.
4. You will notice the care plan added to the bottom of the OV note in the lower right corner on the patient's chart.
5. Print the OV Note by clicking on the [Print] button in the lower right. Submit the document to your instructor.
6. Close the patient chart.

Drug Interaction and Allergy Checking button

LO 7.7 DRUG AND ALLERGY INTERACTION

The *Drug Interaction and Allergy Checking* feature of SpringCharts is a web-based interface with *NewCrop Rx*™. This service provides the ability to check any new drug prescribed to a patient against the patient's allergies and current medications for any adverse reactions. It is available throughout the program in any window where medication can be prescribed.

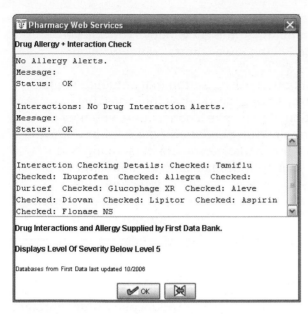

Figure 7.14 Drug interaction from Pharmacy Web Service.

Once activated, the resulting window, seen in Figure 7.14, shows the details of the drugs checked against the patient's current medications and allergies. Any potential allergic reactions or drug interactions are listed in this window; for drug-drug interactions, the severity level of the interaction and discussion are shown. If the drug and allergy check locates a current medication in the patient's chart that is not indexed, the user is alerted to this fact. The information in the resulting window enables the physician to determine if the prescribed medication should be given to the patient. The information cannot be printed out and the program allows the physician to prescribe the medication even if there is an alert.

Concept Checkup 7.6(LO 7.7)

A. The drug and allergy checking feature in SpringCharts evaluates any new patient prescription against that patient's

_____.

B. If a drug-to-drug adverse interaction is discovered, the Pharmacy Web Service window will display

_____.

Focal Point

SpringCharts accesses a web service in order to conduct a drug interaction analysis with the prescribed medication and the patient's current medications and allergy list.

Exercise 7.7 Operating the Drug and Allergy Checking Feature (LO 7.7)

1. Let us check for any drug allergies in a medication that we have prescribed. Open your patient chart. Locate the OV note for allergies. Open the OV window.

2. Select the [Rx] navigation button in the OV window. You will see the medications prescribed in the lower central window: allegra, Flonase, and deconsal.

3. If the *Drug Allergy/Interaction Checking* button (pill bottle) to the left of the prescription window is not grayed out, it indicates that you have an Internet connection. If you have a connection, you may click on this icon and the Pharmacy Web Service will check for any known allergic reactions between the medicine you are prescribing and your listed allergies and your current medications. It appears that there are no allergies. If you were successful logging into this data, you may now close this window. This information cannot be printed out; it is for the provider's eyes only. Close the OV note.

LO 7.8 DRAW PROGRAM

Focal Point

The draw program within the OV screen enables the provider to use basic templates or elaborate illustrations to indicate the specific information.

SpringCharts' *Office Visit* screen provides access to a rudimentary draw program that enables the provider to indicate the procedure that was conducted by drawing on inbuilt templates. Within an opened *Office Visit* screen the provider will access the *Tools* menu and select the *Draw* option. From the *Template* menu within the Draw program the user selects the desired body section and then uses the draw tools on the left to mark the illustration, shown in Figure 7.15. Only one draw item can be added to each office visit note. The *Edit* menu inside the draw program enables for the cutting, copying, pasting, and clearing of the *Simple Draw* screen.

More elaborate illustrations can be quickly imported into the draw program, seen in Figure 7.16, by selecting *Background Image* on the menu bar and then selecting a .jpg image from within the computer or a computer on the network. A digital photo can even be taken of the patient's body area and imported to the draw program so the physician can indicate the specific work that was done. The text box [T] is set at a 10-point plain font. To increase the size or "bold" the

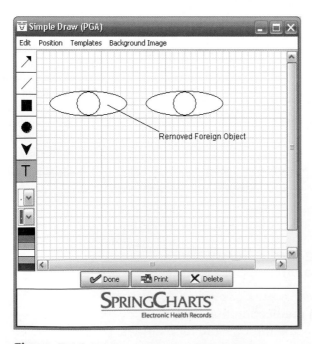

Figure 7.15 Basic templates in draw program.

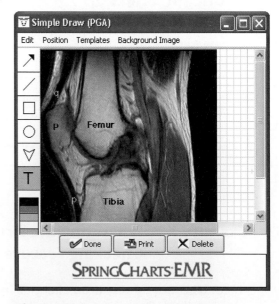

Figure 7.16 Imported images into draw program.

font, set the font size and style before selecting the [T] button. The font size and style buttons are located below the [T] button.

The draw item is stored with the office visit note. The *Follow-Up* segment on the note is stamped with the word: *Graphic*. To view the attached graphic from within the patient's chart without opening up the office visit, the user would simply click on the specific office visit in the care tree, then click the word: *****Graphic***** in the lower right detail panel of the chart; the draw item window will display along with the accompanying office visit note.

C·C

Concept Checkup 7.7(LO 7.8)

A. The *Draw* feature is located in the _____ menu of the *Office Visit* screen.

B. Images can be imported into the draw program from

_____

_____.

LO 7.9 IMPORTING DOCUMENTS

Three options are available to import a file into the patient's chart. We have already mentioned two of these options in Chapter 5 when we discussed importing items to the electronic chart. *Import New Text File* and *Import Picture* actually store the file in the patient's chart and that can slow performance of the program over a period of time. However, *Import File Cabinet Document* enables the user to attach the file to the patient's chart while the file is stored in a separate file cabinet folder in SpringCharts Server directory. This will not affect the performance of SpringCharts.

The *File Cabinet Document* window, seen in Figure 7.17, is located in the *New* menu of the patient chart, under the *Import Items* sub-menu. It is a powerful feature that allows the user to add any type of document to a chart, including .doc, .xls, .html, .xml, .pdf, .jpg, .tiff, and DICOM. Since this third option is designed to store the documents in a database folder separate from the patients' charts, the user can import multiple documents and extensive graphics without compromising the performance of SpringCharts. When the document is accessed within the patient's chart, it is opened in the original program.

When selecting the import feature, *File Cabinet Document,* a dialog window appears in which the user will need to record three pieces of information. In the first field the document is named. The patient's name is automatically added because this window was accessed from the patient's chart. If the document is to be stored in the *File Cabinet* section of the care tree, then an appropriate file cabinet folder needs to be selected for storage of the document.

> Note: A new folder category can be created by accessing SpringCharts Server and adding a new item to the *File Cabinet Folders* list in the *Category Preference* window.

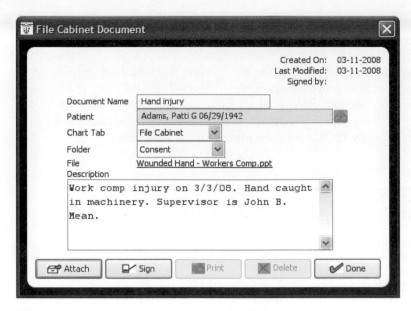

Figure 7.17 Import file cabinet document window

Some medical offices will store imported documents under a different tab in the care tree. They may do this if the document is accessed often, so that they can find it more speedily.

Third, a description of the document is added in the *Description/Summary* field. The user should always select the [Sign] button to time- and initial-stamp the operation. The user then selects the [Attach] button and chooses the *Existing* option. A standard file dialog will appear for users to select a document stored on the network. The file name will appear in blue in the import window as indicated in Figure 7.17. Once the document is attached, the user selects the [Done] button to store the document into the patient's file cabinet.

The program creates a copy of the original file and attaches the copy to the patient's chart. The original document is still available on the network to be copied to other patient's charts.

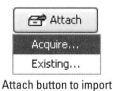

Attach button to import document

The second option for importing a document into the patient's file cabinet is through the TWAIN device interface. In this case the user would select the [Attach] button and choose the *Acquire* option. This technology enables communication between image-capturing devices such as scanners, cameras, webcams, and computer programs. After selecting the *Acquire* option the operator will choose the appropriate interface TWAIN source in the *Morena source selector* window, seen in Figure 7.18.

Note: TWAIN technology has been incorporated into equipment manufactured since the year 2000 and operates in Windows™ and Macintosh OS™ environments.

The *Source Selector* window lists the equipment that is connected to the user's computer. It could be a scanner, Webcam, or other TWAIN device. When the device is selected, the appropriate *Graphic User Interface* (GUI) dialog box will open, illustrated in Figure 7.19. From this window the user will be able to activate the scanner or extract the image from the appliance.

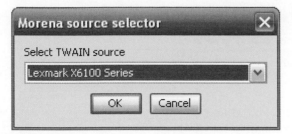

Figure 7.18 TWAIN source selection window

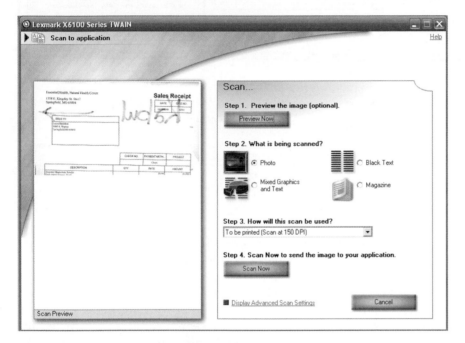

Figure 7.19 Specific operating window of TWAIN device

The GUI screen will look different for each of the devices that it is connected to. This one-touch scanning feature enables the user to operate the scanner directly from SpringCharts. The scanned document can be resized before attaching into the patient's care tree. The user will select the [Done] button to store the document in the patient's chart, seen in Figure 7.20.

To open the newly attached document in the patient's care tree, the user will highlight the appropriate document and click the [Doc] button. The document opens the native program in which the file was originally created.

Button to open attached document

> Note: The native program must be on the Client machine to view the document. For example, if the document is an Excel spreadsheet, then Microsoft Excel must be on that workstation to open the document.

Note the summary of the document in the lower right-hand window of Figure 7.20. As much detail as necessary can be added into the summary, enabling the provider to view information at a glance without opening the document. Once opened within the patient's chart, any dynamic document can be edited and resaved. It is dated by SpringCharts and can be signed by the doctor.

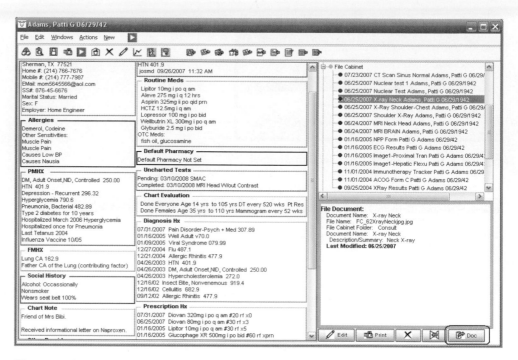

Figure 7.20 File document in care tree of patient's chart

Figures 7.21 and 7.22 illustrate two different file types that can be imported through the *Import File Cabinet Document* window and opened in the original programs.

Stored documents can be managed in the *File Cabinet Documents* window, Figure 7.23, located in the *Productivity Center* menu or the *Edit* menu. From this file cabinet document manager, global database searches can be conducted for documents filtered by document name, saved date range, patient range, and folder range.

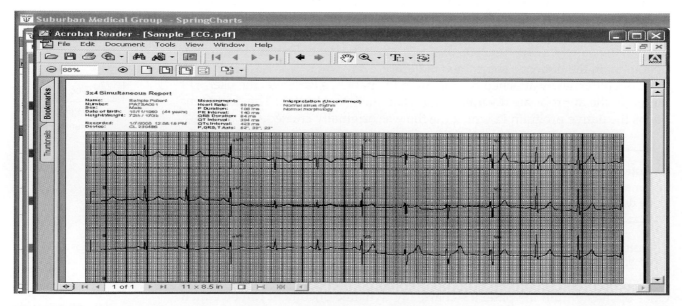

Figure 7.21 A scanned document as a .pdf file is opened in Acrobat Reader

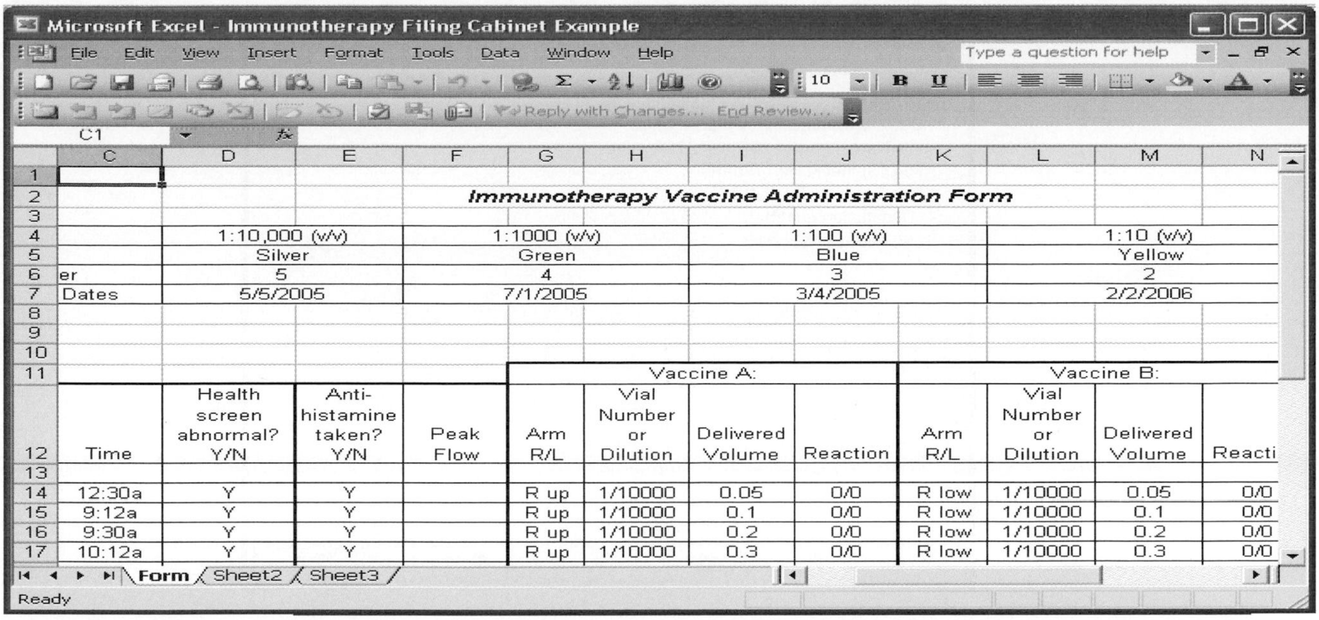

Figure 7.22 An attached .xls document is opened in Microsoft Excel

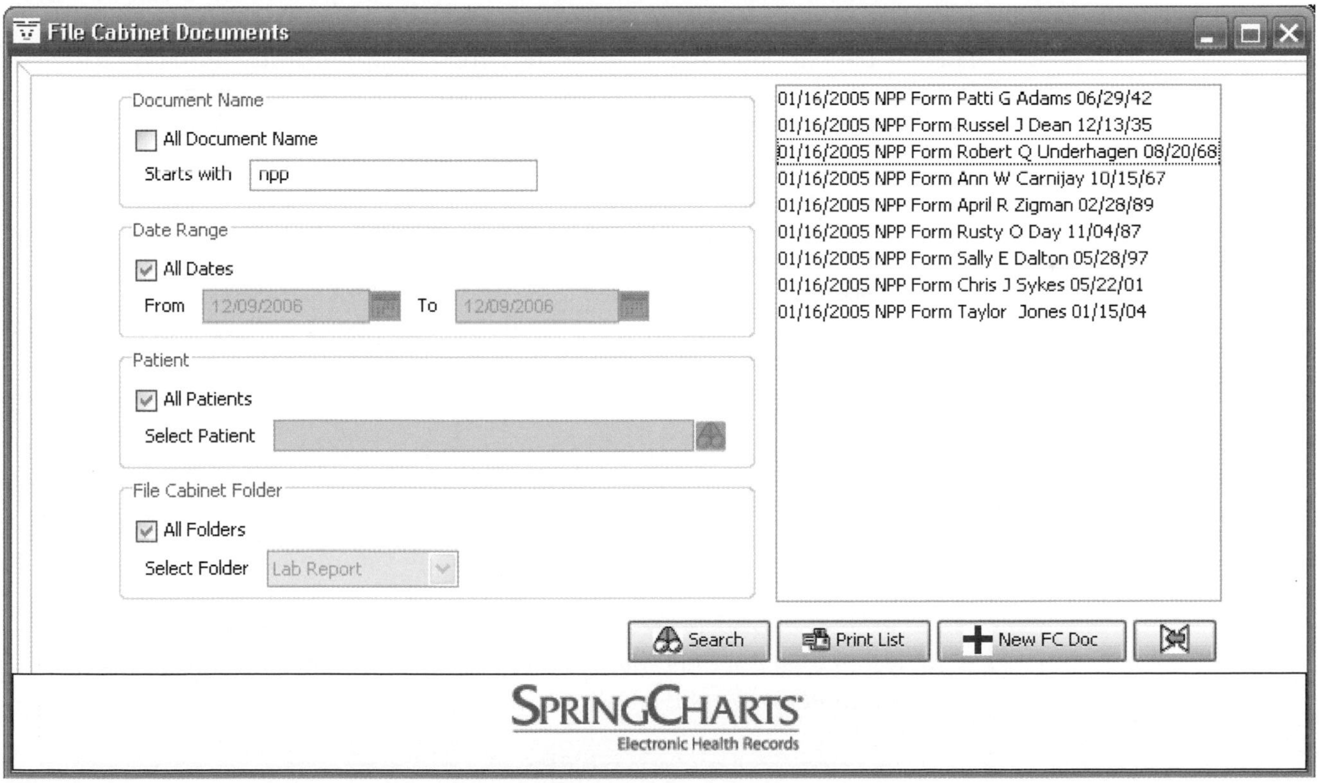

Figure 7.23 Search results in *File Cabinet Documents* window

An item may be highlighted from the filtered list and the summary window will be displayed, shown in Figure 7.24, giving the provider useful information regarding the document. The buttons presented at the bottom of the window give the user the ability to open the document, open the patient's chart, or print the summary.

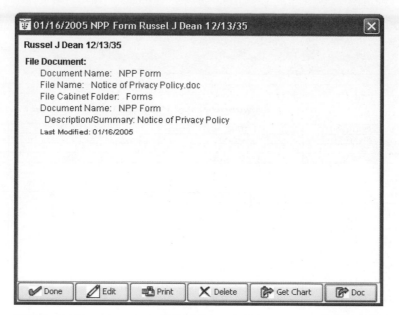

Figure 7.24 Document summary window

From the master *File Cabinet Documents* window, documents can be stored in SpringCharts that are needed for clinic use but not necessarily related to a specific patient. This feature gives the clinic the opportunity to have a truly paperless office. When adding a new file cabinet document from this window, the user will be presented with the option of relating the item to a patient or not. If a patient is not selected, the document is not stored in a patient's chart, but rather stored in the general SpringCharts directory. These non-patient documents may be accessed from the master *File Cabinet Documents* window by searching in the specific folder in which it was originally stored. Non-patient documents may include original forms that need to be printed out for patients to sign. It is helpful if the medical office creates a folder that can be specifically used for these non-patient forms.

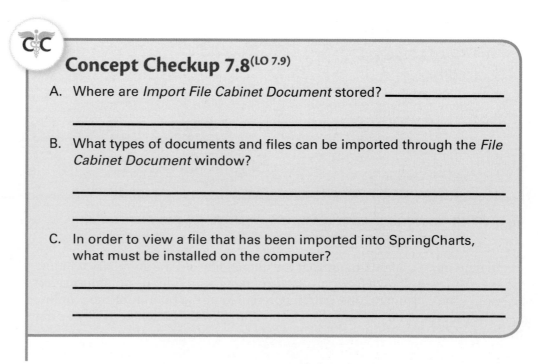

Concept Checkup 7.8(LO 7.9)

A. Where are *Import File Cabinet Document* stored? _____

_____

B. What types of documents and files can be imported through the *File Cabinet Document* window?

_____

_____

C. In order to view a file that has been imported into SpringCharts, what must be installed on the computer?

_____

_____

Exercise 7.8 Importing A Document (LO 7.9)

1. Open your patient's chart and select *Import Items* from the *New* menu. Select the *Import File Cabinet Document* option.
2. Let's import a patient's insurance card. It will be helpful to have a copy in the chart. Fill out the document name in the *File Cabinet Document* window. Select the chart tab: *Insurance Card.* In the description box type: *Galaxy Health Network—Primary Ins.*
3. Click the [Sign] button to add your initials only.
4. Click on the [Attach] button and choose the *Existing* option (because your computer is not attached to a scanner).
5. Maneuver in the *Open* dialogue box to find your *EHR Material* folder. Your instructor will inform you where the *EHR Material* folder is located. Open the folder and select the *Ins Card* file. Make sure the file name shows in the *File name* field. Click the [Open] button to attach the file. If you were successful the file will be shown in blue in the *File Cabinet Document* window.
6. Click the [Done] button. The newly imported file will show up under the Insurance Card tab in the care tree.
7. Click on the [Doc] button in the lower right of your patient's chart to view the document. You may have to expand the window to see the entire image.
8. Print the document. Write your name on it and submit it to your instructor.

Name _____ Instructor _____ Class _____

USING TERMINOLOGY

Match the terms on the left with the definitions on the right.

_____ 1. Superbill

_____ 2. Wellness screenings

_____ 3. Care plans

_____ 4. Chart evaluations

_____ 5. E&M coder

_____ 6. Patient instruction
manager

_____ 7. NGC

_____ 8. NewCrop RX

_____ 9. Well woman visit

_____ 10. Encounters

_____ 11. Draw program

_____ 12. RTF

A. Determines the correct evaluation and management CPT code for office visit encounters.(LO 7.3)

B. In this feature patient instructions can be modified and new ones created.(LO 7.5)

C. A comprehensive database of evidence-based practice guidelines known as the National Guidance Clearinghouse.(LO 7.6)

D. The drug interaction and allergy checking feature is a SpringCharts interface with this web-based company.(LO 7.7)

E. Practice guidelines are specific documents that provide a "road map" to guide all who are involved with a patient's care.(LO 7.6)

F. Chart evaluation summaries are automatically recorded in the care tree under this category.(LO 7.1)

G. Periodical medical checkups to test for or inoculate against significant diseases.(LO 7.1)

H. A feature in the *Tools* menu of the *office* visit screen that enables the provider to illustrate procedures on built-in templates.(LO 7.8)

I. A SpringCharts feature used to establish criteria for medical checkups and appraise patients' charts for needed health screenings and test.(LO 7.1)

J. When a new patient instruction is needed it must be created in this format to save into SpringCharts.(LO 7.5)

K. An annual pap smear would be included in this encounter and recorded in an office visit note.(LO 7.2)

L. In SpringCharts this panel contains additional codes that can be added to the routing slip for the purposes of billing(LO 7.4)

CHECKING YOUR UNDERSTANDING

Write "T" or "F" in the blank to indicate whether you think the statement is true or false.

_____ 13. Patient instructions can be created in SpringCharts then accessed in the *Office Visit* screen to print or e-mail the patient.(LO 7.5)

_____ 14. The customized superbill may display procedures and codes such as vehicle-punctures, shunts, and other billable and non-billable items.(LO 7.4)

_____ 15. Some key words in the E&M coder are: review of systology, examine body crustaceans, and organic systems.(LO 7.3)

_____ 16. You cannot set up chart evaluations on SpringCharts Server in a network environment.(LO 7.1)

_____ **17.** SpringCharts chart evaluation function allows users to define preventive health criteria and be proactive in the wellness screening of patients.[LO 7.1]

_____ **18.** In SpringCharts you can make a customized superbill that can contain additional and ancillary codes not usually selected in the office visit.[LO 7.4]

Answer the question below in the space provided.

19. In the chart evaluation setup, the administrator will define what five criteria for wellness screenings?[LO 7.1]

1. _____

2. _____

3. _____

4. _____

5. _____

Choose the best answer and circle the corresponding letter.

20. Once a practitioner attaches a plan of care in the *Office Visit* screen, it becomes:[LO 7.6]
a) A temporary document which deletes after 90 days
b) A permanent part of the office visit note
c) A care plan cannot be attached to an office visit note

21. The National Guidelines Clearinghouse website holds:[LO 7.1]
a) National conference dates per calendar year for physicians
b) Detailed clinical information for nurses only
c) Numerous medical treatment plans

22. The drug/allergy interaction feature of SpringCharts provides:[LO 7.7]
a) The ability to check any new prescription against the patient's current medications and allergies
b) The ability to price drugs in Canada and Mexico
c) The ability for the physician to prescribe experimental drugs for terminally ill patients

23. This feature allows the provider to indicate the procedure that was conducted by drawing on built-in templates:[LO 7.8]
a) The doodle art program
b) The draw program
c) The filing cabinet

24. When creating a new patient instruction the user can choose the "write your own" option. The user can then:[LO 7.5]
a) Type out the instruction
b) Copy and paste the instruction
c) Both a and b

25. SpringCharts enables the user to import what type of document into the patient's file cabinet?[LO 7.9]
a) Only .pdfs
b) Only Microsoft files: .doc, .xls, .jpg, and .tiffs
c) Any type of file

8

Customizing Templates and Pop-up Text

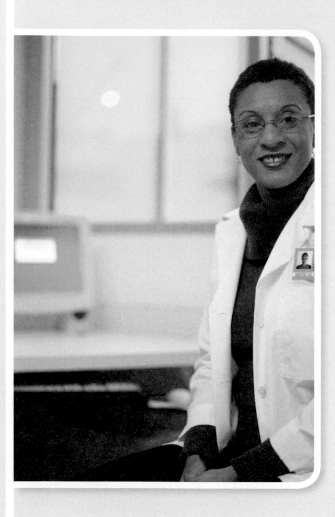

Learning Outcomes

After completing Chapter 8, you will be able to:

LO 8.1 Understand the concept of templates

LO 8.2 Create and use an office visit template

LO 8.3 Describe how to create and use an order template

LO 8.4 Create and use a letter template

LO 8.5 List the steps to create and edit pop-up text

LO 8.6 Demonstrate how to export and import pop-up text

What You Need to Know

To understand Chapter 8 you will need to know how to:

- Open a patient's chart
- Navigate in a patient's chart
- Open a new or established office visit note
- Navigate in an *Office Visit* screen
- Add new pop-up text
- Refresh pop-up text

Key Term

Term you will encounter in Chapter 8:

Templates

LO 8.1 OVERVIEW

Templates are available in SpringCharts that serve as a pattern for letters, order forms, and office visit notes. They can be created and customized to minimize the amount of data that needs to be added when working in the program. SpringCharts templates are easy to set up, edit, and use. The template manager stores three template types for: 1) office visits, 2) orders, and 3) letters.

1. The *Office Visit Templates* are created for the most common types of encounters. They should be designed to fit approximately 90+ percent of the patients with any given ailment and diagnosis. The specific details relevant to each patient will be added in the OV encounter itself. The OV template layout is similar to the navigation categories in the *Office Visit* screen, which makes it easy to build the template. The template layout allows users to free-type text or add pop-up text data into the fields shown on the template.

> Note: In the *Office Visit* screen, data is added to OV templates wherever the cursor is positioned, if the *Insert at Curser* option has been chosen in the *User Preferences* setup.

2. The *Letter Template* allows SpringCharts users to create form letters that will be used as *Letter to the Patient* or *Letter About the Patient*. Only the body of the letter template and the subject line need to be created. SpringCharts will automatically default in the appropriate recipient's name, address, and greeting.
3. The *Orders Template* stores recurring orders to speed documentation. Physician order templates can be created for the most common lab, imaging, and medical tests.

LO 8.2, 8.3, 8.4 CREATING TEMPLATES

To create a new *Template*, the user will select the *New>New Template* from the main *Practice View* screen menu and then highlight the appropriate type of *Template* needed to create, as seen in Figure 8.1. Spring Medical Systems Inc.

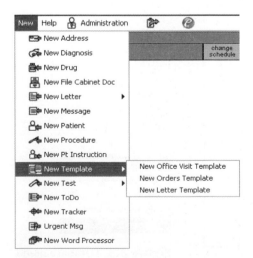

Figure 8.1 New menu in *Practice View* screen.

Template
A document that is predesigned with a set format and structure. It serves as a model for a letter, fax, report, or note that needs to be filled in to be completed.

Focal Point
TemplateWare is an add-on feature for SpringCharts. It is designed to add templates and specific pop-up text to suit different medical specialties.

has developed TemplateWare as an add-on feature for different medical specialists. TemplateWare comes with prebuilt office visit, orders, and letter templates as well as pop-up text tailored to each specialty. TemplateWare saves a tremendous amount of time and enables providers to more rapidly complete patient documentation with a minimum of effort. Available TemplateWare formats include pediatrics, family practice, internal medicine, gastroenterology, psychiatric, and pulmonary medicine.

Office Visits Templates

From the *Practice View* screen, the provider would select *New>New Template> New Office Visit Template.*

In the *Template Name* field, the user inserts the title for the template. This would typically be the chief diagnosis that the office visit is addressing. The provider then completes the template as if performing an office visit. Any form of data input can be used, including selections from pop-up text, typing, handwriting recognition on a Tablet PC, or third-party speech recognition software. The pop-up text is accessed by clicking on each side navigation tab and selecting appropriate text. The OV template is broken into the same segments as the navigation tabs in the *Office Visit* screen in which the OV note is created, illustrated in Figure 8.2. It is important to remember to place the desired text into the proper template section so that it will correspond to the correct navigation tab in the OV screen. There is no place for recording the vitals or the face sheet information in an OV template. The vitals and the face sheet information can be added during the time of the patient's actual visit. If a physician has already created office visit templates in an electronic format, they can be copied and pasted segment by segment into a SpringCharts OV template. Once the [Save] button is clicked, the newly created template will be added to the list of OV templates in the *Templates* window.

A template can also be created by saving an *existing* office visit note as a template. Within the *Office Visit* Screen, the physician will select the *Database* Menu, and then choose *Copy OV to Template*, seen in Figure 8.3. The entire OV note that the provider has created for a real patient is then placed in an OV template

Focal Point

OV templates can be created from scratch on an existing OV note copied into a template.

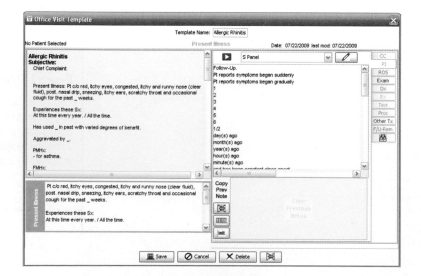

Figure 8.2 New office visit template window.

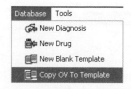

Figure 8.3 Database menu in *Office Visit* screen.

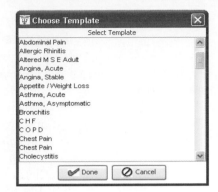

Figure 8.5 List of OV templates accessed in the OV screen.

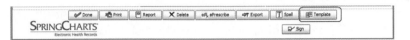

Figure 8.4 Template button inside an *Office Visit* screen.

format with each portion of the note going into the appropriate segment. Once again, the vitals and the face sheet are not copied across to the template. In the *Template Name* field, the user will insert the title of the template. There is no limit to the number of OV templates that can be created.

Office visit templates are used to rapidly populate the *New OV* window. To use an office visit template, a provider will open a patient's chart and select *New>New OV* on the menu to bring up the *New OV* screen. When the practitioner has determined the nature and cause of the chief complaints, the list of OV templates can be accessed by clicking on the [Template] button, seen in Figure 8.4, then selecting the desired template from the list, illustrated in Figure 8.5. The template information will populate all the various segments of the *SOAP* format in the *Office Visit* screen. The provider will then add the vitals and any other modifications specific to the patient. The use of OV templates saves an enormous amount of time in unnecessary redundant documentation.

Concept Checkup 8.1(LO 8.1, 8.2)

A. SpringCharts contains three types of templates:

1. _____

2. _____

3. _____

B. The OV template has the same segments as

_____

_____.

C. In addition to building a template from scratch, the provider can also create an OV template by

_____.

Open a Chart icon

Exercise 8.1 Creating an Office Visit Template (LO 8.2)

1. Open your patient chart (see margin illustration). Open the office visit note that you created dealing with the *allergies, runny nose, itchy eyes, and congestion* complaints. Select the *Database* menu and choose *Copy OV To Template.* Name the new template: *Adult Allergies* and [Save] the template. Close the *Office Visit* screen, skip billing, and close your patient chart.

2. Click on the main *Edit* menu and select *Templates.* Locate your *Adult Allergies* template under the office visit templates list. Click on the *CC* navigation tab on the right. Remove all the chief complaints: allergies, runny nose, etc. in the lower section. Click on the *F/U-Rem* navigation tab. Remove the verbiage in the *F/U-Rem* segment dealing with the patient returning to the clinic as needed. Save the edited template.

Focal Point

Order templates are typically designed to be sent to outside testing facilities. When selected within the OV screen they will automatically contain the diagnoses and tests from the OV note.

Exercise 8.2 Activating an Office Visit Template (LO 8.2)

1. Open Patti Adams' chart. Open a new OV note screen from the *new* menu.

2. Click on the *CC* navigation button. Patti mentions that she has a runny nose and congestion. She believes she has allergies again. You notice in the lower right hand window that Patti was in your office on 12/21/2004 with the same complaints. With your mouse highlight *Allergies, runny nose, congestion.* (Do not highlight the date.) Click on the *copy highlighted text to note* button and the previous chief complaints are added into the new OV note.

3. Enter some vitals in for your patient. Remember she doesn't have an elevated temperature.

4. Knowing that you have a template for adult allergies, click on the [Template] button at the bottom of the window and choose the *Adult Allergies* template. The template will be added into the OV note augmenting the chief complaints and vitals that you have already added.

5. Patti mentions that her cough started about 7 days ago and she tells you she does not have a headache. Click on the [PI] navigation button. This brings the PI text to the lower center text box where it can be edited. Change the cough onset time to 7 days. **Remember to use the [Delete] key on your keyboard, not the [Delete] button in the OV screen.**

6. Perhaps you decide not to give her Flonase, which is in the template. Click on the [Rx] navigation button and highlight *Flonase* in the lower center window and delete the medication.

7. Print the prescription and submit to your instructor.

8. Save the office visit and edit the routing slip. Use the recommended E&M code and [Send] the routing slip. See how the introduction of a template into the OV notes greatly enhances the speed of documentation. You will see the completed OV note saved under the *Encounter* category in the care tree of Patti Adams' chart. Close the chart.

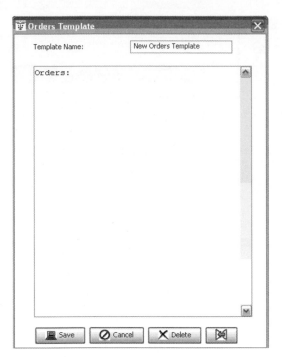

Figure 8.6 New order template window.

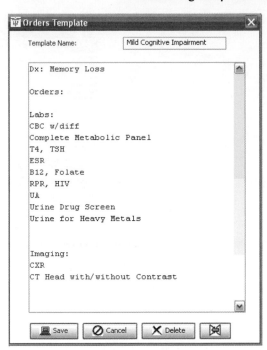

Figure 8.7 Saved order template window.

Order Templates

Order templates are created to provide rapid documentation for the ordering of tests and referrals within SpringCharts. To create an order template, the user will select *New>New Template>New Orders Template* menu from the *Practice View* screen. The window illustrated in Figure 8.6 will appear. The orders information is entered as needed. If the order templates are used in the OV screen the diagnosis(es) and the ordered tests will be automatically added to the order form from the OV note. Therefore, in creating an order template this information does not need to be added. Order templates can be designed with instructions, prompts, and specific questions that will guide the practitioner in providing the necessary information for outside diagnostic testing facilities. Once completed, the order template is given a title in the *Template Name* field, seen in Figure 8.7. The saved new order template is added to the list.

Order templates can be selected from within the patient chart or the *Office Visit* screen. In the patient's chart the user would select the *New>New Excuse/Note/Order>New Orders* menu. The order forms would only be used in the patient's chart if the patient was not being seen as part of a normal office visit. A patient may be seen in a doctor's office to complete a test for which an order form needs to be created without opening an office visit. In an *Office Visit* screen, a blank order form, seen in Figure 8.8, can be created by selecting the *Tools>New Excuse/Note/Order>New Orders* menu. This is the same blank order form that will be created if accessed in the patient's chart.

Clicking the [Template] button will show the available order templates, seen in Figure 8.9. The practitioner will highlight the desired template and the order will be populated. From this window the user may add additional line items from the *PopUp Text* window and add diagnosis from the *Previous DX* window into the order form along with the chosen template. The new order can then be printed and/or charted.

Focal Point

Orders are created from either the patient's chart or an OV screen. Orders created within the patient's chart will not automatically contain diagnoses or medical tests.

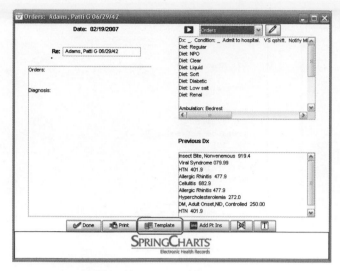

Figure 8.8 New order form window.

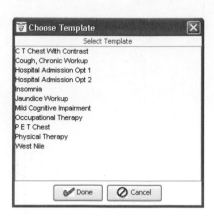

Figure 8.9 Order templates window.

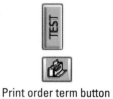

Print order term button

Order templates can be created in such a way as to automatically display the diagnosis(es) and ordered tests from the current office visit note. To create this type of order the practitioner will need to be in the *Test* navigation button window. Once the test(s) have been ordered the user will click on the printer icon located below the [Test] button in the lower left quadrant of the screen. The order window will display showing the diagnosis(es) and test(s) already selected in the OV note, illustrated in Figure 8.10.

Letters Templates

Letter templates are created the same way as the OV and order templates. The user will select the *New>New Template>New Letter Template* menu from the *Practice View* screen and a blank letter format will appear.

The name of the letter template will be typed in the *Template Name* field, the subject of the letter in the *Re:* field, the *Text* or body portion of the letter needs to be completed, as seen in Figure 8.11. The remaining fields will be populated

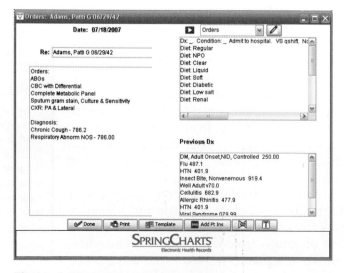

Figure 8.10 Order templates window.

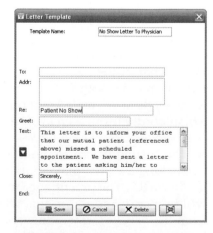

Figure 8.11 New letter template window.

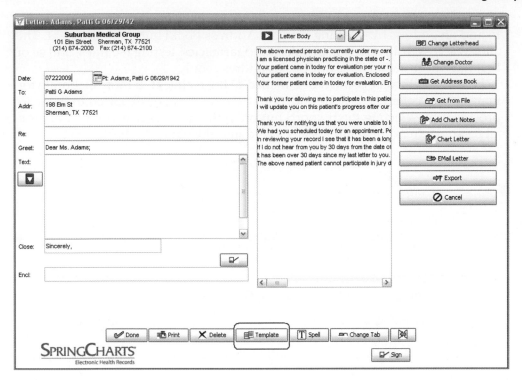

Figure 8.12   New letter window.

by SpringCharts when using this feature. The program will include the word *Sincerely*, as the *Close* unless a different close has been used in the template. Predefined pop-up text is available by clicking on the pop-up text icon. Once completed, the new letter template will be added to the list of program templates. Letter templates to the patient or about the patient are created in this same window.

Letter templates are accessed from within the patient chart. The user will select *New>New Letter To Pt* or *New Letter ABOUT Pt* and the following screen, seen in Figure 8.12, will appear.

When a user needs to generate a letter for which a template letter has already been created, the user will select the [Template] button and choose the desired template from the list, seen in Figure 8.13. The letter may be amended by using line items from the *PopUp Text* window. If selecting a letter template to the patient, the name, address, and greeting portions of the letter are added

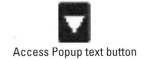

Access Popup text button

Focal Point

Letter templates are a list of all letters that have been created either to or about the patient. They are selected within the patient's chart, modified, printed, or e-mailed, and a copy is saved into the patient's care tree.

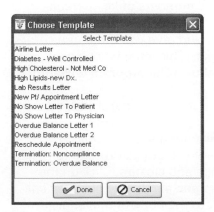

Figure 8.13   List of letter templates.

automatically by the program. If the letter is *about* the patient, the user will need to add an address by selecting the [Get Address Book] button to the right. This allows access to all referring physicians, pharmacies, testing facilities, and so on that have been set up in SpringCharts address book.

Letters can then be printed or e-mailed to the recipient. If more elaborate formatting and color needs to be added to the letter it can be exported to the word processor by selecting the [Export] button in the *New Letter* window. Copies of all created letters are automatically saved into the patient's chart.

C&C Concept Checkup 8.2(LO 8.3, 8.4)

A. When the order templates are used in the OV screen, the _____ and _____ are automatically added from the OV note.

B. When creating a letter template, the user will need to complete the _____, _____, and the _____ portions of the template.

C. Letter templates are available when the user is creating a *New Letter to Pt* and _____ from within the patient's chart.

Exercise 8.3   Creating and Using a Letter Template (LO 8.4)

1. Create a new letter template by accessing the *New* menu in the *Practice View* screen and choosing *New Template>New Letter Template.* In the *Letter Template* window type the subject (*Re*): *Welcome.* In the body of the letter (*Text*) type a letter welcoming the new patient to the clinic that gives the names and phone numbers of key personnel. You may want to start the letter like: *Thank you for your recent visit to our clinic. I want to welcome you and give you the names of a few key contact people here at the clinic.* (This letter will be sent out to all new patients coming into the clinic.) The program will automatically add a 'close' to the letter.

2. Give the letter template the name: *New Patient Letter* and click the [Save] button.

3. Open your patient chart. Click on the *New* menu and select *New Letter to Pt.* You will notice that the letter is already addressed to the patient and is complete with greetings and closure. Click on the [Template] button at the bottom of the screen and locate *New Patient Letter.* Highlighting the item will add it into the body of the letter.

4. To add the signature to the bottom of the letter, click the *signature* icon at the bottom of the letter and select a signature line. (See margin reference.) You will be given the option of your default doctor (this was set up initially under *User Preferences*) or your name. You are logged in as John Smith (demo), that's why you see the name twice.
5. If you used your proper e-mail address when setting up this patient, the letter can be e-mailed to the patient by clicking on the [Email Letter] button to the right or the letter may be printed or faxed by selecting the [Print] button at the bottom.
6. Print the letter. Add the letterhead and electronically sign the letter when prompted. Submit the letter to your instructor.
7. Click the [Done] button and saved the letter under the *Letters* category in the care tree. Save the letter as: *New Patient Letter.* You will notice the letter displayed in the lower right window and stored under the *Letter* category.

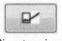

Signature icon

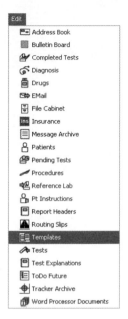

Managing Templates

All three types of SpringCharts templates can be accessed in the same location. The template manager is accessed from the *Practice View* screen by selecting *Edit* menu and choosing the *Templates* option, illustrated in Figure 8.14.

The resulting template manager screen stores a list of templates for each of the three categories. The user selects the appropriate category button to view each list. To edit any of the templates the user simply highlights the desired template. Templates can be created from this window as well by clicking the [New Template] button. A window will be displayed, allowing the user to choose which type of template to create, seen in Figure 8.15. Once selected, the corresponding template window will be shown.

Figure 8.14 Accessing templates in the edit menu.

LO 8.5 CUSTOMIZING POP-UP TEXT

As we have seen in previous chapters, SpringCharts pop-up text can be edited from multiple locations throughout the program. In any dialogue box within SpringCharts that displays pop-up text, the edit icon button will give access to the *Edit PopUp Text* window from where text can be added, deleted, or modified. Pop-up text is stored in SpringCharts by the users; therefore, each user has his or her own set of pop-up text, which can be modified without affecting any other user's pop-up text.

If a user wants to spend some time modifying pop-up text, the *Edit PopUp Text* window, seen in Figure 8.16, can be accessed without being in a specific area of the program. In this case the user would click on *File>Preferences>PopUp Text* on the main *Practice View* screen.

The user would first locate the appropriate category of text in the left column then modify, delete, or add to the existing text.

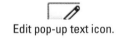

Edit pop-up text icon.

Focal Point

Additional pop-up categories and pop-up text can be added into the program by each user.

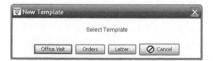

Figure 8.15 Three forms of templates.

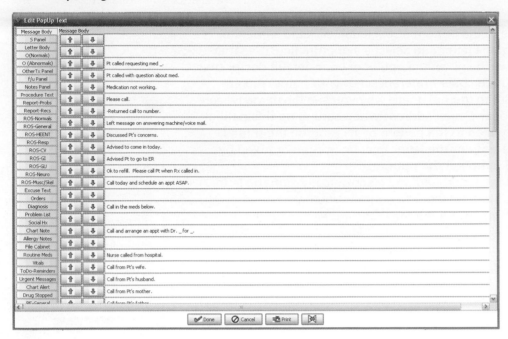

Figure 8.16 Edit PopUp Text window.

Figure 8.17 Customizing pop-up category headings.

Additional categories can be added to the existing pop-up text list. The *Edit PopUp Text* window allows for 60 line items to be added to any pop-up text category. These text lines can be individual words, sentences, or full, complete paragraphs. In addition to the 34 preset category headings that come with the installed program (these cannot be altered), there are 20 customizable categories in the side menu. (Some may already be in use if TemplateWare was installed; however, the category headings and pop-up text can still be edited.)

The customizable category headings are edited from the main menu bar—File>*Preferences*>*My List Names*, seen in Figure 8.17. Once new text has been added in the *Edit PopUp Text* window to a new category, the corresponding category name will need to be created.

The "up" and "down" arrows to the left of the pop-up text enable the user to manipulate the text in any desired order, that is, priority, topic, alphabetized, and so on, for quick selection when working within SpringCharts. If an empty line is needed in the pop-up text listing to divide groups of text, the user will need to move an empty line between text by using the up and down arrows in the *Edit PopUp Text* window. Once an empty line has been positioned, the user will place the cursor on the empty line and hit the space bar. This will add an invisible character to the line, thus displaying a space between text items in the pop-up text list as seen below in Figure 8.18.

Focal Point

Pop-up text can be organized by each user into the desired format by using the up and down arrows.

LO 8.6 EXPORTING POP-UP TEXT

Although pop-up text is user-defined, it can be exported from one user and imported under another user's name. However, in the import operation it will override any existing pop-up text that the user may have already created. Many times a clinic will complete all the initial editing and customizing for the office under *one* user's login name and then export the revised pop-up text to all the other users. Once the master pop-up text has been imported by all users, they can customize their own pop-up text and/or lists names.

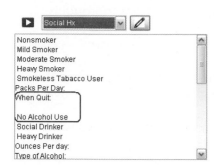

Figure 8.18 **Placing lines between pop-up text.**

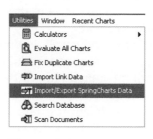

Figure 8.19 **Import/ export utility feature.**

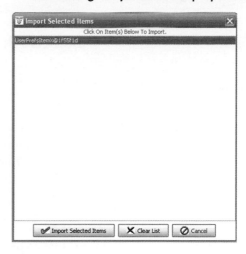

Figure 8.20 **Importing the pop-up text file.**

To export pop-up text, the administrator will select the *Utilities* menu in the *Practice View* screen and choose *Import/Export SpringCharts Data*, seen in Figure 8.19.

The administrator chooses the *Export PopUp Text* option and saves the file to a location on the computer. The administrator logs out of SpringCharts by accessing the *File* menu and choosing *Log Off*. In the displayed *Log In* window, the user logs back into SpringCharts under another user's name and password. Once again, the *Import/Export* feature is selected under the *Utilities* menu and *Import SpringCharts Data* chosen. The pop-up text file that was originally exported is located on the computer and imported under the new user's name. Once selected, the file name needs to be highlighted before clicking the [Import Selected Items] button, illustrated in Figure 8.20.

Focal Point

In the initial process of setting up SpringCharts, pop-up text can be modified and exported to all users who then import the file for their own use.

Concept Checkup 8.3 (LO 8.5, 8.6)

A. ✎ What Is the purpose for this icon?

_____

_____

B. What does this mean? The pop-up text is stored in SpringCharts by user.

_____

_____

_____

C. Although pop-up text is user-defined, it can be

_____

_____

_____

Exercise 8.4 Adding Pop-up Text (LO 8.5)

1. Let's add some pop-up text that will enable us to more thoroughly document the recent office visit of your patient for the regular Pap smear. Click on the *File* menu in the *Practice View* screen and select *Preferences>PopUp Text.*
2. Choose the *S Panel* and scroll down until you find an empty line. Type: *Routine Pap smear exam.* Using the arrows to the left, move the text up until it is placed under the line *Follow-Up.*
3. Because this will be text that is used for a wellness exam, we want to make sure we have appropriate text in the *ROS-Normals* panel. Locate this category. Scroll down in this panel and find an empty line. Type: *Patient denies abdominal pains.* and *Patient states she is not pregnant.* on two separate lines. Using the arrows to the left, move both lines of text up and position them in the *GU/GYN (female):* area under the line beginning: *No urgency, dysuria, nocturia, . . .* You will need to move the lines separately. Click on the [Done] button.

Exercise 8.5 Using Pop-up Text (LO 8.5)

1. Open up your patient chart. Locate the office visit note regarding the Pap smear exam and open the OV note. Click on the [CC] navigation button and select the text: *Routine Pap smear exam* from the *S Panel* pop-up text.

Note: When a user selects a series of pop-up text, the text wraps by default. If the user wants to have each new category of text on a new line, he/she will have to click at the end of the previous line of text in the lower center window and hit the *Enter* key. This will place the cursor on the next line. When selecting new pop-up text it will go to where the cursor is positioned.

2. Click on the [ROS] navigation button. Start each new section on a new line by placing the cursor on a new line in the lower central text box. Select all the *ROS-Normals* text starting with *GENERAL:* down through *GU/GYN (female).*
3. Click on the [Exam] button. Start each new section on a new line and be sure to use the heading names. Again, select all the *O(Normals)* text starting with *GENERAL:* down through *GU/GYN (female).* Your text in the lower center window should finish with *Pap smear performed.*
4. While performing the physical exam, the physician notices several benign lesions on the skin. Start a new line in the lower center text box and then drop down the pop-up text category list and choose *O (Abnormals).* Locate the *Skin* heading and select *SKIN: + maculopapular lesions* and add them into the text box.

5. Notice the enormous amount of text that was effortlessly compiled detailing the patient's review of systems and the physician's exam. Click the [Done] button and the [Save and Edit Routing Slip] button. Notice in the *Routing Slip* window that the E&M code recommendation is now 99215. Even though your diagnosis code and text code remained the same, a great volume of documentation was added to the OV note to indicate the thoroughness of the exam. This is now indicated by pressing the [Details] button.

6. Let us assume this patient is a Medicaid recipient. Rather than choosing the recommended E&M code, you will choose a preventive E&M code that we listed in the superbill earlier. Highlight the *EP 18–39 yrs old* for an established patient wellness visit.

7. Print the routing slip and submit it to your instructor.

8. [Send] the routing slip and close your patient chart.

chapter 8 review

Name _____ Instructor _____ Class _____

CHECKING YOUR UNDERSTANDING

Write "T" or "F" in the blank to indicate whether you think the statement is true or false.

_____ 1. A template is a file that is predesigned with a set format and structure.(LO 8.1)

_____ 2. Order templates are created to provide rapid documentation for the ordering of supplies within SpringCharts.(LO 8.3)

_____ 3. Pop-up text is stored in SpringCharts by users; therefore, each user has his or her own set of pop-up text.(LO 8.5)

_____ 4. Pop-up text is user-defined but it can be exported from one user and imported under another user's name. It will not override any *existing* pop-up text.(LO 8.6)

_____ 5. The export pop-up text feature is located in the *Database* menu in the *Office Visit* screen.(LO 8.5)

_____ 6. Pop-up text can be edited from the file menu.(LO 8.5)

Answer the question below in the space provided.

7. The template manager stores three template types. They are:(LO 8.1)

 1. _____

 2. _____

 3. _____

Choose the best answer and circle the corresponding letter.

8. A SpringCharts template is best described as:(LO 8.1)
   a) A preset pattern for letters, order forms, and office visit notes
   b) A medical vocabulary resource
   c) A series of pop-up texts

9. SpringCharts has an add-on template feature for specialists called:(LO 8.1)
   a) TemplatePro
   b) TemplateWare
   c) TemplateSOAP

10. The letter templates allow the user to create form letters that will be used as:(LO 8.4)
    a) Letters to patients or about patients
    b) Letters from patients or referring physicians
    c) Letters not regarding patients

11. Office visit templates are used to rapidly populate the:(LO 8.2)
    a) New patient window
    b) New office visit window
    c) Both a and b

12. Order templates are created to provide rapid documentation for the ordering of:(LO 8.3)
    a) Fast food that can then be faxed automatically
    b) Tests
    c) Prescription drugs

13. The *Edit PopUp Text* window allows you to:(LO 8.5)
    a) Modify text
    b) Delete error codes
    c) Add and send personal messages to other users

Fill in the blanks.

14. To create a new template select the *new>new template* from the _____ screen and select the appropriate type of template you want to create.(LO 8.1)

15. TemplateWare was developed by Spring Medical Systems as an add-on feature for specialists. Available TemplateWare formats include such medical specialties as:(LO 8.1) (three points)

    1. _____

    2. _____

    3. _____

    4. _____

    5. _____

    6. _____

16. When you select the [Get Address Book] in the new letter window, it accesses the addresses of all referring physicians as well as:(LO 8.4)

    _____ and _____.

17. The template manager that houses all three template types is accessed from the *Practice View* screen by selecting the _____ menu and choosing the _____ option.(LO 8.1)

18. To export pop-up text, select the _____ menu in the *Practice View* screen and choose _____ SpringCharts data.(LO 8.6)

9

Tests, Procedures, and Diagnosis Codes

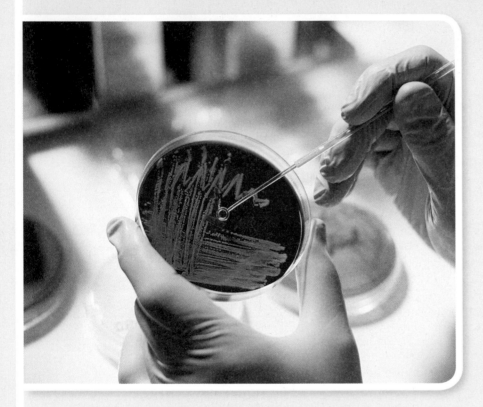

What You Need to Know

To understand Chapter 9 you will need to know how to:

- Open a patient's chart
- Navigate in a patient's chart
- Open a new and an established office visit note
- Navigate in an *Office Visit* screen
- Navigate in the *Practice View* screen
- Use pop-up text

Key Terms

Terms you will encounter in Chapter 9:

Analyte
Reference Labs
SpringLabs

Learning Outcomes

After completing Chapter 9, you will be able to:

LO 9.1   Discuss how to order a lab, imaging, and medical test

LO 9.2   Process Reference Lab results

LO 9.3   Process and chart tests manually

LO 9.4   Create a test report

LO 9.5   Understand test status alerts

LO 9.6   Describe how to create a lab, imaging, and medical test

LO 9.7   Create and document procedures and diagnoses

OVERVIEW

SpringCharts comes installed with a limited activated list of the current year's diagnosis and procedure codes as well as a comprehensive list of lab, imaging, and medical tests. It may be necessary at times for additional codes and tests to be added to the system. The entire ICD-9 and CPT dictionaries are part of the installed database; however, if additional codes need to appear in the program they need to be activated from these dictionary files. This chapter deals with the creation and use of lab, imaging, and medical tests and the activation of diagnosis and procedure codes.

LO 9.1 ORDERING A TEST

In SpringCharts, the term "tests" includes lab tests, imaging tests, and medical tests. Although the test description and the code may be in the CPT code book, it is classified as a test (not a procedure) in SpringCharts because it requires a result. When a test is ordered it is stored in the *Pending Tests* area of SpringCharts. When data is received the results can be entered manually into the *Pending Tests* and then sent to the *Completed Tests* area of the program for the physician's viewing. Once the tests have been viewed by the physician, they are permanently filed in the patient's chart under the category for one of these three types of tests in the care tree diagram. Lab results can also be entered automatically from the lab company through the electronic interface module, **SpringLabs,** and the pending test sent directly into the patient's chart. Tests are ordered from within the *Office Visit* screen or within the *Patient's Chart* screen.

Office Visit Order: On the side navigation tab of the *New OV* window the physician will find the *Test* tab. Once the tests have been selected the user will click the [Order Selected Tests] button, seen in Figure 9.1, to move the tests into the office visit note. At this time the tests are sent to the *Pending Tests* area of the program. The printer icon will enable the provider to print an order form for these selected tests.

Patient Chart Order: The alternative way to order a test is from within the patient chart. The user will click the *Actions* menu, select *Lab, Imaging,* or *Med Test,* illustrated in Figure 9.2. An *Order Test* window, seen in Figure 9.3, will be

Focal Point

SpringCharts comes equipped with the entire dictionaries of the current year's ICD-9 and CPT codes.

Focal Point

Lab results may be entered manually into the program or automatically entered through the SpringLabs interface.

SpringLabs
SpringCharts feature that provides the capability of automatically receiving lab test results directly from the reference lab by using Electronic Data Interchange (EDI) standards and protocols over a secure Internet connection.

Printer icon

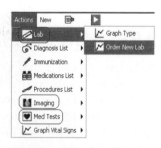

Figure 9.1 Ordering of test in *Office Visit* screen.

Figure 9.2 Three types of tests to order in the patient chart.

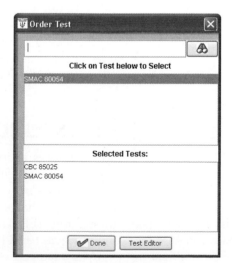

Figure 9.3 *Order Test* window.

displayed where a user can search for and select a particular test. When the first few letters of the test are entered and the search feature activated, a matching list will appear in the top portion of the window. The appropriate test is then selected. Repeat searches can be conducted for other tests while remaining in this window. The bottom list will contain all the tests that are being ordered. The test's name can be selected in the lower window to remove it from the orders.

When the selection of tests has been completed, the [Done] button is clicked. Once the tests have been selected they are sent to the *Pending Test* area to await data entry of the results. Tests ordered within the patient's chart *are not* sent to the Routing Slip.

C&C

Concept Checkup 9.1 (LO 9.1)

A. The three types of tests that can be ordered in SpringCharts are:

1. _____

2. _____

3. _____

B. Tests can be ordered from the _____ screen

and the _____ screen.

C. Lab results can be entered into SpringCharts manually or electroni-

cally via _____.

Exercise 9.1 Ordering a Lab Test (LO 9.1)

1. Open Patti Adams' chart. In the *Actions* menu of the chart select: *Lab>Order New Lab*.
2. Order a CBC (complete blood count) for the patient. Conduct a search, select the item, then press the [Done] button.
3. Access the *Edit* menu on the *Practice View* screen and locate the CBC test under the *Pending Tests* option.
4. Close the *Pending Tests* window.

LO 9.2 SPRINGLABS™ AND REFERENCE LAB RESULTS

Reference Labs
Specific lab companies that transmit electronic data to SpringCharts using HL7 language and protocols. Some of the many reference lab companies are LabCorp, Quest, Spectrum, Carilion, WestCliff, and Antek.

SpringLabs is an optional lab interface that provides the capability for practices to automatically receive test results directly from lab companies such as Quest, Lab Corp, Spectrum, and many others. Lab results are sent directly into SpringCharts over a secure Internet connection using Electronic Data Interchange (EDI) standards and protocols. The results can then be reviewed by the physician and placed directly into a patient's chart.

Once received electronically, the lab test results are automatically imported into a staging area called *Reference Lab* for processing. **Reference Lab** is a secured area within SpringCharts. Users must have appropriate security permission to view or process the information within the Reference Lab section.

Users who have the access level of *Get Pending Tests* (set up in user's profile on SpringCharts Server) are notified of newly received results by a *LAB* icon next to the user's login name in the upper left-hand corner of the main *Practice View* screen, shown in Figure 9.4.

Authorized users can access and process the received results by clicking on *Reference Lab* in the main *Edit* menu, seen in Figure 9.5.

The *Reference Lab* results screen, illustrated in Figure 9.6, shows the tests that have been sent directly from the lab company; it details the date of the test, the test description, the associated patient's name, and the name of the lab company.

The user will view the detailed results by clicking on any test. The data that is sent securely from the lab company, displayed in Figure 9.7, will include the patient's name and date of birth, the lab items (indicating the "in range" and "out of range" results), and the acceptable range established by the lab company. This may differ from the range the clinic may have set up on the pending test; however, the imported lab's ranges will be used when storing the completed test in the patient's chart so that the test results reference the ranges from the original source.

Access Stored Data: All imported labs are stored permanently in the repository within SpringLabs. By selecting the [Access Stored Data] button in the *Imported Reference Lab Tests* window the user can conduct global searches for stored tests by test name, date of test, or by patient name, illustrated in Figure 9.8. Although a copy of each imported reference lab is placed in the patient's chart when the provider "matches" it to the ordered pending test, the original imported lab test is kept in SpringLabs for research purposes.

Manage Test Name Synonyms: A unique feature of SpringLabs is its ability to "learn" the way a practice prefers to receive results. After a short time,

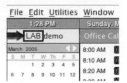

Figure 9.4 Visual indication of reference labs.

> **Focal Point**
>
> Reference Lab results are sent directly into the patient's chart after they are viewed in the Reference Lab area of the program.

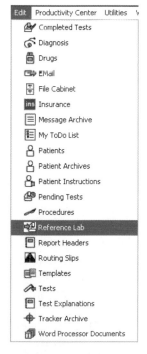

Figure 9.5 Accessing Reference Lab in the edit menu.

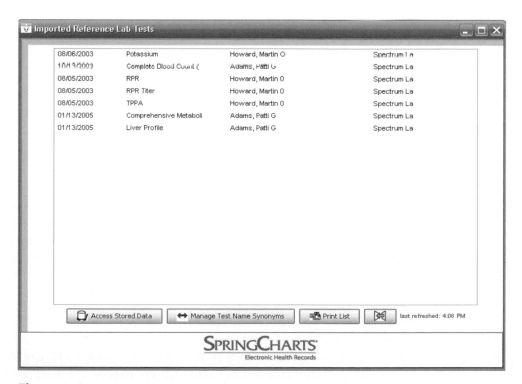

Figure 9.6 Imported Reference Lab list.

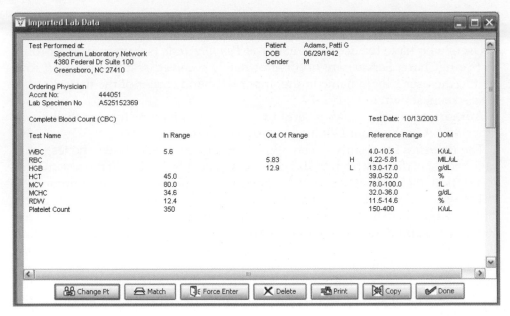

Figure 9.7 Reference Lab results.

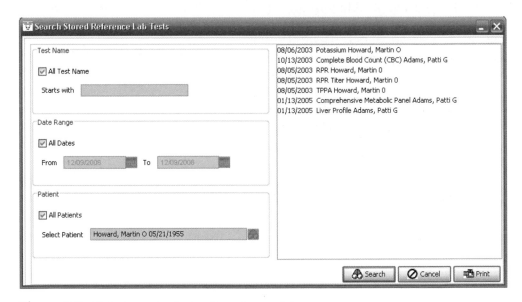

Figure 9.8 Global search window for reference labs.

SpringLabs will "know" the practice's lab item terminology and will be able to automatically match the terminology of the incoming lab test to the appropriate line item of the test that has been ordered and is pending within SpringCharts.

When the lab's test name differs from the name used in SpringCharts (e.g., *Protein, Total,* used by a lab company, and *Total Protein,* used by SpringCharts) SpringCharts will ask the user to match the test item name and then remember these synonyms for subsequent test matching. The list of test name synonyms can be viewed and deleted in the *Imported Lab Test Synonyms* window, seen in Figure 9.9, by accessing the [Manage Test Name Synonyms] button in the *Imported Reference Lab Tests* window (refer to Figure 9.6). If any lab item name match is deleted, SpringLabs will request another name match the next time a lab is matched to a pending test that includes that lab item name.

Focal Point

SpringCharts has the unique ability to learn lab items that are matched to pending test items for quick import to the patient's chart.

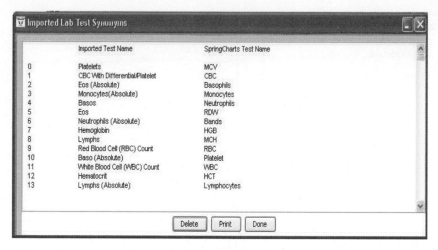

	Imported Test Name	SpringCharts Test Name
0	Platelets	MCV
1	CBC With Differential/Platelet	CBC
2	Eos (Absolute)	Basophils
3	Monocytes(Absolute)	Monocytes
4	Basos	Neutrophils
5	Eos	RDW
6	Neutrophils (Absolute)	Bands
7	Hemoglobin	HGB
8	Lymphs	MCH
9	Red Blood Cell (RBC) Count	RBC
10	Baso (Absolute)	Platelet
11	White Blood Cell (WBC) Count	WBC
12	Hematocrit	HCT
13	Lymphs (Absolute)	Lymphocytes

Delete   Print   Done

Figure 9.9 Manage *Test Name Synonyms* window.

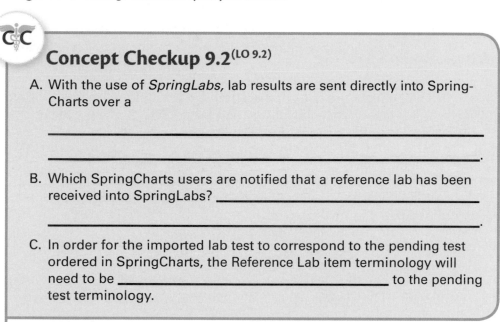

Concept Checkup 9.2(LO 9.2)

A. With the use of *SpringLabs,* lab results are sent directly into SpringCharts over a

_____

_____.

B. Which SpringCharts users are notified that a reference lab has been received into SpringLabs? _____

_____.

C. In order for the imported lab test to correspond to the pending test ordered in SpringCharts, the Reference Lab item terminology will need to be _____ to the pending test terminology.

Focal Point

Among other matching criteria, an imported reference lab may have to be associated with the patient's name and test item name.

Processing the Received Test Result

Once a test is selected in the *Imported Reference Lab Tests* window, the *Imported Lab Data* screen (Figure 9.7) allows the user to process the lab test results into SpringCharts. There are three choices:

Match: The provider will select the [Match] button to begin the process of reconciling the received lab result with an ordered pending test. Matching a lab test result can consist of one or more of the following tasks:

1. **Identify Patient:** SpringLabs is able to automatically match an imported reference lab result to a SpringCharts patient by using multiple data fields, including name and date of birth, so the need to manually identify a patient will be a rare occurrence. If the patient was not automatically identified by SpringLabs, the user must search for and identify the matching patient in the patient search window, shown in Figure 9.10. After this match is made SpringLabs will "remember" this link and when this particular lab company sends another lab result for this patient, the match will not need to be made again.

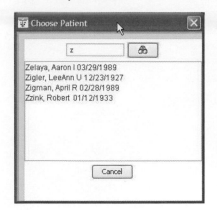

Figure 9.10 Matching the reference lab to a SpringCharts patient.

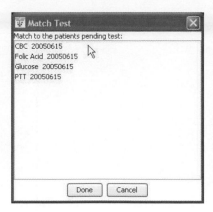

Figure 9.11 Matching the reference lab to the patient's pending tests.

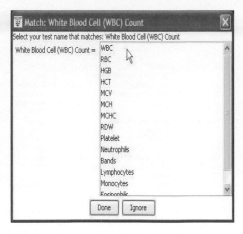

Figure 9.12 Matching reference lab analytes to pending text analytes.

Lab Analyte

Blood test compound that is the subject to its own specific chemical analysis. A lab panel is composed of multiple analytes that will undergo analysis.

2. **Match Test:** SpringLabs will automatically match an imported lab test with a patient's pending test. If, however, SpringLabs is not able to recognize the lab name, the user must match the test by selecting from a window displaying a list of pending tests for that specific patient, shown in Figure 9.11. SpringCharts stores the test name association and will not require the user to identify this test name in future instances.

3. **Match Test Analyte:** If the imported lab result is a lab panel with a series of **lab analytes,** SpringLabs will need to match those on the imported test to those on the pending test in order for the results and ranges to go to the appropriate places. (Analytes are individual test components within a given test panel.) Any unrecognized test analyte will activate a screen requiring the user to manually match the lab's analyte name with one defined within the chosen SpringCharts pending test, seen in Figure 9.12. Each time an analyte is matched the link is stored in SpringLabs' synonym list. This process will only be conducted the first time SpringLabs receives a result with an unknown analyte. Subsequent occurrences are automatically matched using the created synonym list.

4. **Review Match Results:** The final matched test data is shown in the window displaying a SpringCharts pending test side-by-side with the imported lab, illustrated in Figure 9.13. The clinician may now want to send a *ToDo/Reminder* to the physician, giving notice of the new lab results. The [Make ToDo] button is for this purpose. If the data match is accurate and the administration of the test is complete the user will click the [Done] button. The imported lab results along with the imported normal ranges are sent immediately to the patient's chart from where the assigned provider will view the test results. The reference lab has now been removed from the imported list; however, a permanent copy is stored in the test repository area of SpringLabs. These tests can be viewed by accessing them through the [Access Stored Data] button in the *Imported Reference Lab Tests* window (Figure 9.6).

Force Enter: The [Force Enter] button in the *Imported Lab Data* window is used when SpringLabs does not recognize any patient or test name in the *Pending Test* area. Perhaps a test was not ordered through SpringCharts; therefore, the test is not in the *Pending Test* list. *Force Enter* requires the user to choose a patient's name and enter a CPT code for this test (or accept the

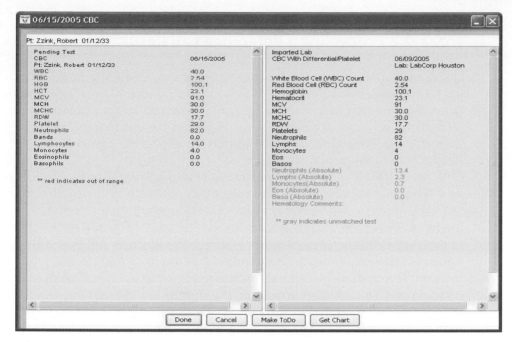

Figure 9.13 Results of matching analytes in a lab panel.

default code of 000). This creates a one-time lab type and places the data into the *Completed Test* list. The lab results will be placed in the patient's chart once it is viewed by the physician. Force enter will not add the test name or any of the analytes into the list of test name synonyms.

Delete: The [Delete] button removes the test from the *Reference Lab* list, but still stores a copy in the test repository. This data will not go into a patient's chart but can be searched for through the [Access Stored Data] button.

Focal Point

A user may have to "force enter" an imported reference lab into a patient's chart if the pending test is not found in SpringCharts.

Concept Checkup 9.3 (LO 9.2)

A. In order to reconcile the imported lab test results with the pending test in SpringCharts, the provider may have to match the results by what three criteria?

1. _____

2. _____

3. _____

B. When the imported lab test is successfully matched with the patient's pending test it is sent to

_____ .

C. Why would an imported lab need to be *force entered* into Spring-Charts instead of matching it to a pending test? _____

_____

Exercise 9.2 Processing a Reference Lab Result (LO 9.2)

1. Under the *Edit* menu on the *Practice View* screen, locate the *Reference Lab* option.
2. Open the *Imported Reference Lab Tests* window and locate the complete blood count lab for Patti Adams. Highlight the test to open the *Imported Lab Data* window. The imported lab shows the patient's results both in range and out of range.
3. Click on the [Match] button to match this test to a SpringCharts patient. Type in Patti's last name and select this patient.
4. You will be presented with a window displaying Patti Adam's pending tests. Select the CBC to link the imported complete blood count to this test. Drag the smaller window in front to the side and you will notice in the larger comparison window that the imported lab on the right has already placed the analyte results into a SpringCharts pending test. The lab item in gray on the right side indicates an unmatched test analyte. The smaller *Match* window is asking you to match the *Platelets* to an item in the pending test. Select *Platelet* to complete the match. Confirm the match. You will notice that there are additional items that are listed on the imported test that are not listed on the pending test. Many times lab companies will test for more or less items than what the physician needs. This is based upon the lab companies' protocols. Click on the [Ignore] button to ignore the additional items on the imported lab.
5. Click the [Make ToDo] button and send a *ToDo/Reminder* to the physician alerting him or her to the completed test. Use your pop-up text.
6. Click the [Done] button and the CBC is removed from the reference lab list.
7. Close the *Imported Reference Lab Test* window. Open the *Pending Test* window. You will notice the pending CBC test for Patti Adams is missing. Once the match was completed with the imported reference lab the test was sent automatically to the patient's chart.
8. Open Patti's chart. Locate the newly added lab in the care tree.
9. Print out the lab and submit to your instructor.

LO 9.3 PROCESSING AND CHARTING TESTS

Once a test (lab, imaging, and other medical tests such as EKG, stress test, and so on) is ordered, it is sent into the *Pending Tests* list. When the test results come back from the testing facility, or when the results are processed in the clinic, the results will be either manually entered into the pending test or the lab results will be automatically entered via the *SpringLabs* reference lab interface. After results are entered manually, the test moves into the *Completed Tests* list. The test results are viewed by the physician and then stored in the patient's chart.

If manually entering lab results or entering imaging and medical tests results, the user will select *Pending Tests* from the main *Edit* menu, illustrated in Figure 9.14.

The *Pending Tests* window, Figure 9.15, appears, showing all tests ordered in SpringCharts that are still outstanding.

Figure 9.14 Accessing pending tests through the edit menu.

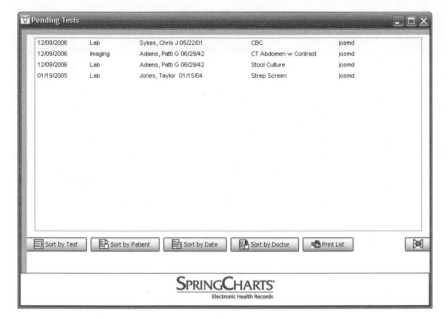

Figure 9.15 Pending Tests window.

The user will then select the specific ordered test that is awaiting the results. Some results require simply clicking the radio button to enter a *Positive* or *Negative* test result. Others will require clicking the [Normal Test] button and other tests may require more elaborate text to define the results. If the clinic is receiving an extensive evaluation from the testing facility, the document may be copied and pasted into the *Results* area of the *Pending Test*. In order to paste an imaging or medical test evaluation into the pending test window, the test evaluation would have to be received electronically by the clinic. The electronic mode may have been via e-mail or electronic fax. (If the test result arrives at the clinic in a paper format, the evaluation will need to be scanned into an electronic file.) When the electronic file is opened, the clinician will highlight the evaluation, copy it, and then paste it into the text field of the pending test, as seen in Figure 9.16.

> **Focal Point**
>
> Incoming test data is entered into the outstanding pending test and then sent to the completed test area for the physician's viewing before being stored in the patient's chart.

> Note: Because SpringCharts is an Apple Macintosh program, the right-click function of the mouse is not activated. Therefore the user may not be able to *paste* into SpringCharts using the mouse. To paste text into SpringCharts the keyboard may be used by selecting the keys [Ctrl] + [V].

If the clinic is not using SpringLabs, the lab results will need to be entered manually, shown in Figure 9.17.

The technician will click the [Tech Sign] button to indicate the source of the data entry and then click the [Testing Facility] button to choose the appropriate originating facility, illustrated in Figure 9.16 and Figure 9.17. If the facility is not listed, it must be set up in the address book under the *New* menu or the *Productivity Center* menu. The data entry technician may use the [ToDo] or [Message] buttons to send a ToDo or message to the physician or another colleague. The clinician then clicks the *Complete* radio button on the right side of the screen and then the [Done] button to move the *Pending Test* to the *Completed Test* list.

The physician will either receive the internal notice regarding the completed test or routinely check the system for any completed tests. When ready to evaluate a completed test, the physician opens the *Completed Test* window, seen in

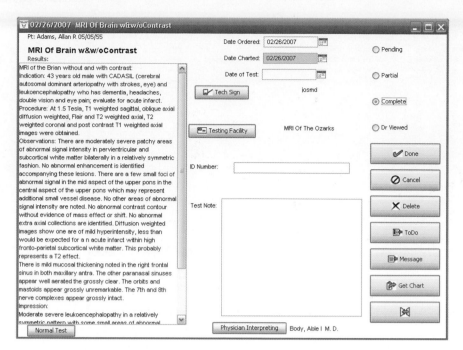

Figure 9.16 Text results copied and pasted into pending test.

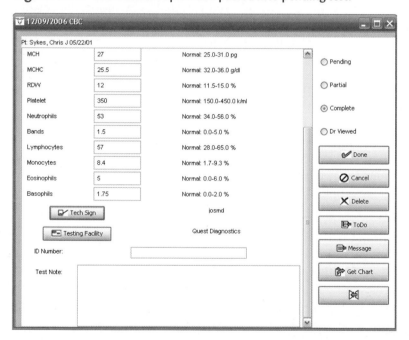

Figure 9.17 Results being entered into the pending test.

Figure 9.18, from the *Practice View* screen by selecting *Edit>Completed Tests*. The *Completed Tests* window will display all the *Pending Tests* in which results were entered. The list of tests can be organized by the test name, patient name, test order date, or ordering physician. In a large practice with multiple physicians this sort feature will enable a physician to quickly find his or her tests within a long list of completed tests.

When a completed test is selected a window will display the test results. Any abnormalities in the outcome (e.g., those outside the normal range) will be highlighted in a color bar to alert the physician, seen in Figure 9.19. From this screen, the doctor can perform all the administrative functions necessary to

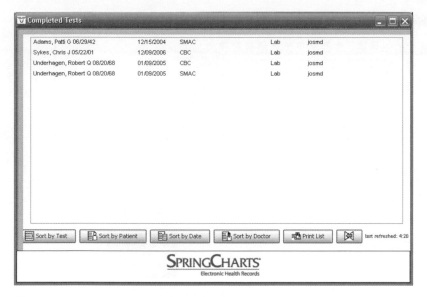

Figure 9.18 List of completed tests.

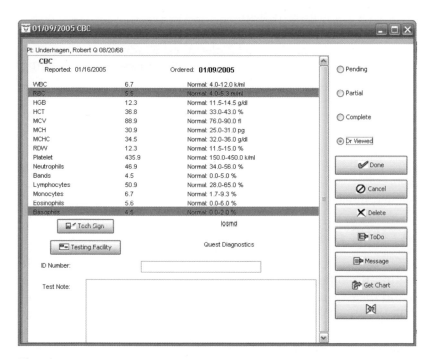

Figure 9.19 Completed test results.

process the test. He or she can open the patient's chart to look for other medical information, send a *ToDo/Reminder* to himself/herself or another coworker to follow up on a needed assignment or send a *Message* to another user. Free text can be typed in the *Test Note* window where the physician may want to record an observation or a plan of care.

When the results have been evaluated, the practitioner selects the *Dr. Viewed* radio button on the right side of the screen, and then clicks the [Done] button. The tests are not charted until the *Dr Viewed* button is selected. If the physician clicks the [Done] button without first selecting *Dr Viewed* the completed test will remain in the *Completed Test* window awaiting further analysis.

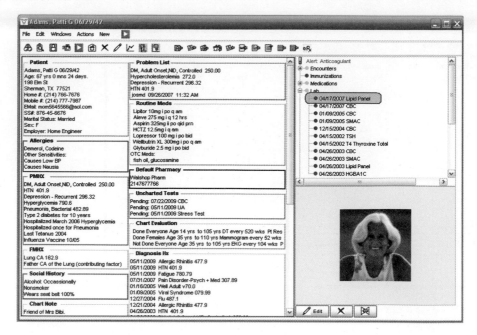

Figure 9.20 Test result stored in patient's chart.

Note: The *Dr. Viewed* radio button in the completed test window is only available if the user is logged on as a doctor. This ensures that a completed test will not enter a patient's chart unless the physician first views it.

When the physician has completed the test analysis, as described above, the test result is automatically removed from the *Completed Tests* window and is placed into the patient's chart along with any test notes the doctor has made. There are three categories in the care tree under which tests are stored: *Lab*, *Imaging*, and *Medical Tests*. SpringCharts automatically stores the tests under the appropriate category, illustrated in Figure 9.20.

LO 9.4 CREATING A TEST REPORT

Once a test is entered into the chart, it is final and cannot be edited. If the tests were ordered within the office visit encounter, then the results will appear in the *H&P* report and the *Examination Report*, which are both created from within the office visit. Because test results were entered in this manner, rather than imported from a static scanned document, SpringCharts can now use the data to create trend analyses, reports, and add test results into letters and e-mails.

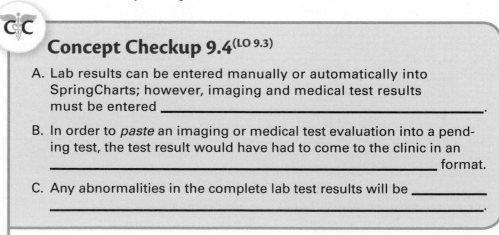

Concept Checkup 9.4(LO 9.3)

A. Lab results can be entered manually or automatically into SpringCharts; however, imaging and medical test results must be entered _____.

B. In order to *paste* an imaging or medical test evaluation into a pending test, the test result would have had to come to the clinic in an _____ format.

C. Any abnormalities in the complete lab test results will be _____ _____.

Exercise 9.3 Ordering and Processing a Lab Test (LO 9.3)

1. Open your chart and order a new lab from the *Action* menu within the chart. In the order test window type "lip" and search with the icon (see margin reference). Select "Lipid Panel," then click the [Done] button.
2. Select "Pending Tests" from the main *Edit* menu. Highlight the "Lipid Panel" just ordered for your chart.
3. Enter in some lab results in the various fields. Check the normal ranges to the right. Place some results in range and some out of range. Click on the [Tech Sign] button and then select an appropriate [Testing facility]. Enter an ID number for the incoming lab.
4. Send a *ToDo* to Dr. S. Finchman indicating that a lab result is ready to be looked at. Select "Check Lab" from the available pop-up text. Send the *ToDo*.
5. Click the "Complete" radio button then click the [Done] button. Close the *Pending Test* window.
6. Let us now assume you are Dr. Finchman. Under the *Edit* menu open the *Completed Test* window.
7. Select the "Lipid Panel" test that was just completed for your chart. Notice the lab items that are outside the normal ranges. Open the patient's chart by clicking the [Get Chart] button (see margin reference). Look in the Routine Meds section of the face sheet and note that the patient is on the cholesterol-lowering drug Lipitor.
8. Close the chart and send a message (see margin reference) to Jan requesting that she call the patient and schedule an appointment ASAP. Place your curser in the body of the message and start a new line by pressing the [Enter] key. Now choose the appropriate pop-up text. Initial the message by clicking the [init] button. Send the message to Jan.
9. Check the *Dr. Viewed* radio button in the completed lipid panel test and click the [Done] button. Close the *Completed Test* window.
10. Open your chart and notice the "+" expand sign added to the *Lab* category of the care tree. Click on the expand sign and you will see the recently completed lab panel. Highlight the lipid panel and the results can be viewed in the lower right quadrant of the patient's chart.
11. Click on the [Print] button at the bottom and submit a copy of the completed test to your instructor.

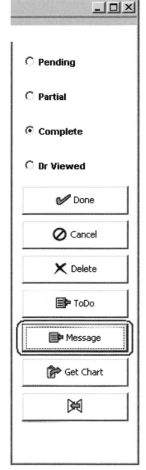

Message button inside completed test window

Exercise 9.4 Processing a Lab Manually (LO 9.3)

1. Locate your pending test for a Pap smear in the *Pending Tests* list of the *Edit* menu in the *Practice View* screen. Highlight the pending test.
2. In the results window type: *Normal* in the upper left window. Click the [Tech Sign] button indicating the inputting clinician. Click the [Testing Facility] button and choose a facility. Click the *Complete* radio button then the [Done] button. The pending test is now removed from the list.

3. Open the same test in the *Completed Tests* area of the *Edit* menu. You will notice it is stamped "Normal." Remember that only those logged on as physicians have the *Dr Viewed* radio button available in this window. The physician has multiple choices for administration in this window including getting the patient's chart. Check the *Dr Viewed* button and then click the [Done] button. The test is removed from the completed list and sent into the patient's chart. Close the *Completed Tests* window.
4. Open your patient chart. Click on the "+" sign beside the lab category in the care tree. Notice the addition of the Pap test.
5. Print out the lab and submit to your instructor.

Focal Point

If test results are entered into SpringCharts through the pending test area, the program is able to create test reports for the patients.

A *Test Report* can be run utilizing these lab results by accessing *New Test Report* in the *New* menu of the patient's chart. A *Test Report* is designed for the patient and will display the test result and add a description of the various analytes in a lab panel and the purpose for the test. SpringCharts comes with layman's explanations for many of the tests that can also be customized. Identified problem areas and recommendations can be added from the pop-up list to complete the *Test Report*. The completed *Test Report* can be either printed out or e-mailed to the patient.

Exercise 9.5 Creating a Test Report (LO 9.4)

1. Inside your patient chart open a *New Test Report to Pt* under the *New* menu.
2. Select the Pap lab test in the upper right panel. Because this is a "normal" result, we can delete the *Problems* and *Recommendations* headings in the report.
3. Print out the report and submit to your instructor.

LO 9.5 AUTOMATED TEST STATUS ALERTS

SpringCharts automatically scans the "Completed" and "Pending" tests lists when opening a patient's chart and notes the face sheet of any unprocessed pending tests and any uncharted completed tests, illustrated in Figure 9.21. This enables the clinic to keep current on outstanding tests that need to be completed and added to the patient's chart.

This unprocessed tests information is also added to the "Chart Overview" panel in the *Office Visit* window, seen in Figure 9.22. Providers are able to view this information when commencing an office visit note, thus keeping current with uncharted tests.

```
┌─ Uncharted Tests ─────────────────────────────
│ Pending: 07/22/2009 CBC
│ Pending: 05/11/2009 UA
│ Pending: 05/11/2009 Stress Test
│
└───────────────────────────────────────────────
```

Figure 9.21 Pending and completed tests alert.

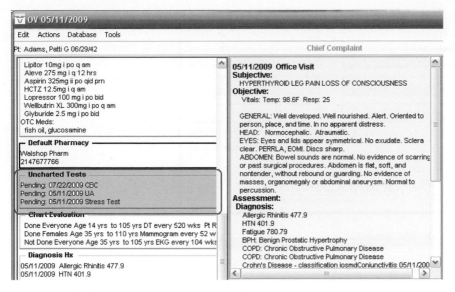

Figure 9.22 Tests alert in chart overview panel of *Office Visit* screen.

Concept Checkup 9.5(LO 9.4, 9.5)

A. The *Test Report* displays the selected test(s) results and a test description. This report is designed to be sent to

_____.

B. The clinician is notified of any unprocessed pending and completed

test when the _____ and the

_____ are opened.

LO 9.6 CREATING A NEW TEST

Lab Tests

Although SpringCharts is installed with a very comprehensive set of labs and imaging and medical tests, additional tests can be added to the program. To do this, the user would select *Tests* from the *Edit* menu on the *Practice View* screen. The *Tests* window, seen in Figure 9.23, enables the user to view all installed tests as well as create new ones.

The following options are displayed in the *Tests* window:

1. *New Lab Test*—creates a new laboratory test or panel.
2. *New Imaging Test*—creates a new x-ray, CT scan, or MRI test.
3. *New Medical Test*—creates any other type of test – non-lab and non-imaging.
4. *List Lab Tests*—shows a list of all current lab tests in the program.
5. *List Imaging Tests*—shows a list of all current imaging tests.
6. *List Medical Tests*—shows all other tests in the program.
7. *List Lab Items*—shows a list of all current analytes that are used to create a lab test or panel.

Focal Point

Outstanding pending and uncharted completed tests are identified by the program and alert the user when the patient's chart is opened and when a new OV note is started.

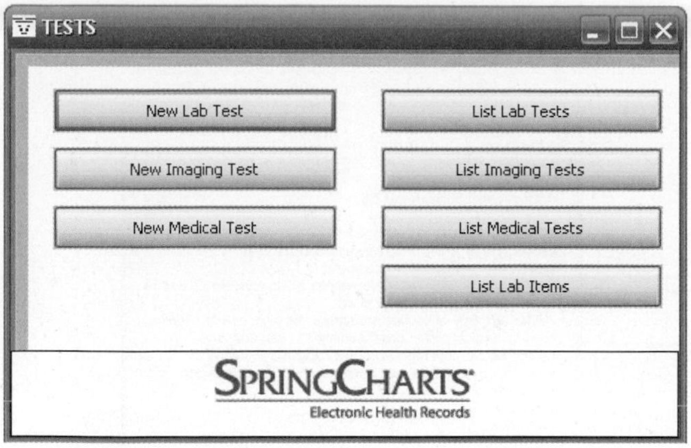

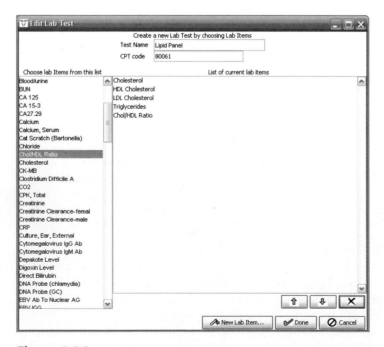

Figure 9.23 Test window.

Before creating any new tests the clinic administrator typically will print the list of lab, imaging, and medical tests from the *Lists* windows. These lists can be examined against the various tests that the clinic regularly orders. Whether the tests are performed within the clinic or sent to an outside testing facility, all tests need to be on these lists so they can be ordered from SpringCharts; this will create a *Pending Test*. Within the *Lists* windows all existing tests can be edited in order to change the test name, CPT code, and/or the panel item on labs.

To create a new lab test, the user will click on the [New Lab Test] button. This displays the *Create a New Lab Test* window, seen in Figure 9.24. Lab tests are created by adding parts called analytes or *lab items*. Lab tests may contain one or more analytes. For example, a serum pregnancy test would consist of one lab item (a serum pregnancy lab), whereas a CBC would contain many lab items (WBC, RBC, HGB, HCT, etc.). With the *Create a New Lab Test* window opened, the user enters a name in the *Test Name* field and enters the CPT code in the *CPT Code* field. The code is important because the test name along with the code will be printed on the routing slip for billing purposes. It will also print on the order form when sent to

Focal Point

To create a new lab test, the user must select at least one lab item to complete the test.

Figure 9.24 Creating a new lab panel.

an outside testing facility, which will also be used by that facility for billing. The user will then select the analyte from the list on the left to include in the lab test. The order in which these lab items are selected is the order that they will appear in the pending lab test. Sometimes it may be helpful for the clinic to have related labs combined together on a single order. To do this the user would create a new lab and select all the analytes that make up the various related labs. By doing so, the provider will only need to order the one lab; however, the pending test will display all the lab items for the related labs. When the user finishes building a lab test, the [Done] button is clicked and the test is saved to the existing lab list.

Creating an Analyte

If an analyte (lab item) does not appear in the resource list on the left side, then it can be created by choosing the [Create New Lab Item] button located in the bottom of the window (Figure 9.24). New lab items are set up based on how the lab item result will be presented (e.g., as a positive/negative, text field, or a minimum/maximum number range), illustrated in Figure 9.25. The user will choose the correct option based on the analyte result display. Once completed the lab item will appear in the list of analytes and can then be added to a *New Lab Test* panel. To edit an existing analyte listed in SpringCharts the user will choose the [List Lab Items] button in the *Tests* window and select the appropriate lab item. The resulting window, seen in Figure 9.26, will allow the user to select and edit ranges and defaults that are displayed for each of the lab items.

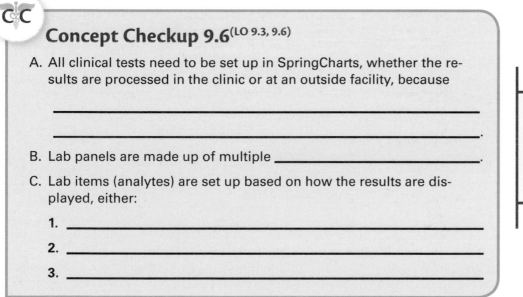

Concept Checkup 9.6(LO 9.3, 9.6)

A. All clinical tests need to be set up in SpringCharts, whether the results are processed in the clinic or at an outside facility, because

_____

_____.

B. Lab panels are made up of multiple _____.

C. Lab items (analytes) are set up based on how the results are displayed, either:

1. _____

2. _____

3. _____

Focal Point

The clinic may have to edit an existing lab item (analyte) in order to modify the normal range.

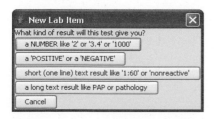

Figure 9.25 Creating a new lab analyte.

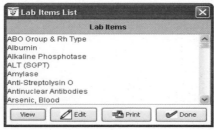

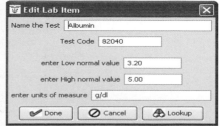

Figure 9.26 Editing an analyte.

Exercise 9.6 Creating a New Lab Test (LO 9.6)

1. Open the *Tests* option in the *Edit* menu of the *Practice View* screen. Click on the [List Lab Tests] button and see if you can locate a complete metabolic panel (CMP) test.

2. Because a CMP is not set up for this medical practice we will need to create a new lab test so the clinic can order the test and so that we can match the results to the pending test. Click on the [New Lab Test] button and fill in the test name and the CPT code. The code for a CMP is 80052.

3. Next we will need to build the analytes that make up the panel. They are listed in alphabetical order in the left side window. When you highlight an analyte it will be added into the right side window. Below is a list of lab components that you will need to select from the list of analytes:

   Glucose, BUN, Creatinine, Sodium, Potassium, Chloride, Bicarbonate (see no. 4 below), Calcium, Total Protein, Albumin, AST, ALT, Alkaline Phosphotase, Total Bilirubin, Globulin, and A:G Ratio (see no. 4).

4. When you cannot find a specific lab item in the left window you will need to create it. Click on the [New Lab Item] button and select one of the four options for the layout of the analyte. Based on the following lab item details below create the new analyte. Once created, it will be added into the resource list in the *Create a New Lab Test* window. It then can be selected for the lab panel that you are building.

   Bicarbonate – a Number, Code – 99999, Low Range – 22, High Range – 32, UOM (Units of Measure) – MMOL/L
   A:G Ratio – a Number, Code – 99999, Low Range – 1.0, High Range – 2.3, UOM – Ratio

5. Now that the CMP panel has been built, click [Done] to save the test. You can now find the CMP listed in the *List Lab Test* window.

Focal Point

All users have access to the entire CPT code dictionary to activate new tests into the program.

Imaging Test or Medical Test

To create a new imaging or medical test, the user will click on the [New Imaging Test] or [New Medical Test] button, respectively. The *New Imaging Test* or *New Medical Test* window appears, as seen in Figure 9.27.

The test name and the CPT code (required) are typed in and the new test is saved. The user can use the [Lookup] button to access the CPT code dictionary database and have this data entered automatically. In the *Lookup* window the test can be searched by either description or code.

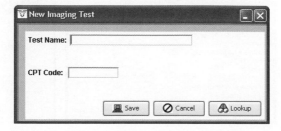

Figure 9.27 Creating a new imaging test.

Exercise 9.7 Creating a New Imaging Test(LO 9.6)

1. Open the *Tests* window in the main *Edit* menu. Click on the [List Imaging Tests] button. Examine the list of imaging tests that are in SpringCharts. Check to see if a test for an x-ray of the larynx with contrast was activated. Close this window.
2. In order to add this imaging test, click on the [New Imaging Test] button. You will notice the [Lookup] button. This will access the CPT dictionary database of SpringCharts. Press *Lookup.*
3. In the *Lookup CPT Code* window type the code: 70373 and hit the search icon. When the new code has been located, highlight it. The description and code are added to the *New Imaging Test* window. Delete the term *Laryngography* and replace it with *Xray Larynx.* Click [Save] and the new code will be added to the list of activated imaging tests. Click on the [List Imaging Tests] button again to view the new test.

LO 9.7 DOCUMENTING AND ACTIVATING PROCEDURE AND DIAGNOSIS CODES

Documenting a Procedure

Procedures are selected from within the *Office Visit* screen. From the patient chart the user will open a new office visit by selecting the *New* menu and clicking *New OV*, as seen in Figure 9.28.

To document procedures, the physician will click on the [Proc] navigation tab in the OV screen. Using the standard search field the provider will type a

Focal Point

Procedures are chosen within the OV screen by either typing the procedure name, selecting from category lists, or selecting from a list of previously used procedures for that patient.

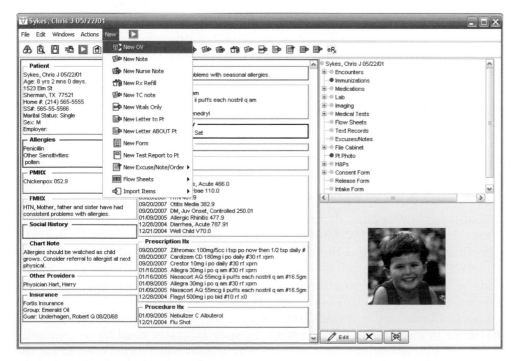

Figure 9.28 Accessing a *New Office Visit* screen.

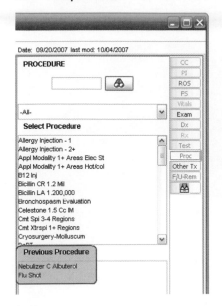

Figure 9.29 Selecting a procedure in the OV note.

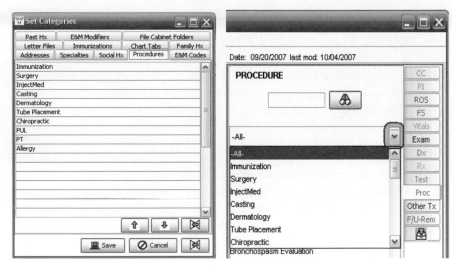

Figure 9.30 Procedure categories in the administration panel and procedure categories listed in the OV screen.

few letters and search for the procedure. The practitioner also has the option to choose a procedure from the *Previous Procedures* window in the lower right section, seen in Figure 9.29. SpringCharts stores all previous procedures performed and lists them in the OV screen for easy access. Many times a patient returns for the same procedure; listing these previous procedures enables the provider quick access to select the procedure rather than conducting another search.

Procedures are also set up under category headings; another way to select a procedure is to first select the category heading from the drop-down category list. Category headings are designed to narrow the search criteria and speed the selection of procedures in the OV note. Once the category heading is selected the provider will choose an activated procedure from the list. The selected procedure(s) are then placed in lower center procedure panel on the *Office Visit* screen.

The procedure categories are set up in the *Category Preferences* window of the *Administrator* menu on SpringCharts Server in a network environment or in the *Administration* menu on a stand-alone version. The clinic administrator can set up to 30 categories based upon the type of procedures that are conducted in your clinic, illustrated in Figure 9.30.

Creating a New Procedure

To add a new procedure, the user selects *New>New Procedure* from the *Practice View* screen. The *New Procedure* window will be displayed, seen in Figure 9.31. The *Procedure Name* and the *CPT Code* fields are completed. It is important to select the correct type of procedure from the *Category* drop-down menu. This will group the procedures in the category drop-down list within the OV screen. The [Lookup] button provides access to all the AMA procedure codes available in the SpringCharts imbedded dictionary. Although the CPT database is installed with SpringCharts, specific codes need to be manually activated in this manner. This enables only the relevant codes needed for the clinic to be sorted and processed in the program. Again, this will speed up

New Procedure

Procedure Name: Dstrj B9 Sk Tgs/cutan Vasc Up 14 <

CPT Code: 17110

Category: Surgery

Procedure Text

Pt was advised of the purpose, benefits, and signif
The patient asked the following questions and was

Pt was advised of the purpose, benefits, and significant risks of this procedure, including but not limited to bleeding, infection, damage to the surrounding tissues, and (other specific risks). Alternative treatments and their risks/benefits were discussed as was the risks of non-treatment. The patient's questions were answered. The patient appears to understand the procedure's risks and possible benefits and has given informed consent.

Save   Cancel   LookUp

Figure 9.31 Creating a new procedure code.

the selection process within the OV screen. The program will automatically populate the code and description fields once the code has been selected in the *Lookup* window.

Procedural text can be chosen from the *PopUp Text* window on the right. It can also be manually typed into the *Procedural Text* window. If the provider consistently has used certain text when administrating a certain procedure, then this is the text that needs to accompany the procedure. Any text added to the setup on a new procedure will be automatically populated in the OV note when the procedure is selected under the [Proc] navigation tab, illustrated in Figure 9.32.

Focal Point

Mini-templates can be created by adding text to the setup of procedure codes. When the procedure is selected in the OV screen, the predefined text is also added to the note.

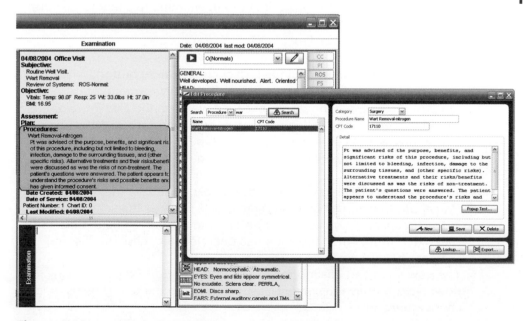

Figure 9.32 Procedure pop-up text automatically added to the OV note when procedure is selected.

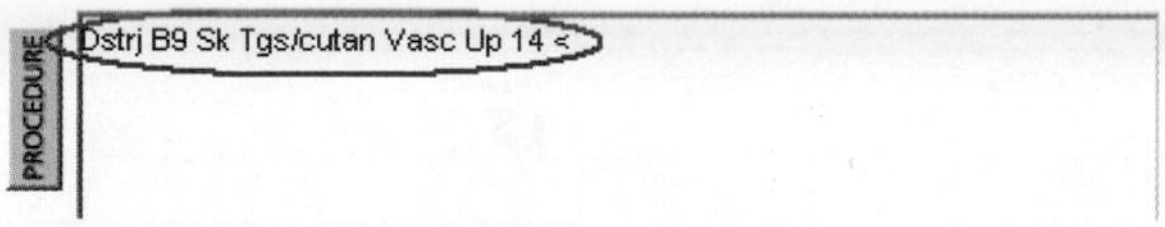

```
Dstrj B9 Sk Tgs/cutan Vasc Up 14 <
```

Figure 9.33 Selecting the procedure to modify the text.

This particular procedural text can be modified for the specific patient in the OV screen by clicking on the procedure in the lower left quadrant, shown in Figure 9.33. Pop-up text that is modified within the OV screen only affects the note for the current patient; it does not change the original text in the procedure setup.

Concept Checkup 9.7(LO 9.7)

A. In the procedure panel on the OV screen, the provider can choose a procedure from either the _____ window or the _____.

B. Where are procedure category headings set up? _____

_____

_____

C. Text that is added to text field when setting up a new procedure will be displayed in the _____ when that procedure is selected.

Exercise 9.8 Creating a New Procedure Code(LO 9.7)

1. Let's create a new procedure code. We need the procedure: Destruction of Benign Lesion – 17111. First of all, we need to check to be sure the code is not already activated. Open the *Edit* menu in the *Practice View* screen and select *Procedures*.

2. In the *Edit Procedure* window select *CPT Code* as the search mode and type 17111 in the search field. Click the [Search] button.

3. A new procedure code can be activated in the *New* menu of the *Practice View* screen; however, because we have the *Edit Procedure* window open we can activate a new code from here. Click the [New] button on the right side. You can either type the procedure name or code in the upper fields or look up the code in the CPT dictionary database.

4. To access the CPT database click the [Lookup] button. In the *Search Procedure Master List* window, select *CPT Code* as the search mode in the first drop down list and type 17111 in the search field. Click the [Search] button. When the code has been located, click the [Select] button.

5. The new code and description is added to the *Edit Procedure* window. Now we have to categorize it. Drop down the *Category* list and choose *Surgery*.

6. There is text that we need to add to this procedure that will be consistent each time the procedure is conducted. Click the [PopUp Text] button. In the *PopUp Text Composer* window select the paragraph that begins with: *Pt was advised of the purpose, benefits*...etc. and click the [OK] button. The text is now added to the *Detail* window and will be associated with this code. Save the new procedure code and close the window.

Creating a New Diagnosis

SpringCharts is installed with the complete library of ICD codes. However, the clinic staff will need to activate the specific codes they intend to use. This method enables the clinic to have a limited number of codes to choose from, thus speeding the selection process. When SpringCharts is initially installed a limited set of diagnosis codes is activated automatically. To activate a new diagnosis the user will select *New Diagnosis* under the *New* menu on the *Practice View* screen. The *New Diagnosis* window will be displayed, shown in Figure 9.34. A new diagnosis can be added directly into the appropriate text and code fields or by selecting the [Lookup] button. The [Lookup] button will give access to the ICD-9 database, enabling the user to search for a new diagnosis by either code or description. When the desired ICD code has been selected the *Dx Brief Name* field will need to be completed. Whatever is typed into this field will determine the text that the practitioner will use when searching for a diagnosis code in the OV screen. If the clinic normally uses the same text as the ICD database, simply check the *Use ICD name for Brief name* box.

Focal Point

Usually during the initial set up of SpringCharts in a doctor's office, additional CPT and ICD-9 codes are added to the activated codes in the program.

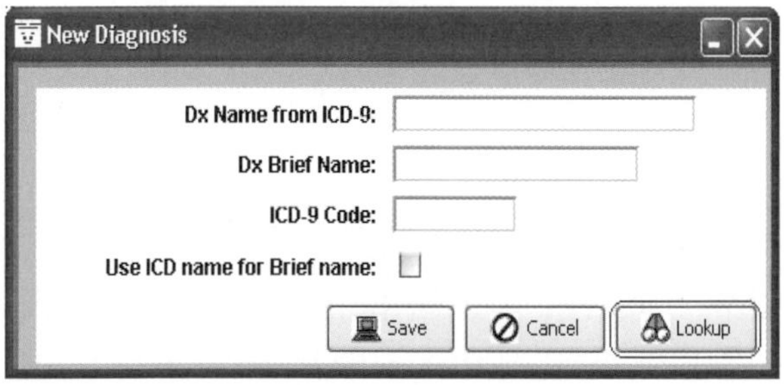

Figure 9.34 Activating a new diagnosis code.

Exercise 9.9 Using Diagnosis and Procedure Codes(LO 9.7)

1. Open your patient chart and launch a new office visit.
2. Under the [CC] navigation button select the pop-up text *Follow-Up*. Because maculopapular skin lesions were discovered during a previous wellness check, this will be a follow-up visit that was scheduled to conduct the removal procedure.
3. Add several normal vitals.
4. Under the [Exam] navigation button, choose the *(O Abnormals)* as the pop-up text category. Scroll down and select the text: *SKIN: + maculopapular lesions*.
5. In the [Dx] navigation area search for any diagnosis starting with *lesion*. Type in *lesion*. The pigmented lesion is not the one we want to use, so

we will need to activate another diagnosis code. In the *Database* menu of the OV screen select *New Diagnosis*. To access the ICD dictionary database click the [Lookup] button. In the *Lookup Dx Code* window search for the main 102 code. From the list select: *Yaws; Other Early Skin Lesions*. The diagnosis description and code is placed in the *New Diagnosis* window. Perhaps the physician does not commonly refer to the diagnosis by this name; rather than selecting the *Use ICD name for Brief name* box, the physician will enter *maculopapular lesions* in the *Dx Brief Name* field and save the newly activated diagnosis.

6. In the diagnosis field of the OV screen, type: *mac* and search for the code. From the presenting list select the new code.

7. Under the [Proc] navigation button click the drop-down list of procedure categories. Select *Surgery* and choose the newly activated CPT code – destruction of benign lesion.

8. Click on the [F/U-Rem] navigation button. You will notice all the text that was associated with this procedure during its creation is now added into the body of the *SOAP* note. Choose a follow-up in 1 week.

9. Click on the "*create a reminder*" icon and send a *ToDo/Reminder* to Jan at the front desk to schedule an appointment on 1 week. Use the appropriate pop-up text and send the ToDo item. Click the [Done] button and create a routing slip.

10. In the *Routing Slip* window bill for the surgical tray that you find itemized in the *Superbill Form* in the right panel. You will *not* need to choose an E&M code because this visit will not be billed as an office visit, rather a procedure.

11. Print the routing slip and submit to your instructor. Send the routing slip and close your patient chart.

Editing Procedures and Diagnoses

To edit procedures and diagnoses the user will select *Edit>Procedures* or *Edit>Diagnosis* on the main *Practice View* screen. To view the complete list of activated codes the user selects the [Search] key without selecting a letter. Figure 9.35 shows a list of activated procedure codes. This list may be printed

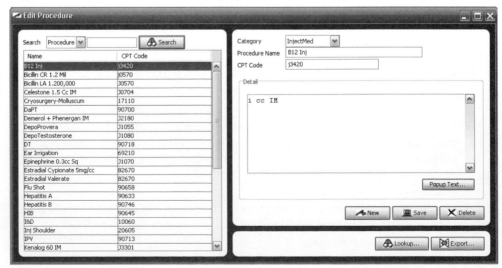

Figure 9.35 Editing a procedure code.

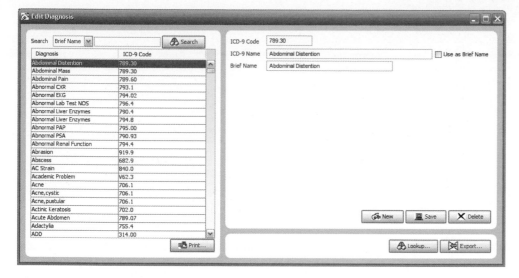

Figure 9.36   Editing a diagnosis code.

out to compare with the list of common codes that the clinic typically uses during the initial setup phase of the program. Codes that are not already activated in SpringCharts can then be created.

Procedures can be searched for by either code or description by selecting the desired search mode in the *Search* field. To edit the procedure, a user will select the desired procedure from the list and the details, including the category heading, will be displayed in the right side panel. The *Edit Procedure* window, seen in Figure 9.36, also presents a text field for describing the details of the procedure. When setting up default text for a procedure code the user will either type in the text field or select the [PopUp Text] button to access preset text. This text is added to the office visit note when the specific procedure code is selected within the *Office Visit* screen. The [Save] button is selected when the modifications are complete. New procedures can also be activated from the *Edit Procedure* window also by selecting the [New] and [Lookup] buttons.

The *Edit Diagnosis* window enables you to search for a diagnosis by either the brief name or the ICD code based upon the selection of the *Search* field. If the code description requires modifying, remember the text that is placed in the *Brief Name* field is the text by which the code is searched for in the *Office Visit* screen. As with procedure codes, new diagnoses can also be activated from the *Edit Diagnosis* window by selecting the [New] and [Lookup] buttons.

Focal Point

Text in the "brief name" field of the *Edit Diagnoses* window determines the description by which the code will be searched for in the OV screen.

Concept Checkup 9.8(LO 9.7)

A. A new diagnosis can be activated through the *New Diagnosis* window under the *New* menu on the *Practice View* screen or under the *Database* menu in the _____ screen.

B. New procedure codes and new diagnosis codes are created under the *New* menu of the *Practice View* screen. They can also be activated from the _____ and the _____ windows, respectively.

chapter 9 review

Name _____ Instructor _____ Class _____

USING TERMINOLOGY

Match the terms on the left with the definitions on the right.

_____ 1. SpringLabs

_____ 2. Reference labs

_____ 3. Analyte

_____ 4. Imported lab data

_____ 5. EDI

A. A blood test compound that is the subject to its own specific chemical analysis.(LO 9.6)

B. Lab results that are received from reference labs over a secure Internet connection.(LO 9.2)

C. Specific lab companies that transmit electronic data to SpringCharts using HL7 language and protocols.(LO 9.2)

D. Electronic data transfer standards and protocols.(LO 9.2)

E. A SpringCharts feature that provides the capability of automatically receiving lab test results directly from the lab.(LO 9.2)

CHECKING YOUR UNDERSTANDING

Write "T" or "F" in the blank to indicate whether you think the statement is true or false.

_____ 6. The entire ICD-9 and CPT dictionaries are part of the installed database.(LO 9.7)

_____ 7. SpringCharts has a feature that enables medical practices to automatically receive test results directly from outside labs.(LO 9.2)

_____ 8. The term CBC on an ordered lab test stands for certified bilirubin count.(LO 9.1)

_____ 9. When a provider opens the patient's chart to conduct a physical exam, he or she will be alerted to any unprocessed medical tests in the face sheet.(LO 9.5)

_____ 10. Once a test is entered into the chart, it is final and cannot be edited.(LO 9.2)

_____ 11. Additional tests cannot be added to the very comprehensive set of labs, imaging, and medical tests in SpringCharts.(LO 9.3)

_____ 12. When working with imported lab results where the reference lab's test name differs from the name used in the pending test, SpringCharts "remembers" the synonym for subsequent test matching.(LO 9.2)

Answer the question below in the space provided.

13. There are three categories in the care tree where tests are stored. They are:(LO 9.2)

1. _____

2. _____

3. _____

208

Copyright © 2011 by The McGraw-Hill Companies, Inc.

Choose the best answer and circle the corresponding letter.

14. A new imaging test creates:^(LO 9.6)
    a) The report produced after a MRI scan
    b) A new x-ray, MRI, or CT scan
    c) A computer-generated body makeover

15. The procedure categories are set up in the *Administrator* menu. The administrator can set up to:^(LO 9.7)
    a) 50 categories
    b) 25 categories
    c) 30 categories

16. The *Edit Diagnosis* window enables you to search for a diagnosis by:^(LO 9.7)
    a) Brief name
    b) ICD code
    c) Either a and b

17. ICD-9 is a term used for a:^(LO 9.7)
    a) Diagnosis code
    b) Procedure code
    c) A British rock group

18. When test data is received through SpringLabs, it goes into this area:^(LO 9.2)
    a) Pending tests
    b) Completed tests
    c) Reference lab

19. When a lab company sends test data, the term "out of range" means:^(LO 9.2)
    a) Abnormal level
    b) The patient couldn't be reached by cell phone
    c) Outside the danger level

20. Users who have access level of *Get Pending Tests* are notified of newly imported lab results by a:^(LO 9.2)
    a) Red flag in the patient's chart
    b) A lab icon next to the user's login name
    c) A pop-up box that appears on the screen when accessing a patient's chart

10

Productivity Center and Utilities

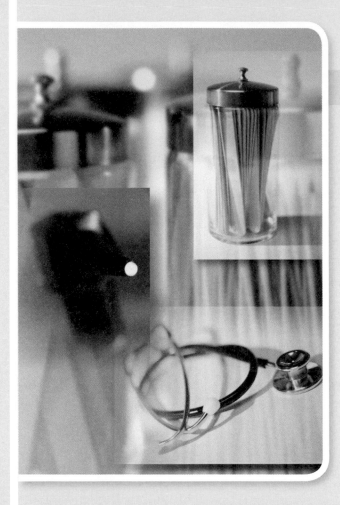

What You Need to Know

To understand Chapter 10 you will need to know how to:

- Navigate in the *Practice View* screen
- Open a patient's chart
- Navigate in a patient's chart

OVERVIEW

The *Productivity Center* menu, seen in Figure 10.1, located on the *Practice View* screen is design to bring together in one place some of the most common functions of SpringCharts. This enables each user access to one menu where regular administrative activities can be performed such as: posting a message on the company's bulletin board, locating and importing file cabinet documents, checking inbound and outbound faxes, creating urgent messages and todo items, and accessing the user's preset favorite websites. The *Utilities* menu, seen in Figure 10.2, is another menu that offers administrative features. Here the user can access various calculators, evaluate medical screenings on the entire patient database, analyze the medical database for reports and form letters, and activate one-touch scanning of documents.

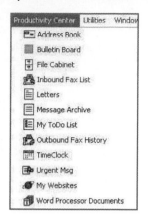

Figure 10.1 Productivity center menu.

LO 10.1 BULLETIN BOARD

The bulletin board located in the *Productivity Center* allows users to place general messages for others in the clinic to see. It replaces the typical bulletin board often seen in the office break room and aids in moving the clinic toward a paperless environment. This feature can also be activated from an icon on the main toolbar. The bulletin board window is network-defined; all users share the same bulletin board. Once opened, the user can select any subject heading on the left, which will then display it on the right, seen in Figure 10.3. Posted bulletins may be printed out. To add a new bulletin to the board the user will click the [New] button. Users will replace the phrase *New Bulletin* with the appropriate subject heading and type the message under the heading. Bulletins can be colored by selecting the [Color] button and choosing from a range of colors. Each user will

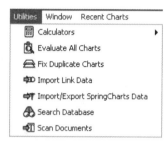

Figure 10.2 Utilities menu.

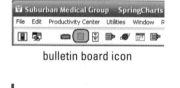
bulletin board icon

Focal Point

The electronic bulletin board in SpringCharts is designed to replace the typical bulletin board in the office.

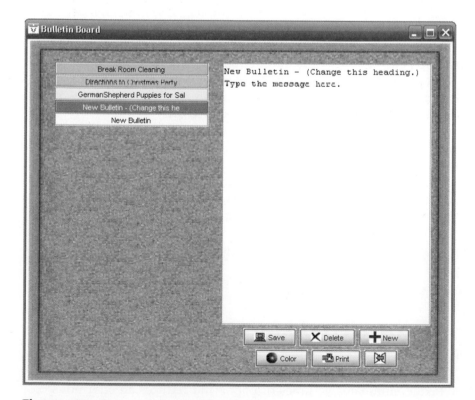

Figure 10.3 Universal clinic bulletin board.

need to routinely check the bulletin board for new messages; there is no automatic announcement when items are placed on the board.

Concept Checkup 10.1(LO 10.1)

A. Name the two menus that enable the user to access regular administrative activities.

1. _____

2. _____

B. What does it mean that the bulletin board is network-defined?

_____

_____.

Focal Point

SpringCharts allows for Internet faxing through a third party company that eliminates the need for a fax line and modem.

Exercise 10.1 Creating a New Bulletin Post(LO 10.1)

1. Click on the bulletin board icon on the tool bar of the main *Practice View* screen. Click on the [New] button to open a new bulletin.
2. Highlight the phrase: *New Bulletin* and replace it with the name of a bulletin you would like to post. Remember the purpose of the bulletin board is to place items for general viewing. If a message or directive needs to be sent to another coworker, the message center or the todo/reminder sections of the program would be used for that purpose. Bulletins could be information and directions about an office gathering, parties, things for sale, and so on.
3. On the next lines of your new bulletin type the details of your message. You can color your bulletin by accessing the color options under the [Color] button. Then click the [Save] button.
4. Once again click on the [New] button and create another bulletin as outlined above. You will notice that as each bulletin is created it is added to the left-hand side for others to view. To view your previous bulletins simply click on the subject on the left side. Select your original bulletin.
5. Print a copy of your original bulletin and submit to your instructor.

LO 10.2 INTEGRATED FAXING

SpringCharts interfaces with *InterFax*™ (www.Interfax.net) to allow users to send and receive faxes to and from any SpringCharts Client computer. Electronic faxing eliminates volumes of paper and reduces an enormous cost for paper, toner, and supplies normally incurred by the clinic. SpringCharts

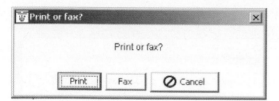

Figure 10.4 Fax option available in the print window.

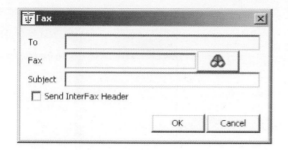

Figure 10.5 Fax dialog window.

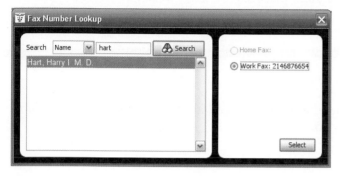

Figure 10.6 Selecting the fax recipient from SpringCharts address book.

faxing requires an Internet connection to the computer; however, no separate analog phone/fax line is required. A new fax number will be assigned to the clinic when establishing an account with InterFax. Once an account is set up and the faxing option activated, the fax feature is available in SpringCharts anywhere the print function is available.

To fax from SpringCharts the user will select the [Print] button from any one of multiple print option windows in the program. The user will then be presented with the choice to print or fax, illustrated in Figure 10.4.

Selecting the [Fax] button takes the user to the fax dialog window, seen in Figure 10.5. Here the recipient's name, fax number, and subject are entered. The *Lookup/Search* icon will access the SpringCharts address book from where the user can quickly select the fax numbers of individuals and businesses on file, seen in Figure 10.6. Once selected, the integrated program will automatically populate the recipient's name and fax number in the fax dialog window. The user will then fill out the subject line. The user can choose whether or not to use the page header that was set up on the account screen at InterFax.

Outbound Fax History

To check the status of sent faxes from SpringCharts the user will select the *Outbound Fax History* item in the *Productivity Center* menu, illustrated in Figure 10.7.

Figure 10.8 shows the *Outbound Fax History* dialog screen, which displays the most recently sent faxes. The *Status* column displays pending, completed, or failed transmissions. The remaining columns display the recipient, the destination fax number, fax subject, the date of original submission, and completion. The [Refresh] button enables the user to update the records in this window to

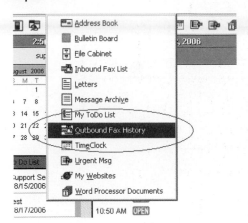

Figure 10.7 Outbound fax history in productivity center.

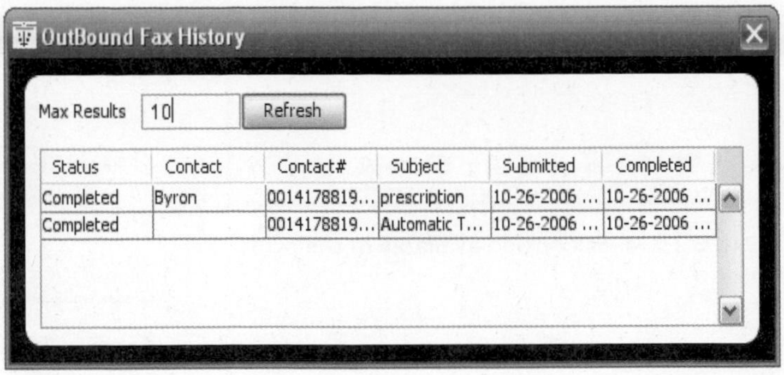

Figure 10.8 *Outbound Fax History* **window.**

the outbound faxes that may have been logged at InterFax while the *Outbound Fax History* window was open.

Inbound Fax List

Checking for received faxes is done by accessing the *Inbound Fax List* dialog from the *Productivity Center* menu. Figure 10.9 shows the *Inbound Fax List* screen displaying the sender's fax number, the time received, and the number of pages. When a fax is received into the clinic's account a corresponding e-mail is sent to the clinic notifying them of the inbound fax. The SpringCharts user who has the security clearance to receive e-mails will receive this notice. By highlighting a fax in the *Inbound Fax List* window and then selecting the [View] button the user can view the actual faxed document on the computer screen. The [Refresh] button refreshes the inbound list retrieving any new faxes that may have come into the InterFax account while the dialog window was open. The [Add to File Cabinet] button allows the user to import the selected faxed document directly into the patient's file cabinet within the chart's care tree. This feature enables the clinic to electronically capture medical information, evaluations, and consultations faxed from external sources. It bypasses the paper fax which normally would have to be scanned back into the electronic health record. The [Delete] button deletes the selected fax; however, it will still be retrievable through the InterFax website for some time.

Focal Point

Both the list of inbound and the list of outbound faxes can be viewed by accessing the Interface website through SpringCharts Productivity Center.

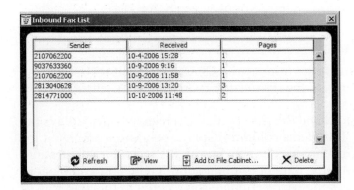

Figure 10.9 *Inbound Fax List* **window.**

Concept Checkup 10.2(LO 10.2)

A. SpringCharts sends and receives electronic faxes by interfacing over the Internet with a web-based company known as:

_____.

B. Both the outbound and inbound fax history windows are located under the _____ menu.

C. Inbound faxes can be added quickly to the patient's chart by selecting the _____ button located in the *Inbound Fax List* window.

Note: In order to fax directly out of SpringCharts you will need to activate the *Interfax* feature. Complete the following steps before beginning Exercise 10.2.

1. Click on the *Administration* menu and select the *InterFax Setup* option.
2. In the *InterFax Setup* window check the *Enable* box. Enter the Username *mnti* and the Password *springmedical*.
3. Click on the [Fax Web Service Key] and enter the number 2036. Click the [OK] button and the [Done] button.
4. Close down SpringCharts and reboot the program.

Exercise 10.2 Faxing a Prescription Electronically(LO 10.2)

1. In the *Productivity Center* menu open the *Address Book* option. Change the search criterion on the right side to *Category*. In the *Find* field type: *pharmacy* and conduct the search.
2. Select the *Walshop Pharm*. In the *Address* window add a fax number to the *Work Fax* field and click the [Save] button. Close the *address* window.
3. Open your patient chart. Select the office visit note under the *Encounter* category of the care tree that deals with the adult allergy symptoms. Click on the [Edit] button to open the OV screen.
4. In the OV screen click on the [Rx] navigation button to display the three prescriptions that were ordered. Click on the printer icon in the lower center section of the screen.
5. In the *Prescription Printing Options* window select *Use Digital Signature* and *Print License No on Rx*. Click on the [Fax] button.
6. In the *Fax* window conduct a search for a pharmacy by clicking on the search icon. In the *Fax Number Lookup* window choose *Category* as the search criterion. In the search field type: *phar* and click the [Search] button. In the list of displayed pharmacies select the Walshop Pharmacy. On the right side the fax number will be displayed that you typed in earlier. Click the radio button beside the fax number and click the [Select] button.
7. Back in the *Fax* window type in the *Subject* field: *Prescription*. Check the box to *Send InterFax Header* and click the [Send] button. The fax will now be transmitted to the pharmacy.

Exercise 10.3 Processing an Inbound Electronic Fax(LO 10.2)

1. If the medical facility had an account set up with InterFax, all inbound faxes to the clinic would be listed in the *Inbound Fax List* of the *productivity Center.* Because we are not currently interfaced with this Web service we will retrieve our fax from the *EHR Material* folder on the desktop. Within this folder, locate the document regarding an *MRI of the Ozarks* and open it.

2. With the left-click of your mouse held down, highlight the document. Or you may simply select the [Ctrl] + [A] buttons to highlight **all** the document. Right-click inside the highlighted area and select *Copy.* Or you may simply select the [Ctrl] + [C] buttons to **copy** the document. Close the fax image and close the *EHR Material* folder *window.*

3. Open the *Pending Tests* window under the *Edit* menu, locate and open the MRI of the brain test for Robert Underhagen. Click in the *Results* text box and press [Ctrl] + [V] on your keyboard to **paste** the document. The MRI evaluation will appear in the pending test.

4. Click the [Tech Sign] button to add your initials and choose the appropriate testing facility. Select the interpreting physician.

5. Send a *ToDo* to Dr. Finchman (scfmd) notifying him of the completed MRI test that he will need to look at. Select the pop-up text: *Check XRay.* You will notice it is already linked to the patient and descriptive text is already applied. Send the item. Click in the *Complete* radio button and click the [Done] button. Close the *Pending Tests* window.

6. Now ask Dr. Finchman to open the *Completed Tests* window in the *Edit* menu. Select the MRI test for your patient. Send a *Message* to Jan to have her call the patient and schedule an appointment. Click on the *Dr. Viewed* radio button and the [Done] button.

7. Open the patient's chart and view the MRI test under the *Imaging* category in the care tree.

8. Click on the MRI item and select the [Print] button in the bottom right window.

9. Print the **MRI** report, write your name on it and submit to your instructor. Close the patient's chart.

LO 10.3 TIME CLOCK

Focal Point

The time clock module in SpringCharts provides the medical staff with another function to move the office toward a paperless environment.

The time clock feature is not activated in SpringCharts by default. Clinics that want to take advantage of this feature will "enable" it from the *Administrator* panel on SpringCharts Server and select the *Time Clock Setup* option. This feature illustrates another way in which medical clinics are moving towards a paperless environment.

The administrator whose name appears within the time clock feature setup, seen in Figure 10.10, is the one who will receive all the employees' time clock information. This person will also be responsible for approving or disallowing requested time clock changes. Once enabled on SpringCharts Server, each

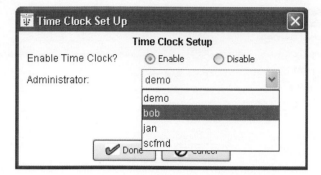

Figure 10.10 *Time Clock Set Up* window.

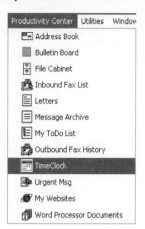

Figure 10.11 Time clock feature in productivity center menu.

Client version will need to be rebooted for the feature to refresh for each user. Figure 10.11 shows the *Time Clock* feature available from the *Productivity Center* menu on the *Practice View* screen once enabled on SpringCharts Server.

The time clock screen on the administrator's login looks a little different from the time clock window on the other users' login. The administrator's *Time Clock* window, seen in Figure 10.12, displays the logged time in and out of all users. This enables the administrator to run time clock reports over a determined period of time in order to do payroll.

If an employee failed to login at the appropriate time, the [Request Change] button can be used to request a time change from the administrator. This request, when sent, activates a *ToDo/Reminder* item in the administrator's *To Do List*.

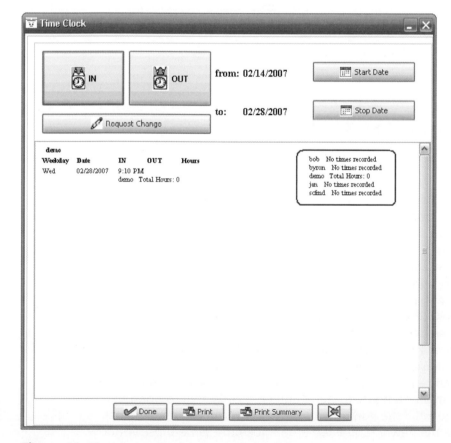

Figure 10.12 *Administrator's Time Clock* window.

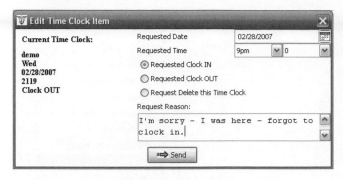
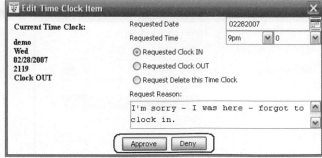

Figure 10.13 *Edit Time Clock Item* windows.

It gives the administrator the opportunity to either approve or deny the request. Once the request is responded to it is sent back to the user's *ToDo List* either as approved or denied. If the request was approved, SpringCharts automatically updates the user's time clock record to the corrected approved time. The *Request Change* window and the administrator's response window are seen in Figure 10.13.

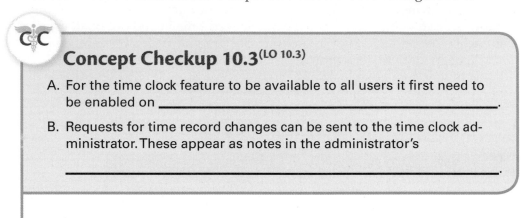

Concept Checkup 10.3(LO 10.3)

A. For the time clock feature to be available to all users it first need to be enabled on _____.

B. Requests for time record changes can be sent to the time clock administrator. These appear as notes in the administrator's

_____.

Exercise 10.4   Working with the Time Clock (LO 10.3)

1. If the *Time Clock* submenu is not visible in the *Productivity Center* menu you will need to activate the feature in SpringCharts.
2. Click on the *Administration* menu on the main screen and select the *Time Clock Setup* submenu.
3. Check the *Enable time clock* box and select *demo* as the administrator. Click the [Done] button.
4. You will now need to close down the SpringCharts program and reboot it for this feature to be activated.
5. Access the *Productivity Center* menu and select *Time Clock.* In the *Time Clock* window click the *In* box and then confirm the clock-in. Your time-in is stamped into the window.
6. You have clocked in after the hour. Let's say that you were actually in the clinic but had forgotten to clock in. Click the [Request Change] button and edit your existing time. Highlight your time and the *Edit Time Clock Item* window will open.
7. On the right-hand side, change the time back to the top of the hour. In the *Request Reason* text box state the reason why you clocked in so late and click the [Send] button.
8. The program has now sent your request to the office administrator as an item in the administrator's ToDo list, marking it with an orange bar. The administrator is able to open the item and either approve or deny the request. If the administrator approves the request, the user's time clock will be adjusted to reflect the newly requested time. Close the *Time Clock* window.

LO 10.4 MY WEBSITES

My Websites is a feature also found in the *Productivity Center* menu, illustrated in Figure 10.14. This window lists websites intended to provide rapid access to Internet-based knowledge systems. Patient educational material can be quickly accessed via this means and printed for the patient. Figure 10.15 shows web addresses of several highly rated knowledge bases that are included with the SpringCharts setup. This feature is user defined so all users can have their own unique list of website links. The user simply clicks on a list item to activate the browser and go immediately to this website from within SpringCharts.

The list can be edited by clicking the [Edit] button. The following window, shown in Figure 10.16 will be displayed. Here the user enters the website name and the URL address in the format indicated. The new website will be added to the list in the *My Websites* window.

> **Focal Point**
>
> The My Website feature is a user-defined function of SpringCharts that contains websites commonly accessed by the user.

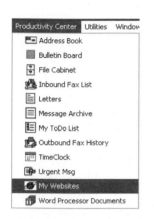

Figure 10.14
Accessing my websites in the *Productivity Center* window.

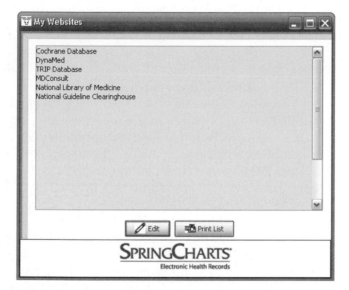

Figure 10.15 List of user-defined websites.

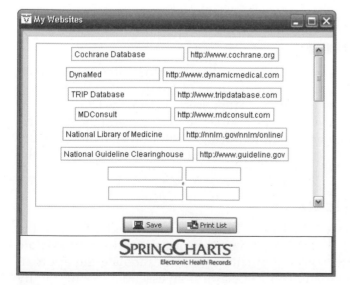

Figure 10.16 My Websites setup window.

Concept Checkup 10.4(LO 10.4)

A. Is the *My Websites* feature user–defined or network-defined?

_____

B. To add additional website locations the *My Websites* feature, each user will need to add both the _____ and the _____ in the *Edit* window.

Exercise 10.5 Adding a New My Website Link (LO 10.4)

1. Under the *Productivity Center* open the *My Websites* option. In the *My Websites* window, click on the [Edit] button.
2. Enter the phrase *Patient Instructions* in the first blank space on the left. Move your cursor to the far left. In the right side field place the curser to the far left of the field and, following the same format as the other links, type in the web address: http://www.familydoctor .org. Save your website addition.
3. In the *My Websites* window click on the newly added *Patient Instructions* link. The Internet browser will be activated and you will access the website directly from SpringCharts. This website has a wealth of patient instructional sheet that can the copied into SpringCharts as patient instructions or printed directly from this website.
4. Close the Internet browser and the *My Websites* windows.

LO 10.5 CALCULATORS

Conversion Calculator

SpringCharts contains a conversion calculator, displayed in Figure 10.17a, which enables the clinical staff to convert imperial units to metric measurements and vise versa. To activate the conversion calculator, users click on the *Utilities* menu and select *Calculator>Conversion Calculator*. First the user will add the measurement in the weight, length, or temperature field, select the originating units of measure, and then click on the [Convert] button to translate the units to the alternate measurements.

Pregnancy EDD Calculator

The pregnancy calculator, seen in Figure 10.17b, is useful in determining the estimated date of delivery. Simply select the LMP (last menstrual period) date from the supplied calendar and the calculator will extrapolate the approximate fetal age and delivery date. This calculator is an essential tool for family physicians and OB/GYNs.

Focal Point

SpringCharts contains three types of calculators: conversion, pregnancy, and simple calculators.

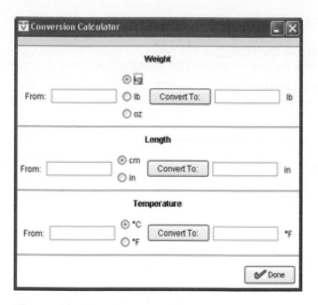

Figure 10.17a Conversion calculator.

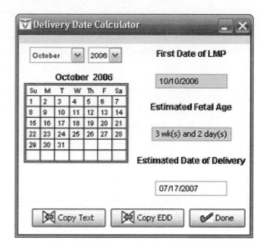

Figure 10.17b Pregnancy calculator.

Simple Calculator

SpringCharts also provides the user with a basic calculator to process simple algorithms.

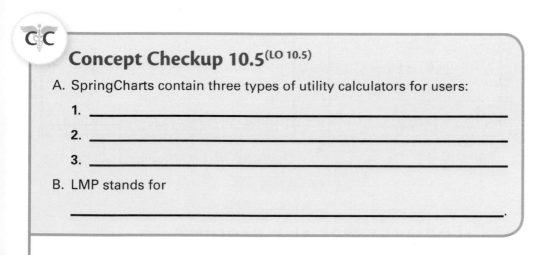

Concept Checkup 10.5(LO 10.5)

A. SpringCharts contain three types of utility calculators for users:

   1. _____

   2. _____

   3. _____

B. LMP stands for

   _____.

Exercise 10.6 Calculating an Estimated Delivery Date (LO 10.5)

1. Open the pregnancy calculator under the *Utility* menu.
2. Let us assume your last menstrual period was 6 weeks ago. Select that date from the calendar. The date will be automatically entered into the LMP field and the estimated age of your baby calculated along with the estimated date of delivery. Congratulations!

LO 10.6 PATIENT DATABASE

Users wanting to conduct a database search will select *Utilities>Search Database*, as seen in Figure 10.18a. SpringCharts users can search the entire database of patient charts listing patients by diagnoses, medications, procedures, tests, insurance companies, employers, and providers, illustrated in Figure 10.18b.

> Note: All users must be logged out of *SpringCharts* for this database search function to be conducted.

Once the search criterion has been selected, the *Search Results* window displays a list of qualifying patients, seen in Figure 10.19. If the user wants to review more information on any of these patients, the user would simply highlight the desired patient and a *Patient Data* window will be displayed. From the *Patient Data* window the patient demographics can be edited and printed and the patient's chart accessed. In the *Search Results* window the user may print the list, create a form letter, or create a report.

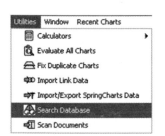

Figure 10.18a Accessing search database menu.

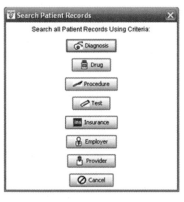

Figure 10.18b The search criteria.

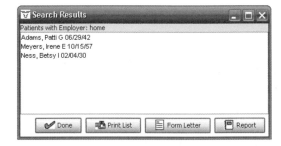

Figure 10.19 List of qualifying patients.

LO 10.7 FORM LETTERS AND REPORTS

Form Letters

To send a form letter to the list of selected patients the administrator would select the [Form Letter] button and enter the subject and text of the proposed letter.

Figure 10.20 illustrates a completed form letter. Once the [Done] button is selected the administrator will be given several options for mass mailing or e-mailing the letters.

The *Actions* available are:

1. *Print* letters to all patients on the list
2. *Email* patients who have e-mail addresses recorded in SpringCharts and print letters to all others
3. Only send the letter to patients with *e-mail* addresses registered in SpringCharts.

> **Focal Point**
>
> Form Letters and reports can be created from patient lists generated through the Search Database feature.

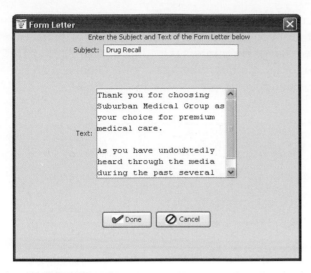

Figure 10.20 Create a form letter from the database search results.

SpringCharts will prompt the user to choose whether or not to print the letterhead on the letters and whether or not to include a copy of the letter in each of the patient's chart. Physicians processing these letters will be given the option to sign the letters electronically. If this option is chosen the system will print the phrase: *Signature electronically verified* along with the doctor's name in the signature line.

Reports

Data reports can be created based on the list of patients identified by the *Search Database* criteria. To create a report the administrator will select the [Report] button in the *Search Results* window. From the *Include in Report* window, seen in Figure 10.21, the user can select various patient demographic items that will

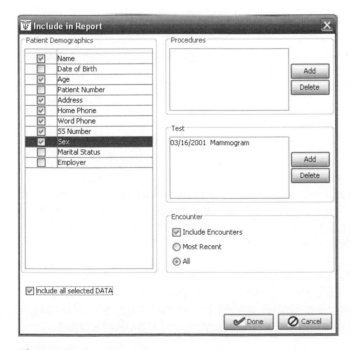

Figure 10.21 *Report Options* window.

be included in the report and cross reference the list of patients to specific procedures and/or diagnoses that are recorded in the patients' charts. The user is also given the option to include a list of encounters (i.e., date and title), that are recorded in the chart's care tree under the *Encounters* category. The user can list all the encounters or the most recent one.

Concept Checkup 10.6 (LO 10.6; 10.7)

A. Name three of the criteria by which the patients can be searched in SpringCharts database?

1. _____

2. _____

3. _____

B. What two options are given to the user once the list of patients have been created?

1. _____

2. _____

C. What three items can be included in the patient report?

1. _____

2. _____

3. _____

Exercise 10.7 Searching the Medical Database (LO 10.6, 10.7)

1. Under the *Utilities* menu select the *Search Database* option. Click [Yes] to "Search all patient records now" and "Yes" in the next window.
2. Select the [Drug] button as the criterion to search by. Type *Lipitor* in the *Select Drug* window and conduct a search. The program will display all strengths of the drug Lipitor; click on all of the medications one by one to add them to the *Selected Drug* window. Click the [Done] button and the program will begin searching the patient database for patients who have been prescribed with the medication Lipitor.
3. Click the [Form Letter] button. In the *Form Letter* window type in the subject: *Drug Recall*. In the text field type the body of the letter informing the patients about the drug recall and the need to contact the doctor's office to schedule a visit. When completed click the [Done] button.
4. In the *Choose Action* window select the [Print Letters] button. Choose "Yes" to chart the letters, "Yes" to print the letterhead, and "Yes" to sign the letters electronically. Print the letters.
5. Open Russel Dean's chart. Under the *Encounters* category in the care tree you will find a copy of your letter saved in the patient's chart. Close the chart.
6. Submit the letter to your patient to your instructor.

LO 10.8 PATIENT ARCHIVE

The patient archive feature allows an administrator to remove a patient from the current patient list into a new "archived patient" list but still retain access to the patient's records. Under the main *Edit* menu the user would select the *Patient* option and search for the patient that needs to be archived, as seen in Figure 10.22. The administrator would then click on the [Archive] button to remove the patient from active lists within SpringCharts.

Once archived the patient's data can be viewed and the patient's record can be reactivated if needed. In the main *Edit* menu, the user would select *Patient Archives*. The patient can be located by various criteria: last name, first name, middle initial, birth date, address, city, state, zip code, SS number, patient number, or date archived. Figure 10.23 reveals that the patient's chart information

Focal Point

Patients who are no longer active in the clinic may be archived from the main database of SpringCharts. Although the patient will no longer be viewed in the program, the medical records can be viewed and reactivated if necessary.

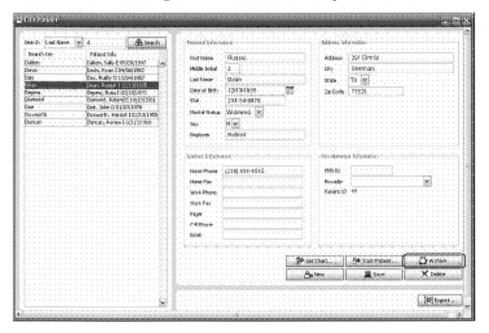

Figure 10.22 *Edit Patient* window.

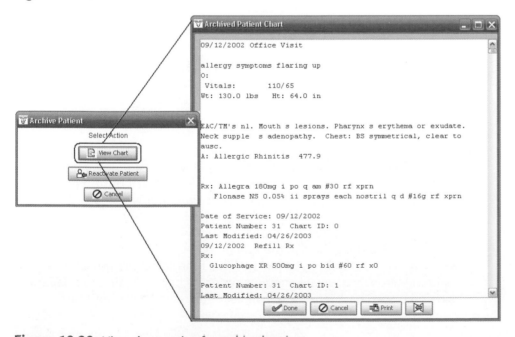

Figure 10.23 View chart option for archived patient.

can be viewed without reactivating the patient into the current data set. This is done by selecting the [View Chart] button. The subsequent window will display a text record of all items within the chart. The information is displayed by chronological order based on when the item was originally added to the chart. The oldest added information will at the top with the patient's demographics at the bottom of the documentation. Information in the *Archive Patient Chart* window cannot be altered. It can, however, be printed by using the [Print] button. When the chart record is displayed for an archived patient, the user can export these old records as a .txt file by using the *Export* icon and then open the file in another program or send it to a PDA and iPod folder.

Documents that were stored in the chart's *File Cabinet* prior to archiving the patient will not be seen in the *Archive Patient Chart* window. However, when the patient is reactivated these former *File Cabinet* documents will also be reactivated into the patient's care tree. Reactivated patients will have a new patient ID number assigned by SpringCharts.

Concept Checkup 10.7(LO 10.8)

A. The patient archive feature allows the user to remove the patient's name and chart from the main program but still

_____.

B. An archived patient's information can be viewed without needing to

_____

_____.

Exercise 10.8 Archiving a Patient's Record (LO 10.8)

1. Select the *Edit* menu of the *Practice View* screen and then the submenu *Patients*. In the *Edit Patient* window select locate the patient: Rusty Day.
2. Archive Rusty by pressing the [Archive] button in the lower right. You will see his name disappear from the patient list. Close the *Edit Patient* window.
3. Open the *Edit* menu once again and select *Patient Archives*. In the *Patient Archive* window search for Rusty Day by last name. Highlight the patient in the list and select the [View Chart] button in the *Archive Patient* window. The *Archive Patient* window will also enable you to reactivate the patient into the active lists in SpringCharts if necessary. Close the *Patient Archive* window.
4. Let's reactivate Rusty Day. In the *Edit* menu open the *Patient Archives* window. Locate the archived patient. This time select the [Reactivate Patient] button. You will be shown a progress bar indicating the patient is being placed back into the active list of patients in SpringCharts.

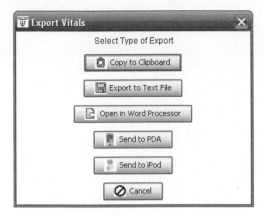

Figure 10.24 Universal export feature.

LO 10.9 UNIVERSAL EXPORT FUNCTION

The *Universal Export* icon is available in all areas of the program. The *Export* window enables the user to copy the specific data from the opened window and manipulate it into other programs and devices, illustrated in Figure 10.24. The data can be:

Universal Export

a. Copied to the internal clipboard then pasted into another program
b. Exported as a .txt file then opened in a text program or sent as an e-mail attachment
c. Opened directly in the computer's default word processor, or
d. Stored in synchronized folders for portable viewing through a PDA and iPod

LO 10.10 PROGRAM INFORMATION AND HELP

The main *Help* menu provides an Internet link to tutorial information about many features of SpringCharts through the *SpringCharts Help* option, shown in Figure 10.25. This feature is available on all Client computers. Users can readily access this tutorial knowledge base and search for areas of interest.

About SpringCharts option in the *Help* menu displays program information which may be important when discussing issues with SpringCharts technicians including:

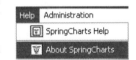

Figure 10.25
SpringCharts help menu.

a. The current version of SpringCharts
b. Operating system
c. The feature options activated
d. Number of user licenses
e. IP address of the user's computer.

Concept Checkup 10.8 (LO 10.9; 10.10)

A. Where is the *Universal Export* feature located in SpringCharts?

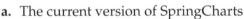

B. Where will one need to look to locate tutorial information about many features of SpringCharts?

Name _____ Instructor _____ Class _____

USING TERMINOLOGY

Match the terms on the left with the definitions on the right.

_____ 1. Conversion calculator

_____ 2. Pregnancy EDD calculator

_____ 3. Patient archive

_____ 4. Bulletin board

_____ 5. Productivity center

A. Located in the *Productivity Center,* this feature allows users to place general messages for others in the clinic to see.(LO 10.1)

B. On the main menu this feature is designed to bring the most common functions together in one place.

C. This enables the clinical staff to change imperial units to metric measurements and vice versa.(LO 10.5)

D. This feature allows an administrator to remove a patient from the current list but still retain access to the patient's records.(LO 10.8)

E. In this feature by selecting the LMP date, the program will extrapolate the estimated date of delivery.(LO 10.5)

CHECKING YOUR UNDERSTANDING

Write "T" or "F" in the blank to indicate whether you think the statement is true or false.

_____ 6. The bulletin board feature in SpringCharts will replace the typical bulletin board in the break room and will help the clinic move toward being paperless.(LO 10.1)

_____ 7. InterFax™ allows users to send and receive faxes to and from any company in the world from their Client computer.(LO 10.2)

_____ 8. The outbound fax history status displays only failed transmissions.(LO 10.2)

_____ 9. The time clock feature in SpringCharts is activated by default. No setup is required.(LO 10.3)

_____ 10. The administrator's *Time Clock* window displays the logged in and out time of all users.(LO 10.3)

_____ 11. My Websites is a feature that lists websites intended to provide rapid access to Internet-based knowledge systems.(LO 10.4)

_____ 12. By using the pregnancy EDD calculator you can determine the baby's approximate fetal age.(LO 10.5)

Answer the question below in the space provided.

13. In the productivity center the users have access to one menu where regular administrative activities can be performed such as:

1. _____

2. _____

3. _____

4. _____

Choose the best answer and circle the corresponding letter.

14. The *Universal Export* window enables the user to:(LO 10.9)
    a) Copy data from an Internet clipboard then paste it into another program
    b) Export data as a .hbo file then open it in a text program
    c) Store in a synchronized folder for portable viewing on an Ipod

15. The SpringCharts Help option will give the user access to:(LO 10.10)
    a) A psychiatrist
    b) A tutorial knowledge base
    c) Contact information for the maker of the PC or laptop

16. Data reports can be created based on the list of patients identified by:(LO 10.6)
    a) The patient archive criteria
    b) The encounters criteria in the care tree
    c) The search database criteria

17. One of the options for sending form letters to a list of selected patients from the database is:(LO 10.7)
    a) Mail the letter to patients with e-mail addresses registered in SpringCharts
    b) E-mail patients who have e-mail addresses recorded in SpringCharts and print letters to the others
    c) The program only mails reports to patients

18. SpringCharts users can search the entire database of patient charts for:(LO 10.6)
    a) Medications and allergies
    b) Diagnoses and procedures
    c) Both a and b

19. With the SpringCharts simple calculator users can:(LO 10.5)
    a) Count simple sugar grams for diabetic patients
    b) Process simple algorithms
    c) Have medication dosages broken down into simple compounds

20. If employees fail to login on their time clock at the appropriate time they can:(LO 10.3)
    a) Reset their time clock to the appropriate time
    b) Send a request to the administrator to request a time change
    c) Beg not to be fired

Applying Your Knowledge

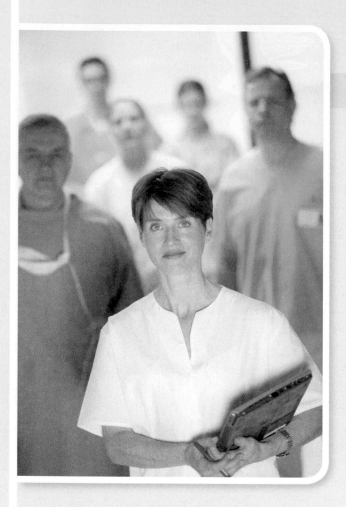

Learning Outcomes

After completing Chapter 11, you
will be able to:

LO 11.1   Successfully function in all aspects of
the SpringCharts program

What You Need to Know

To understand Chapter 11 you will need to
know how to:

- Navigate in the *Practice View* screen
- Navigate in the *Patient Chart* screen
- Navigate in the *Office Visit* screen

A. PRACTICE VIEW SCREEN

1. Office Schedule

Exercise 11.1

1. Let's set up a new patient:
Dustin J. Eatman
6021 Hodges Place
Mansfield, TX 76063
DOB: 10/5/73
SS#: 456-78-2371
Home Phone: (817) 473-0328
Work Phone: (817) 966-2484
Cell Phone: (817) 504-0903
E-mail: dustine@nofencedland.net
Employer: No Fenced Land Company

Dustin is married to Carrie and has two children, Dillon and Emma.
He carries insurance on the family. His assigned doctor is
Dr. Finchman, the family's primary care physician.

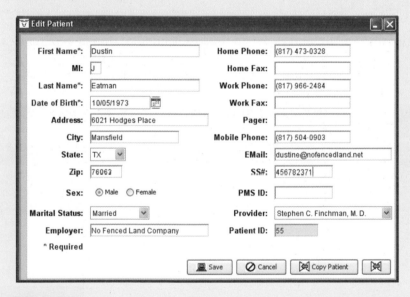

Figure 11.1

2. Let's set up another patient, Dustin's son, Dillon.

Remember, to add family members of the same household you can use
the [Copy Patient] button in a *New Patient* window. Locate *Eatman* and
Dustin's address and home phone will be copied into the new patient
record.

Dillon Eatman was born on October 16, 1998. He does not have an
e-mail address. His Social Security number is: 456-67-9451.

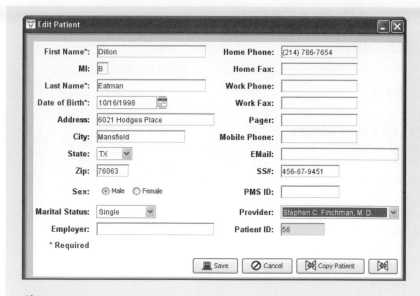

Figure 11.2

Exercise 11.2

1. Add both Dustin and Dillon to today's schedule. Dustin is presenting for a routine well visit and Dillon is presenting for diarrhea.
2. On today's schedule block out the last hour of the day for a staff meeting.

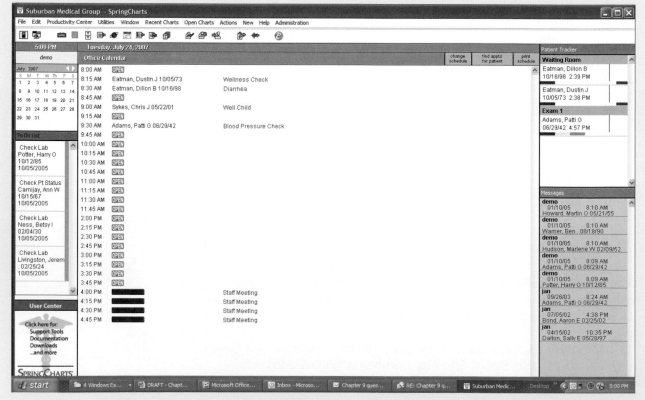

Figure 11.3

3. Dustin indicates on the Sign-in sheet that his cell phone number has changed to (214) 766-8271. Update the patient's record under the *Edit* menu.

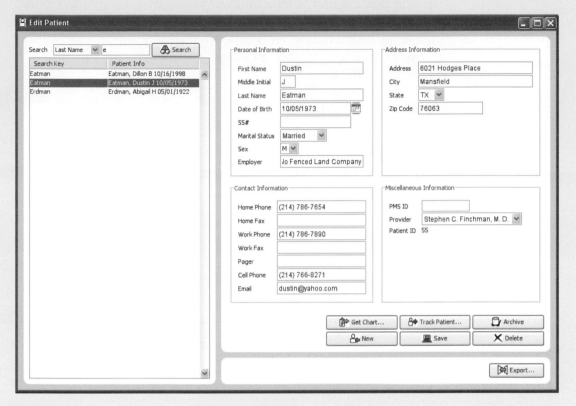

Figure 11.4

2. Patient Tracker

Exercise 11.3

1. Add Dustin and Dillon to the *Waiting Room* in the patient tracker by clicking on their name in the schedule.

2. The clinic has assigned the following *Patient Tracker* colors and their associative usage:

Blue – Dr. Finchman
Yellow – Dr. Smith
Green – Self Pay
Red – Lab Work
Black – Procedures
Fuchsia – Commercial Insurance

Assign Dustin and Dillon the appropriate colors.

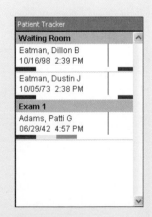

Figure 11.5

Exercise 11.4

1. Add Dustin's and Dillon's following insurance information to the program and the patients' charts.

Insurance Company: Prudential Financial Group
Mail Claim To: NFL Group Claims
Address: PO Box 18974
City: Plano
State: TX
Zip: 56781
Phone: (800) 281-9823
Group Name: NFL Claims
Group Number: 10978NFL
OV Co-Pay: $25
Guarantor: Dustin J. Eatman

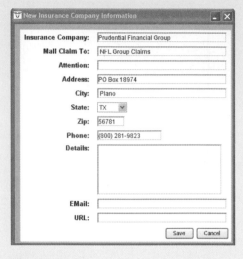

Figure 11.6

Make a note in the *Details* box of Dillon's *Edit Patient Insurance* window: *Insurance Confirmed*.

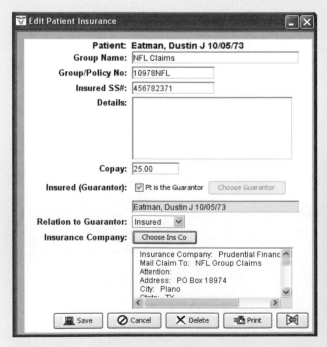

Figure 11.7

Exercise 11.5

1. Set up the patient tracker as the main view.

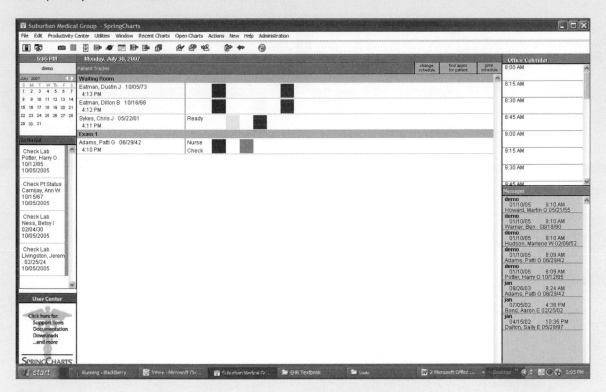

Figure 11.8

2. Move Chris Sykes into exam room 2 and change the status to *Nurse Check*.

3. Add "Doctor Ready" to the *Tracker Status* section of the *Tracker Setup Window* on the *Administration* menu.

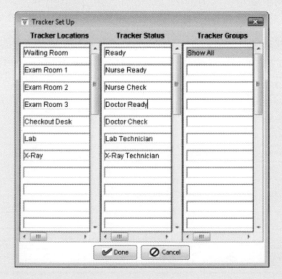

Figure 11.9

4. Close down SpringCharts and restart the program. This will activate the new material added to the *Administration* menu. When SpringCharts reopens, change the status of Patti Adams to *Doctor Ready*.

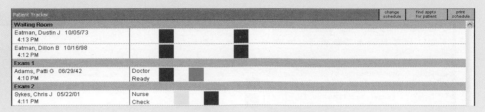

Figure 11.10

3. ToDo List

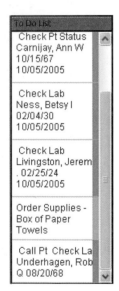

Figure 11.11

Exercise 11.6

1. Send yourself a *ToDo* message to *Order Supplies – Box of Paper Towels*. Use both pop-up text and typing.
2. Send yourself a *ToDo* message to call a patient and check the patient's lab. Use existing pop-up text and link to the patient: Robert Underhagen.

Exercise 11.7

1. Open the *Edit PopUp Text* window and add the sentence: "*Remind patient about scheduled labs*" in the *ToDo/Reminders* category.

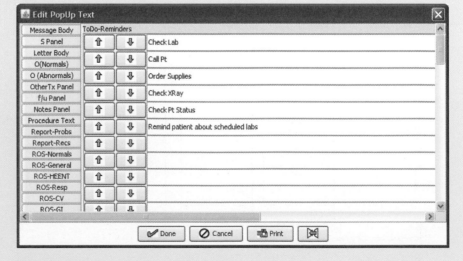

Figure 11.12

2. Send yourself a *ToDo* message to call a patient and remind the patient about scheduled labs. Select the patient: Taylor Jones. Send the *ToDo* item to yourself in two weeks. Check *My ToDo List* and find the future item in the *Edit ToDo* window.

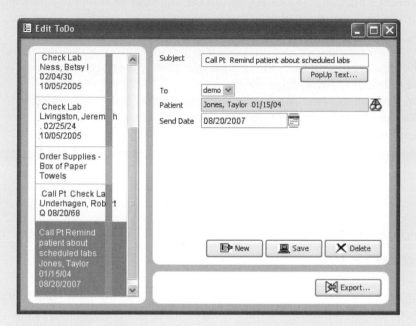

Figure 11.13

4. Message

Exercise 11.8

1. Mr. Dean has called the doctor's office to request some samples of the medication Lipitor. The medical staff is not available so a message is created at the front desk. Open a *New Message* window linked to the patient: Russel Dean. Create pop-up text that indicates that the patient called wanting medication samples. Use the new pop-up text in the body of the message.
2. Mr. Dean had requested some drug samples of Lipitor. From the [Rx] button in the *New Message* window, select Lipitor from the *previous Prescription* list. Save the medication to the note.
3. While you have Mr. Dean on the phone, you notice that you do not have a work phone or a cell phone number for him. Mr. Dean informs you that he is retired but he gives you a mobile phone number: (214) 766-8272 and an e-mail address: russeldean201@aol.com. Update his demographics by selecting the [Pt Info] button. While in the *Edit Patient* window, update the patient records to show Dr. Finchman as his assigned provider.
4. Since you can't log in as the doctor, send the message to yourself.

Exercise 11.9

1. Locate the message regarding Russel Dean in the *Messages*. In the patient's message window change the number of refills on the medication to 0 and the quantity to 15.
2. Add new pop-up text to the *Message Body* category: *OK to give patient sample medication.* Click the [Done] button, and then select the newly created text. Make sure the doctor's response goes on a new line in the message window.
3. On a new line in the message body, time-stamp and initial the note. Click on the [Send Back] button to send the message back to the sender.

Exercise 11.10

1. Select the message in the *Messages* center recently sent back to you from Dr. Finchman.
2. Add the following pop-up text to the *Message Body* category: *Called patient and advised to pick up sample medication.* By using the up and down arrows in the *Edit PopUp Text* window position the new text above the line: *Let Pt know that we are out of samples.*
3. Save and use the new pop-up text on a new line in the message body window.

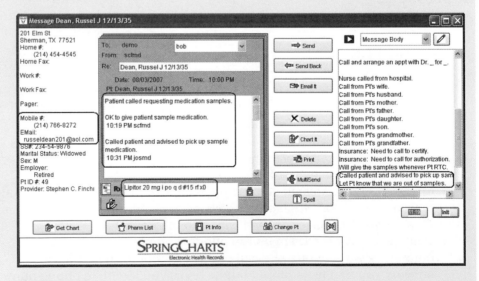

Figure 11.14

4. Time-stamp and initial your note on a new line in the message body window.

5. Using the printer icon below the Rx section of the message window, print a copy of the prescription. Because this prescription is not being sent to the pharmacy, it will not require the doctor's license and DEA number.

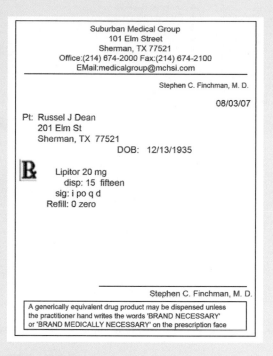

Suburban Medical Group
101 Elm Street
Sherman, TX 77521
Office:(214) 674-2000 Fax:(214) 674-2100
EMail:medicalgroup@mchsi.com

Stephen C. Finchman, M. D.

08/03/07

Pt: Russel J Dean
201 Elm St
Sherman, TX 77521
DOB: 12/13/1935

Lipitor 20 mg
disp: 15 fifteen
sig: i po q d
Refill: 0 zero

Stephen C. Finchman, M. D.

A generically equivalent drug product may be dispensed unless the practitioner hand writes the words 'BRAND NECESSARY' or 'BRAND MEDICALLY NECESSARY' on the prescription face

Figure 11.15

6. Chart the message in the patient's chart. Add to the message heading: *Lipitor Samples*.
7. Open Mr. Dean's chart. Locate the charted message under the *Encounters* category in the care tree. Notice the new prescription in the *Prescription History* of the face sheet.

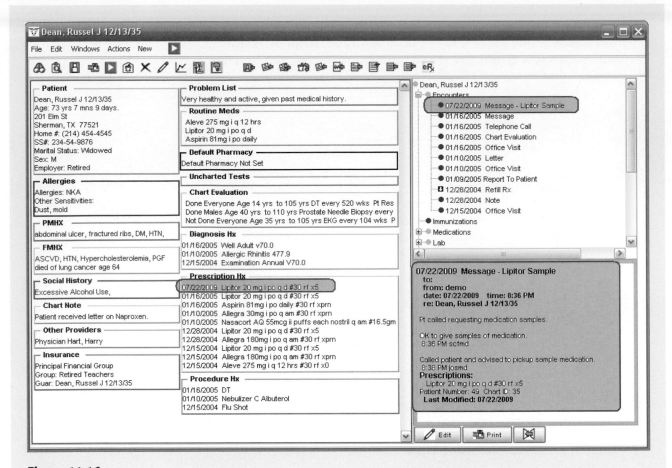

Figure 11.16

B. PATIENT CHART SCREEN

1. Face Sheet

Exercise 11.11

1. Open Dustin Eatman's chart. Open the face sheet window of the chart. Build the following entries in to the face sheet.

Allergies: Mold extracts and latex. In the *Other Sensitivities* window type: *Cat hair,* then select: *causes hives* from the pop-up text list.

Social History: Using the existing *Preferences* list and the *Social Hx* PopUp Text, create the following social history. You will only need to add the occupation by free typing.

Tobacco Use: Nonsmoker.

Alcohol Use: Social Drinker.

Caffeine Use: Yes. Cups Per Day: 4.

Marital Status: Married.

Occupation: Sales.

Education: College.

<u>Past Medical History:</u> Choose asthma and bronchitis from the *Prefer-ences* list. Search for *Fracture of Rib* in the upper *Dx* search window.
<u>Family Medical History:</u> Using the *Preferences* list build the follow-ing family medical history data:
Brother: Heart Disease
Mother: Hypercholesterolemia
Father Died At Age: 59
Cause of Death: Heart Disease
<u>Referred By:</u> This patient was referred by Dr. Able Body.
<u>Chart Note:</u> Click on the edit icon for the pop-up text. In the *Edit PopUp Text* window select the *Chart Note* category and add the following hospitals: *St. Johns Hospital, Cox Medical Centers*, and *Physicians Hospital* – indent each line three spaces. Using the up and down arrows position the new text under the *Prefers Hospital* line. Now move an empty line between the list of hospi-tals and the line *Religion*. Click the space bar to add an invisible character on the empty line. This will create a space between the text lines. Save the material in the *Edit PopUp Text* window. In the face sheet window check your results with Figure 11.18.

Select the text: Prefers hospital

   St. Johns Hospital

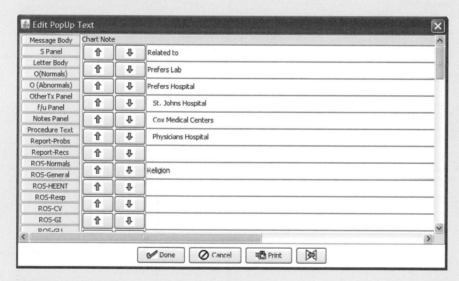

Figure 11.17

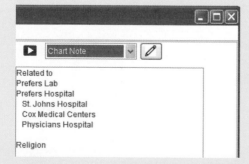

Figure 11.18

Routine Meds: Select the following medications:
    Aleve – 275 mg
    Lipitor – 20 mg
    Aspirin – 81 mg
Edit the Lipitor entry and change the number of refills to 0.
In the *Notes and OTC Meds* window select: *Omega-3*
Problem List: Select *Allergic Rhinitis 477.9* and *Bronchitis 466.0* from the pop-up text list. In the upper *Dx* search area, search for and select *Abdominal Pain*.
Chart Alert: In the *Edit PopUp Text* window select the *Chart Alert* category and add the following sentence: *Insurance approval needed for elective surgery.* Save and select the new text.

    Click on the [Back to Chart] button and check your work with Figure 11.19.

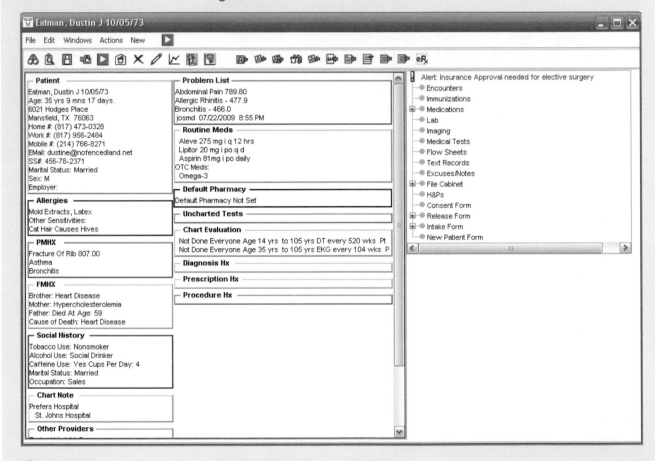

Figure 11.19

2. Patient Chart Activities

Exercise 11.12

1. On the *Patient Tracker* move Mr. Eatman into exam room 3 and change his "status" to *Nurse Check.*

2. Run a Chart Evaluation of Dustin Eatman's chart by accessing the *Evaluate Chart* feature. Record Mr. Eatman's response that he will get a DT shot today. Mark the recommendation as "Completed." You will not be recommending the EKG today so you will **not** check the radio button *Mark this 'Completed.'* Save the evaluation. Check your results in the patient's chart under the *Encounter* tab in the Care Tree.

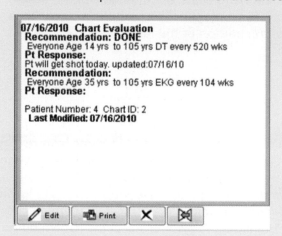

07/16/2010 Chart Evaluation
Recommendation: DONE
 Everyone Age 14 yrs to 105 yrs DT every 520 wks
Pt Response:
Pt will get shot today. updated:07/16/10
Recommendation:
 Everyone Age 35 yrs to 105 yrs EKG every 104 wks
Pt Response:

Patient Number: 4 Chart ID: 2
 Last Modified: 07/16/2010

✏ Edit   🖶 Print   ✕   ⋈

Figure 11.20

Exercise 11.13

Check the *Household List* located in the *File* menu of Mr. Eatman's chart. This list will provide access to the other patient charts of the same household.

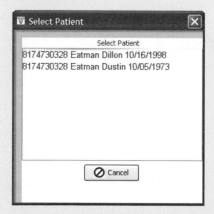

Select Patient
    Select Patient
8174730328 Eatman Dillon 10/16/1998
8174730328 Eatman Dustin 10/05/1973

⊘ Cancel

Figure 11.21

Exercise 11.14

The following pharmacy normally used by Mr. Eatman will need to be added to SpringCharts' address book.

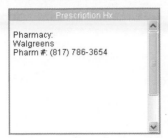

Figure 11.22

Walgreens Pharmacy
Crn Campbell Av. & Battlefield St.
Mansfield, TX 76063
Ph: (817) 786-3654
Fx: (817) 786-9785

Under the *Edit* menu in Mr. Eatman's chart, add this new pharmacy as the patient default pharmacy. The patient's preferred pharmacy will be displayed in the *Prescription Hx* portion of the face sheet.

Exercise 11.15

1. Add Dustin's photo to his chart by accessing the *Pt Photo* feature under the *Edit* menu. Select the [Edit] button in the *Photo* window and click the [OK] button in the *Picture Size* window. Direct your research in the *Open* dialogue window through the *"Desktop"* access to locate the folder titled: *EHR Material.* Double-click on this folder and locate the file: *Dustin's Photo.* Highlight the file and select the [Open] button. Now select the [Done] button back in the *Photo* window.
2. Click on the *Pt Photo* category in the patient's care tree to view Mr. Eatman's photo below.

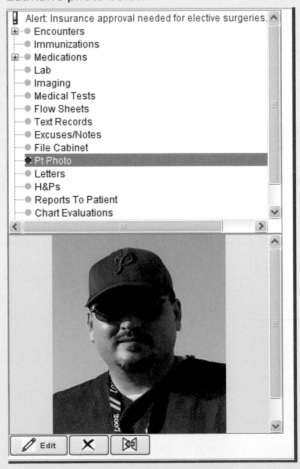

Figure 11.23

Exercise 11.16

1. Mr. Russel Dean has called on the telephone and has requested a list of medications prescribed for him at your office. By using both pop-up text and typing record the details of the conversation by accessing the *New TC Note* under the *New* menu in Mr. Dean's chart. Initial- and time-stamp the note by using the [Sign] button. Save the telephone note and skip billing.

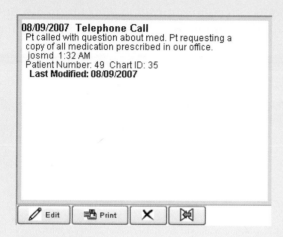

Figure 11.24

2. In Mr. Dean's chart print out the list of all medications prescribed to him by accessing the *Medications List* under the *Actions* menu.

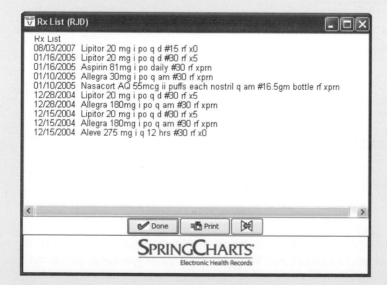

Figure 11.25

Exercise 11.17

1. Open a *New Nurse Note* under the *New* menu of Mr. Eatman's chart. Choose a *Well Adult* diagnosis and record the inoculation of a DT shot. You will need to select the *Immunization* category under the *Choose Procedure* window to locate the DT procedure. Once selected, click on the DT procedure and change the procedure detail to lot number 2695A. Add your initials and time by selecting the [Sign] button. Save the nurse note under the *Encounters* tab and send a routing slip.

2. In the *Routing Slip* window select *Immunization 90471* from the *Superbill Form* for the administration of the injection. Send the routing slip. Check the details of the *Nurse Note* in the patient's chart.

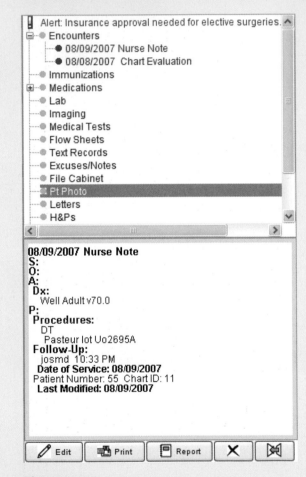

Figure 11.26

Exercise 11.18

Open Patti Adam's chart. Patti is diabetic and she comes into the clinic on a regular basis to have her vitals taken. Under the *New* menu in her chart complete a *Vitals Only* panel. Mrs. Adams is 5 ft 4 in, and weighs

156 pounds. You can complete the other vitals yourself. Remember BMI is calculated automatically from the height and weight. Head circumference (HC) is only used in a pediatric situation for head growth of infants. By using pop-up text found under the *Notes* tab indicate that Mrs. Adams' blood pressure was taken on her right arm. Save the new vitals under the *Encounter* tab and skip billing.

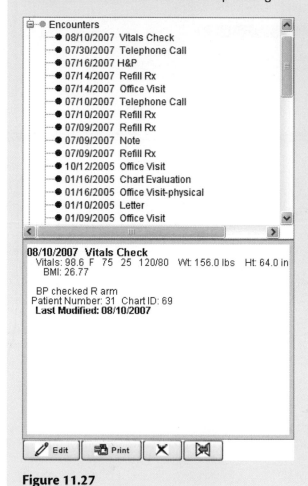

Figure 11.27

C. OFFICE VISIT SCREEN

1. Office Visit Note

Exercise 11.19

1. In Dustin Eatman's chart open a *New OV* window under the *New* menu. Mr. Eatman has come to the doctor's office for his annual well checkup. Under the chief complaint (CC) navigation button select: *Routine Well Visit*. Using the time and initial icon buttons in the lower middle of the OV screen, time- and initial-stamp the chief

complaint note. Under the [Vitals] button complete the well vitals for Mr. Eatman.

2. Save the office visit under the encounter tab and skip billing. Close Mr. Eatman's chart and update the patient's status on the Patient tracker to "Doctor Ready."

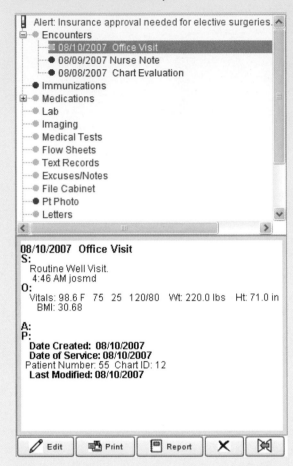

Figure 11.28

Exercise 11.20

1. Reopen the patient's chart and highlight the partially completed office visit note. Click on the [Edit] button to open the *Office Visit* screen.
2. Under the review of systems (ROS) navigation button select the following:
ROS-Normal:
GENERAL: No weight change, fever, chills, night sweats, generalized weakness.

HEENT: No headache, dizziness, lightheadedness, diplopia, tearing, eye pain, blind spots, excessive blinking, tinnitus, ear pain or discharge, nose bleeding, nasal obstruction, nasal discharge, gingival bleeding, dental problem, sore throat, hoarseness, difficulty swallowing, neck stiffness, neck pain.

PULMONARY: No wheezing, cough, congestion, hemoptysis, respiratory infections, tuberculosis, chest wall pain.

CV: No chest pain, arrhythmia, syncope, dyspnea, exertional dyspnea, orthopnea, paroxysmal nocturnal dyspnea, intermittent claudication, dependent edema, varicose vein, phlebitis, heart murmur, hypertension.

GI: No change in appetite, difficulty swallowing, indigestion, heartburn, belching, nausea, vomiting, hematemesis, hematochezia, abdomen pain, flatulence, changes in bowel habits, constipation, diarrhea, abnormal stools, incontinence, hemorrhoids, jaundice.

3. Under the [Exam] button select the following pop-up text:
GENERAL: Well developed. Well nourished. Alert. Oriented to person, place, and time. In no apparent distress.

HEAD: Normocephalic. Atraumatic.

EYES: Eyes and lids appear symmetrical. No exudate. Sclera clear. PERRLA, EOMI. Discs sharp.

EARS: External auditory canals and TMs normal. Hearing normal as tested by whisper and Rinne/Weber.

MOUTH/THROAT: Dentition good. Normal mucosa, tongue, gingiva, and oropharynx. Palate elevates in midline. No thrush, erythema, or exudate.

CV: RRR, normal S1 S2, no S3/S4, murmur, gallop, rub, arrhythmia, or heave. PMI normal in location and character.

ABDOMEN: Bowel sounds are normal. No evidence of scarring or past surgical procedures. Abdomen is flat, soft, and nontender, without rebound or guarding. No evidence of masses, organomegaly, or abdominal aneurysm. Normal to percussion.

MUSCULOSKELETAL: Posture normal. Pulses normal and symmetrical. Motor strength normal. Sensory normal and symmetrical to soft touch and pin prick. Joints show normal range of motion and are without erythema or effusions. Nails: Normal capillary filling and appearance w/o clubbing or pitting. No masses or dependent edema noted.

RECTAL: No mass palpable. Prostate normal in size, shape, and consistency for age. Guaiac negative.

4. Select the [Dx] button and choose the *Well Adult* code from the *Previous Diagnosis* window.

5. Order a CBC and a SMAC under the [Test] button. Because these tests will be conducted at an outside testing facility you will want to print a physician's order form and save a copy in the patient's chart under the *Notes* category in the care tree. Add the patient's primary insurance to the order form. Print the order form and compare with Figure 11.29.

6. The doctor decides to give Mr. Eatman a flu shot during the office visit because of the upcoming flu season. Under the procedure button type: *flu,* search for and select flu shot. Highlight the flu shot

Suburban Medical Group
101 Elm Street
Sherman, TX 77521
(214) 674-2000   Fax (214) 674-2100

Date: 08/10/07
Pt: Eatman, Dustin J 10/05/73
Address: 6021 Hodges Place   Mansfield, TX 76063

Physician Order

Orders:
CBC 85025
SMAC 80054

Diagnosis:
Well Adult v70.0

_____

Patient Insurance Info
Group Name: NFL Claims
Group/Policy No: 10978NFL
Guarantor: Eatman, Dustin J 10/05/73
Certif No: 456782371
Insured
CoPay: 25.0

Insurance Company: Prudential Financial Group
Mail Claim To: NFL Group Claims
Attention:
Address: PO Box 18974
City: Plano
State: TX
Zip: 56781
Phone: 8002819823
Details:
EMail:
URL:

Prepared by
SpringChartsEMR

Suburban Medical Group

Figure 11.29

procedure and change the Aventis Pasteur number to UO701BA, and the vaccine date to today's date, for example, 30JUNE08. Date-, time-, and initial-stamp the procedure note.

7. Under the [Other Tx] button select the counseling notes: *Discussed weight loss strategies. Encouraged pt to exercise 30 minutes 5 times a week.*

8. Plan a follow-up for 1 year. Select the *Create a Reminder* icon and send a *ToDo/Reminder* note to Jan to call the patient and check the lab work (use pop-up text). Send it to her so that she will receive it in 3 business days.

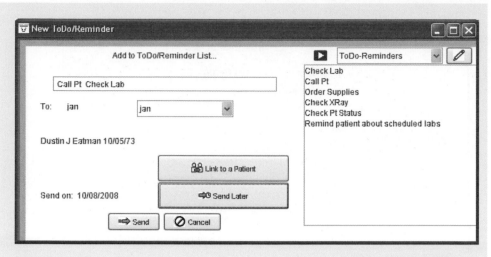

Figure 11.30

9. Save the office visit note and create a routing slip. From the superbill form select the CPT code 90472 because of the additional inoculation that was done. (These additional codes are added to the routing slip at this time rather than in the OV note because they are essential for billing purposes, even though they are not critical to the note.) Depending of whether you did Exercise 11.17 (the nurse note) on the same day or a different day from this exercise, the E&M coder will recommend either a new or established patient visit E&M code. Let us assume this office visit note was created on the same day as the nurse note. If the E&M coder recommendation is not for a new patient you will need to choose the appropriate E&M code for a new patient from the drop down list at the bottom of the routing slip. Send the routing slip.

10. Under the main *Edit* menu locate the routing slip just generated. Print the routing slip. Compare your results with Figure 11.31.

11. Print the routing slip.

Suburban Medical Group
101 Elm Street
Sherman, TX 77521
(214) 674-2000   Fax (214) 674-2100

Eatman, Dustin J 10/05/73
6021 Hodges Place
Mansfield, TX 76063
Home #: (817) 473-0328   Home Fax:
Work #: (817) 966-2484   Work Fax:
Pager: Mobile #: (214) 766-8271
EMail: dustine@nofencedland.net
SS#: 456-78-2371   Marital Status: Married
Sex: M   Pt ID #: 55
Employer: No Fenced Land Company

Date of Service: 08/10/2007
Doctor: Stephen C. Finchman, M. D.   Patient Insurance Info
    99205 NP-Comprehensive   Group Name: NFL Claims
Diagnosis: Group/Policy No: 10978NFL
    Well Adult v70.0   Guarantor: Eatman, Dustin J 10/05/73
Tests: Certif No: 456782371
    CBC 85025   Insured
    SMAC 80054   CoPay: 25.0
Other Procedures:
    Immunization 90471   Insurance Company: Prudential Financial Group
    additional Immunization 90472   Mail Claim To: NFL Group Claims
    Venipuncture 36415   Attention:
                                                Address: PO Box 18974
    Flu Shot 90658   City: Plano
Discussed weight loss strategies. Encouraged   State: TX
pt to exercise 30 minutes 5 times a week.   Zip: 56781
    Followup: Phone: 8002819823
    1 year   Details:
                                                EMail:
                                                URL:

prepared by
gChartsEMR

Figure 11.31

2. Office Visit Activities

Exercise 11.21

In Mr. Eatman's chart print a copy of the recent office visit note.

Suburban Medical Group
101 Elm Street Sherman, TX 77521
(214) 674-2000

08/10/2007 Office Visit
S:

CC:Routine Well Visit.
4:46 AM josmd
PI: Routine Well Visit.
ROS: ROS-Normal:
GENERAL: No weight change, fever, chills, night sweats, generalized weakness.
HEENT: No headache, dizziness, lightheadedness, diplopia, tearing, eye pain, blind spots, excessive blinking, tinnitus, ear pain or discharge, nose bleeding, nasal obstruction, nasal discharge, gingival bleeding, dental problem, sore throat, hoarseness, difficulty swallowing, neck stiffness, neck pain.
PULMONARY: No wheezing, cough, congestion, hemoptysis, respiratory infections, tuberculosis, chest wall pain.
CV: No chest pain, arrhythmia, syncope, dyspnea, exertional dyspnea, orthopnea, paroxysmal nocturnal dyspnea, intermittent claudication, dependent edema, varicose vein, phlebitis, heart murmur, hypertension.
GI: No change in appetite, difficulty swallowing, indigestion, heartburn, belching, nausea, vomiting, hematemesis, hematochezia, abdomen pain, flatulence, changes in bowel habits, constipation, diarrhea, abnormal stools, incontinence, hemorrhoids, jaundice.

O:

Vitals: 98.6 F   75   25   120/80   Wt: 220.0 lbs   Ht: 71.0 in
BMI: 30.68

GENERAL: Well developed. Well nourished. Alert. Oriented to person, place, and time. In no apparent distress.
HEAD: Normocephalic. Atraumatic.
EYES: Eyes and lids appear symmetrical. No exudate. Sclera clear. PERRLA, EOMI. Discs sharp.
EARS: External auditory canals and TMs normal. Hearing normal as tested by whisper and Rinne/Weber.
MOUTH/THROAT: Dentition good. Normal mucosa, tongue, gingiva, and oropharynx. Palate elevates in midline. No thrush, erythema, or exudate.
CV: RRR, normal S1 S2, no S3/S4, murmur, gallop, rub, arrhythmia, or heave. PMI normal in location and character.
ABDOMEN: Bowel sounds are normal. No evidence of scarring or past surgical procedures. Abdomen is flat, soft, and nontender, without rebound or guarding. No evidence of masses, organomegaly or abdominal aneurysm. Normal to percussion.
MUSCULOSKELETAL: Posture normal. Pulses normal and symmetrical. Motor strength normal. Sensory normal and symmetrical to soft touch and pin prick. Joints show normal range of motion and are without erythema or effusions. Nails: Normal capillary filling and appearance w/o clubbing or pitting. No masses or dependent edema noted.
GU (male): RECTAL: No mass palpable. Prostate normal in size, shape, and consistency for age. Guiaic negative.

A:
Dx:

Well Adult v70.0

P:

Patient: Eatman, Dustin J 10/05/73   Page 1 of 2
Prepared by
SpringChartsEMR   Suburban Medical Group

Figure 11.32a

Tests:
   CBC
   SMAC
Procedures:
   Flu Shot
      Aventis Pasteur UO701BA x 30JUNE08 Fluzone
      0.5 IM
      08/10/2007 5:38 AM josmd
Other Tx:
   Discussed weight loss strategies. Encouraged pt to exercise 30 minutes 5 times a week.
Follow-Up:
   1 year
   Date Created: 08/10/2007
   Date of Service: 08/10/2007
Patient Number: no Patient reference Chart ID: not Charted
   Last Modified: 08/10/2007

Patient: Eatman, Dustin J 10/05/73

Prepared by
SpringChartsEMR

Page 2 of 2
Suburban Medical Group

Figure 11.32b

Exercise 11.22

1. Mr. Eatman is requesting a history and physical report of his medical encounter to take with him. Open the current office visit note and select the H&P report from the *Tools* menu.
2. Print the report. Save the H&P report under the *H&Ps* category in the care tree. Close the *Office Visit* screen.

History and Physical
  Patient: Eatman, Dustin J 10/05/73
  Date of Service: 08/10/2007
Chief Complaint:
  Routine Well Visit. 4:46 AM josmd
Present Illness:
  Routine Well Visit.
Allergies:
  Mold Extracts, Latex
  Cat Hair causes hives
Current Medications:
  Aleve 275 mg i q 12 hrs
  Lipitor 20 mg i po q d
  Aspirin 81mg i po daily
  Omega-3
Past Medical History:
  Fracture Of Rib
  Asthma Bronchitis
Family Medical History:
  Brother: Heart Disease Mother: Hypercholesterolemia Father Died At Age: 59
  Cause Of Death: Heart Disease
Social History:
  Tobacco Use: Nonsmoker. Alcohol Use: Social Drinker. Caffeine Use: Yes. Cups
  Per Day: 4 Marital Status: Married. Occupation: Sales Education: College.
Review Of Systems:
  ROS-Normal: GENERAL: No weight change, fever, chills, night sweats,
  generalized weakness. HEENT: No headache, dizziness, lightheadedness,
  diplopia, tearing, eye pain, blind spots, excessive blinking, tinnitus, ear pain or
  discharge, nose bleeding, nasal obstruction, nasal discharge, gingival bleeding,
  dental problem, sore throat, hoarseness, difficulty swallowing, neck stiffness, neck
  pain. PULMONARY: No wheezing, cough, congestion, hemoptysis, respiratory
  infections, tuberculosis, chest wall pain. CV: No chest pain, arrhythmia, syncope,
  dyspnea, exertional dyspnea, orthopnea, paroxysmal nocturnal dyspnea,
  intermittent claudication, dependent edema, varicose vein, phlebitis, heart
  murmur, hypertension. GI: No change in appetite, difficulty swallowing, indigestion,
  heartburn, belching, nausea, vomiting, hematemesis, hematochezia, abdomen
  pain, flatulence, changes in bowel habits, constipation, diarrhea, abnormal stools,
  incontinence, hemorrhoids, jaundice.
Examination:
  Vitals: Temp: 98.6 Pulse: 75 Resp: 25 BP: 120/80 Wt: 220.0 Ht: 71.0
  GENERAL: Well developed. Well nourished. Alert. Oriented to person, place, and
  time. In no apparent distress. HEAD: Normocephalic. Atraumatic. EYES: Eyes and
  lids appear symmetrical. No exudate. Sclera clear. PERRLA, EOMI. Discs sharp.
  EARS: External auditory canals and TMs normal. Hearing normal as tested by

Suburban Medical Group
H&P for Pt: Eatman, Dustin J 10/05/73   Page 1 of 2

Figure 11.33a

whisper and Rinne/Weber. MOUTH/THROAT: Dentition good. Normal mucosa, tongue, gingiva, and oropharynx. Palate elevates in midline. No thrush, erythema, or exudate. CV: RRR, normal S1 S2, no S3/S4, murmur, gallop, rub, arrhythmia, or heave. PMI normal in location and character. ABDOMEN: Bowel sounds are normal. No evidence of scarring or past surgical procedures. Abdomen is flat, soft, and nontender, without rebound or guarding. No evidence of masses, organomegaly or abdominal aneurysm. Normal to percussion. MUSCULOSKELETAL: Posture normal. Pulses normal and symmetrical. Motor strength normal. Sensory normal and symmetrical to soft touch and pin prick. Joints show normal range of motion and are without erythema or effusions. Nails: Normal capillary filling and appearance w/o clubbing or pitting. No masses or dependent edema noted. GU (male): RECTAL: No mass palpable. Prostate normal in size, shape, and consistency for age. Guiaic negative.
Tests:
CBC pending
SMAC pending
Flu Shot
Aventis Pasteur UO701BA x 30JUNE08 Fluzone 0.5 IM 08/10/2007 5:38 AM josmd
Impression:
Well Adult v70.0
Plan:
Discussed weight loss strategies. Encouraged pt to exercise 30 minutes 5 times a week.
1 year

John O. Smith, M. D.

Suburban Medical Group
H&P for Pt: Eatman, Dustin J 10/05/73   Page 2 of 2

Figure 11.33b

2. Close Dustin Eatman's chart. Update the patient tracker to reflect Mr. Eatman being sent to the *Checkout Desk* with a status of *Ready*. Save the *Edit Tracker* window. Reopen it and click on the [CheckOut] button. The patient tracker will show Dustin Eatman in the "Done" section with the *Routing Slip* stamp.

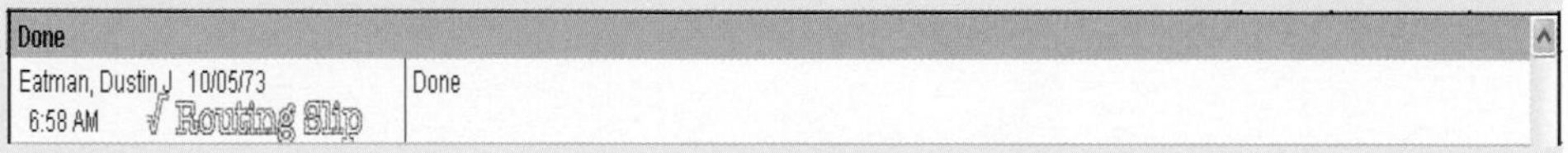

Done	
Eatman, Dustin J 10/05/73 6:58 AM √ Routing Slip	Done

Figure 11.34

12

Electronic Recording

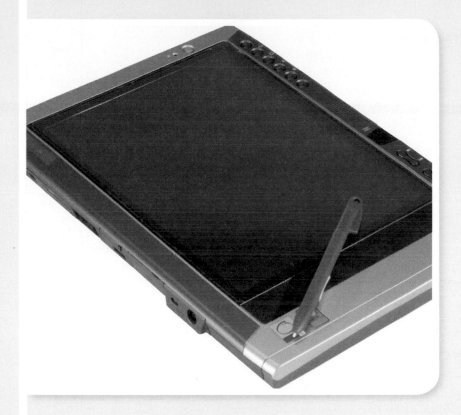

What You Need to Know

To understand Chapter 12 you will need to know how to:

- Navigate in the *Practice View* screen
- Navigate in the *Patient Chart* screen
- Navigate in the *Office Visit* screen

Learning Outcomes

After completing Chapter 12, you will be able to:

LO 12.1 Successfully function in all major aspects of SpringCharts

Exercise 12.1

Using *Source Document 1—Patient Information Sheet (See Appendix B, page 278)*, complete a *New Patient* profile. Click on the *Universal Export* button and Open in Word Processor. Print patient's information.

Exercise 12.2

Using *Source Document 2—Primary Insurance Card Information (See Appendix B, page 279)*, set up a new insurance company in SpringCharts. Save the new company. Click on the *Universal Export* button and Open in Word Processor. Print insurance information.

Exercise 12.3

Using *Source Document 2—Primary Insurance Card Information (See Appendix B, page 279)*, add the primary insurance details to the patient's Face Sheet. Print out the patient's primary insurance information and submit to your instructor.

Exercise 12.4

Using *Source Document 3—Patient Intake Sheet (See Appendix B, page 280)*, add a new doctor's address entry to SpringCharts' address book. Print the address card and submit to your instructor.

Exercise 12.5

Using *Source Document 3—Patient Intake Sheet (See Appendix B, page 280)*, complete the face sheet of the patient's chart. Print the face sheet and submit to your instructor.

Exercise 12.6

Using *Source Document 4—Default Pharmacy Information (See Appendix B, page 281)*, add a new address entry to the Address Book in SpringCharts. Click the [Print Card] button and submit the pharmacy information to your instructor.

Exercise 12.7

Using *Source Document 4—Default Pharmacy Information (See Appendix B, page 281)*, set up the patient's default pharmacy.

Exercise 12.8

Import the patient's photo into the patient's chart through the chart's *Edit* menu. Remember to access this material through the *"Desktop"* and locate the folder titled: *EHR Material*.

Exercise 12.9

Using *Source Document 5—Immunization Record Card (See Appendix B, page 281)*, update the patient's immunization archive in the patient's chart. View the immunizations and print the record. Submit to your instructor.

Exercise 12.10

In the patient's chart perform a Chart Evaluation and record the patient's agreement to have the indicated items conducted.

Exercise 12.11

Using *Source Document 6—Office Visit Notes (See Appendix B, page 282)*, record the notation into a *New OV* window in the patient's chart. Complete Exercises 12.12 and 12.13 from within the OV note. Create a Routing Slip. Go to the *Edit* menu. Locate *Routing Slips* and print the routing slip. Submit to your instructor.

Exercise 12.12

Create a *Prescription Form* from within the OV note for the medication prescribed to the patient. Print the script and submit to your instructor.

Exercise 12.13

Create a *Order Form* from within the OV note for the tests that are ordered. Print order form and submit to your instructor.

Exercise 12.14

Using *Source Document 7—Patient Excuse Note (See Appendix B, page 283)*, create an excuse note for the patient within the patient's chart. Print excuse note and submit to your instructor.

Exercise 12.15

Using *Source Document 8—Letter to Primary Care Physician (See Appendix B, page 284)*, create a letter about the patient in the patient's chart. Save it under the *Letter* category. Print letter and submit to your instructor.

Exercise 12.16

Using *Source Document 9—Letter to Patient (See Appendix B, page 285)*, create a letter to the patient in the patient's chart. Save it under the *Letter* category. Print letter and submit to your instructor.

Exercise 12.17

Using *Source Document 10—Patient Lab Results (See Appendix B, page 286)*, record the lab results into the patient's *Pending Test*. Process the *Pending Test* into the *Completed Tests* area from where you will save it into the patient's chart. From the patient's chart print the lab results and submit to your instructor.

Exercise 12.18

Create a *New Test Report* from within the patient's chart. Remove the *Problems* and *Recommendations* headings from the report. Print the test report and submit to your instructor.

appendix A

Sample Documents

Sample 1   Prescription Forms

Suburban Medical Group
101 Elm Street
Sherman, TX 77521
Office:(214) 674-2000 Fax:(214) 674-2100
EMail:doc@sfischermd.com

John O. Smith, M. D.
Lic: J87877   DEA: AJ3434343
11/27/06

Pt: Patti G Adams
     198 Elm St
     Sherman, TX 77521
                    DOB: 06/29/1942

    Allegra 180mg
            disp: 30 thirty
            sig: i po q am
        Refill: prn

John O. Smith, M. D.
**** Electronic Signature Verified ****

John O. Smith, M. D.

A generically equivalent drug product may be dispensed unless
the practitioner hand writes the words 'BRAND NECESSARY'
or 'BRAND MEDICALLY NECESSARY' on the prescription face

Suburban Medical Group
101 Elm Street
Sherman, TX 77521
Office:(214) 674-2000 Fax:(214) 674-2100
EMail:doc@sfischermd.com

John O. Smith, M. D.
Lic: J87877   DEA: AJ3434343
11/27/06

Pt: Patti G Adams
     198 Elm St
     Sherman, TX 77521
                    DOB: 06/29/1942

Rx   Tamiflu 75mg
            disp: 10 ten
            sig: i po bid
        Refill: 0 zero

John O. Smith, M. D.
**** Electronic Signature Verified ****

John O. Smith, M. D.

A generically equivalent drug product may be dispensed unless
the practitioner hand writes the words 'BRAND NECESSARY'
or 'BRAND MEDICALLY NECESSARY' on the prescription face

Suburban Medical Group
101 Elm Street
Sherman, TX 77521
Office:(214) 674-2000 Fax:(214) 674-2100
EMail:doc@sfischermd.com

John O. Smith, M. D.
Lic: J87877   DEA: AJ3434343
11/27/06

Pt: Patti G Adams
     198 Elm St
     Sherman, TX 77521
                    DOB: 06/29/1942

Rx   Ibuprofen 400mg
            disp: 120 one hundred twenty
            sig: i po q 6 hr
        Refill: 5 five

John O. Smith, M. D.
**** Electronic Signature Verified ****

John O. Smith, M. D.

A generically equivalent drug product may be dispensed unless
the practitioner hand writes the words 'BRAND NECESSARY'
or 'BRAND MEDICALLY NECESSARY' on the prescription face

Sample 2   Selected Items from Patient's Chart

Suburban Medical Group
101 Elm Street Sherman, TX 77521
(214) 674-2000

04/28/2003 Office Visit
   S:
      Needs medications refilled. Follow-Up.
   O:
      Vitals: 97.5 F   80   14   130/74   Wt: 180.0 lbs   Ht: 64.0 in
       BMI: 30.89

      EAC/TM's nl. Pharynx nl. Neck supple s adenopathy. Thyroid normal to palpation. Chest
      clear to auscultation. Heart rrr s m or g. Abdomen: BS nl. nontender no organomegaly or
      masses. Extremities: pulses symmetrical UE and LE's. motor strength normal extrem x 4.
      cap refill < 2 sec extrem x 4. Neurological: CN II - XII nl. DTR's symm no sens defects. Gait
      nl.
   A:
    Dx:
      HTN 401.9
      DM, Adult Onset,NID, Controlled 250.00
      Hypercholesterolemia 272.0
   P:
    Rx:
      Diovan 80mg i po q am #30 rf x3
      Glucophage XR 500mg i po bid #60 rf xprn
      Lipitor 10mg i po q am #30 rf x5
    Tests:
      CBC
      SMAC
      Lipid Panel
      HGBA1C
    Procedures:
      Ear Irrigation

    Other Tx:
      ref to ophth for yearly checkup
    Follow-Up:
      3 months.
      ***** Graphic *****
      Date Created: 04/26/2003
      Date of Service: 04/28/2003
    Patient Number: 31 Chart ID: 12
      Last Modified: 11/22/2006

04/26/2003 CBC
      WBC   6.0
       Normal:4.0-12.0 k/ml
      RBC   5.0   Normal:4.0-5.3 m/ml
      HGB   13.0
       Normal:11.5-14.5 g/dl

Patient: Adams, Patti G 06/29/42

HCT	39.0	Normal:33.0-43.0 %
MCV	85.0	Normal:76.0-90.0 fl
MCH	30.0	Normal:25.0-31.0 pg
MCHC	34.0	
Normal:32.0-36.0 g/dl		
RDW	12.0	Normal:11.5-15.0 %
Platelet	200.0	
Normal:150.0-450.0 k/ml		
Neutrophils	45.0	Normal:34.0-56.0 %
Bands	0.0	Normal:0.0-5.0 %
Lymphocytes	39.0	Normal:28.0-65.0 %
Monocytes	2.0	Normal:1.7-9.3 %
Eosinophils	0.0	Normal:0.0-6.0 %
Basophils	0.0	Normal:0.0-2.0 %

Note:
Tech: scfmd
ID#:
Test Facility:
Reported: 04/26/2003 Last Modified: 04/26/2003

04/26/2003 SMAC

Glucose	112.0	
Normal:70.0-125.0 mg/dl		
BUN	14.0	
Normal:7.0-30.0 mg/dl		
Creatinine	1.0	
Normal:0.5-1.4 mg/dl		
Sodium	140.0	
Normal:135.0-146.0 meq/l		
Potassium	4.0	
Normal:3.5-5.3 meq/l		
Chloride	100.0	
Normal:95.0-108.0 meq/l		
CO2	20.0	Normal:18.0-26.0
Calcium	9.8	
Normal:8.5-10.3 mg/dl		
Total Protein	7.0	Normal:5.8-8.1 g/dl
Albumin	4.0	Normal:3.2-5.0 g/dl
Globulin	4.0	Normal:2.2-4.2 g/dl
Total Bilirubin	1.0	
Normal:0.0-1.3 mg/dl		
Alkaline Phosphotase	45.0	Normal:20.0-125.0 u/l
AST (SGOT)	25.0	Normal:0.0-55.0 u/l
ALT (SGPT)	20.0	Normal:0.0-48.0 u/l

Note:
Tech: scfmd
ID#:
Test Facility:
Reported: 04/26/2003 Last Modified: 04/26/2003

Patient: Adams, Patti G 06/29/42

Sample 3   Patient's Face Sheet

Suburban Medical Group
101 Elm Street Sherman, TX 77521
(214) 674-2000

Name: Patti G Adams 06/29/42
Address: 198 Elm St Sherman, TX 77521
Home Phone: (214) 766-7676
Home Fax:
Work Phone:
Work Fax:
Pager:
Mobile Phone: (214) 777-7987
EMail: mom5645566@aol.com
SS#: 876-45-6676
Marital Status: Married
Sex: F
Pt ID #: 31
Employer: Home Engineer
Date Entered: 04/02/2002
Last Modified: 04/02/2002
Allergies:
Codeine   entered 04/26/2003 1507:39 PM   by demo note:
Patient Number: 31 Chart ID: 3
Last Modified: 11/18/2006
Other Sensitivities
erythromycin causes nausea
Patient Number: 31 Chart ID: 4
Last Modified: 04/26/2003
Social History
Tobacco Use: Moderate Smoker
Alcohol Use: Social Drinker
Patient Number: 31 Chart ID: 11
Last Modified: 11/27/2006
PMHX
HTN 401.9
DM, Adult Onset,NID, Controlled 250.00
HTN 401.9
cholecystectomy 1998, TAH BSO 1999
Patient Number: 31 Chart ID: 5
Last Modified: 12/15/2004
FMHX
HTN 401.9
F died of MI age 48. PGF died of MI age 53.
Patient Number: 31 Chart ID: 6
Last Modified: 04/26/2003
Problem List
Dx:

Patient: Adams, Patti G 06/29/42

Page 1 of 2

Prepared by
SpringChartsEMR

Suburban Medical Group

HTN 401.9
DM, Adult Onset,NID, Controlled 250.00
Hypercholesterolemia 272.0

Patient Number: 31 Chart ID: 7
Last Modified: 04/26/2003

Routine Meds

Diovan 80mg i po q am
Glucophage XR 500mg i po bid
Lipitor 10mg i po q am
Aleve 275 mg i q 12 hrs
Aspirin 325mg ii po qid prn

OTC Meds:

fish oil, glucosamine
Patient Number: 31 Chart ID: 8
Last Modified: 01/16/2005

Referring Dr:

Physician Body, Able
Patient Number: 31 Chart ID: 9
Last Modified: 04/26/2003

Chart Notes

Friend of Mrs Bibi.
Received informational letter on Naproxen.
Patient Number: 31 Chart ID: 10
Last Modified: 01/16/2005

Patient Insurance Info

Group Name: Retired Teachers Association
Group/Policy No: 78329
Certif No: 876456676
Insured's relation to patient: Insured
CoPay: 10.0

Patient: Adams, Patti G 06/29/42

Prepared by
SpringChartsEMR

Page 2 of 2

Suburban Medical Group

Sample 4   Printed Immunization Record

Suburban Medical Group
101 Elm Street
Sherman, TX 77521
(214) 674-2000   Fax (214) 674-2100

Immunizations for Sykes, Chris J 05/22/01
DPT 04/08/2002
MMR 04/08/2002
HepatitisB 02/15/2002
HepatitisB 04/17/2002
DaPT 03/15/2002
HFlu 03/15/2002
IPV 03/15/2002
Pneumococcus 05/18/2002
HFlu 05/18/2002
IPV 05/18/2002
DaPT 07/16/2002
HFlu 07/16/2002
Pneumococcus 07/16/2002
Varicella 01/08/2003
MMR 01/08/2003
Flu Shot 12/21/2004
date printed: 11/27/06

Prepared by
SpringChartsEMR

Suburban Medical Group

Sample 5   Letter to a Patient

Suburban Medical Group
101 Elm Street
Sherman, TX 77521
(214) 674-2000   Fax (214) 674-2100

November 30, 2009

Patti G Adams
198 Elm St
Sherman, TX 77521

Re: New Appointment

Dear Ms. Adams;

An appointment has been scheduled for you on 12/15/09. Please contact our office as soon as possible if you need to change this appointment.

Please arrive at your appointment 10 minutes early in order to complete your new patient forms. You will need to bring all medications that you are currently taking with you.

If you have any questions regarding this appointment, please call our office at (214) 881-3516

Sincerely,

Sample 6   Letter About a Patient

Suburban Medical Group
101 Elm Street
Sherman, TX 77521
(214) 674-2000   Fax (214) 674-2100

November 27, 2006

Harry I Hart M. D.
220 Elm St
Sherman, TX 77521

Re: Chris J Sykes 05/22/01

Dear Dr. Hart;

Thank you for allowing me to participate in this patient's care. If you have any questions or observations for me, please do not hesitate to call.

I will update you on this patient's progress after our next appointment.

Below please find a copy of the patient's recent lab results.

01/09/2005 Strep Screen

Strep Screen   negative   Normal: negative

  ID:
  Note:
  Tech: josmd
  Test Facility: Quest Diagnostics
  Reported: 01/09/2005 Last Modified: 01/09/2005
  ID#:
Note:

Sincerely,

Sample 7   **Test Report to Patient**

Suburban Medical Group
101 Elm Street
Sherman, TX 77521
(214) 674-2000   Fax (214) 674-2100

November 30, 2009

Patti G Adams
198 Elm St
Sherman, TX 77521

Dear Ms. Adams

This report is intended to review the results of your recent lab test. Your test result is printed
next to the name of the test and the normal range is printed to the right of your result.

11/30/2009 Lipid Panel
Cholesterol: 250.0   Normal:0.0-180.0 mg/dl
HDL Cholesterol: 85.0   Normal:40.0-100.0 mg/dl
LDL Cholesterol: 135.0   Normal:0.0-130.0 mg/dl
Triglycerides: 206.0   Normal:0.0-180.0 mg/dl
Chol/HDL Ratio: 4.1   Normal:0.0-4.0

Test Description: These four tests measure different fats in the bloodstream. Their main
importance is in determining the risk of blood vessel disease. Elevated Cholesterol, LDL
cholesterol and Triglycerides are all associated with increased risk of heart disease and strokes.
A high HDL cholesterol is currently thought to be protective against heart disease and strokes.

The ratio of total cholesterol to HDL cholesterol (also called the coronary risk factor) is a
calculation which yields a number useful in prediction overall risk from abnormal tests.

Problems:
Elevated Cholesterol.

Recommendations:
Low cholesterol diet.
Regular exercise program.
Please make an appointment to see the doctor as soon as possible.

Report for Pt: Adams, Patti G 06/29/42   Page 1 of 1
Suburban Medical Group

Prepared by
SpringChartsEMR

Sample 8   Patient's Excuse Note

Suburban Medical Group
101 Elm Street Sherman, TX 77521
(214) 674-2000

11/27/2006 Excuse/Note
   Order
   To: Walmart
   Re: Adams, Patti G 06/29/42
      Please excuse this employee's absence today due to our office visit from 1:00pm
      to3:00pm.
   Patient Number: no Patient reference Chart ID: not Charted
      Last Modified: 11/27/2006

Patient: Adams, Patti G 06/29/42   Page 1 of 1

Sample 9   Test Order Form

Suburban Medical Group
101 Elm Street
Sherman, TX 77521
(214) 674-2000   Fax (214) 674-2100

Date: 11/27/06
Pt: Adams, Patti G 06/29/42
Address: 198 Elm St   Sherman, TX 77521

Physician Order

Orders:
CBC 85025
SMAC 80054

Diagnosis:
HTN 401.9

Patient Insurance Info
Group Name: Retired Teachers Association
Group/Policy No: 78329
Guarantor: Adams, Patti G 06/29/42
Certif No: 876456676
Insured
CoPay: 10.0

Insurance Company: United Healthcare
Mail Claim To: Claims
Attention:
Address: 19900 Molson Dr.
City: San Antonio
State: TX
Zip: 77890
Phone: 8008880404
Details:
EMail:
URL:

Prepared by
SpringChartsEMR

Suburban Medical Group

Sample 10   Report to Patient

Suburban Medical Group
101 Elm Street
Sherman, TX 77521
(214) 674-2000   Fax (214) 674-2100

November 27, 2006

Patti G Adams
198 Elm St
Sherman, TX 77521

Dear Ms. Adams

This report is intended to review the results of your recent physical examination. Your test
result is printed next to the name of the test and the normal range is printed to the right of your
result. Identified problems and recommendations are at the end of the report.

Examination:
Vitals: Temp: 97.5 Pulse: 80 BP: 130/74 Wt: 170.0 Ht: 64.0
GENERAL: NAD, A/O X 4.

Tests:
CBC pending
SMAC pending

Problems
Hypertension

Recommendations
Diovan 80mg i po q am #30 rf x3
Glucophage XR 500mg i po bid #60 rf xprn
Lipitor 10mg i po q am #30 rf x5
Advised to lose weight with goal of 200 minutes exercise each week with heart rate elevated
to 70% of age from 220 and a daily consumption of 1200 - 1500 kcal. 1:46 PM josmd
3 months

Sent 11/27/2006

Prepared by
SpringChartsEMR

Suburban Medical Group
Report for Pt: Adams, Patti G 06/29/42   Page 1 of 1

Sample 11   Office Visit Report

Suburban Medical Group
101 Elm Street Sherman, TX 77521
(214) 674-2000

04/28/2003 Office Visit
  S:
     Needs medications refilled. Follow-Up.
  O:
     Vitals: 97.5 F   80   14   130/74   Wt: 180.0 lbs   Ht: 64.0 in
       BMI: 30.89

     EAC/TM's nl. Pharynx nl. Neck supple s adenopathy. Thyroid normal to palpation. Chest
     clear to auscultation. Heart rrr s m or g. Abdomen: BS nl. nontender no organomegaly or
     masses. Extremities: pulses symmetrical UE and LE's. motor strength normal extrem x 4.
     cap refill < 2 sec extrem x 4. Neurological: CN II - XII nl. DTR's symm no sens defects. Gait
     nl.
  A:
    Dx:
        HTN 401.9
        DM, Adult Onset,NID, Controlled 250.00
        Hypercholesterolemia 272.0
  P:
    Rx:
        Diovan 80mg i po q am #30 rf x3
        Glucophage XR 500mg i po bid #60 rf xprn
        Lipitor 10mg i po q am #30 rf x5
    Tests:
        CBC
        SMAC
        Lipid Panel
        HGBA1C
    Procedures:
        Ear Irrigation

    Other Tx:
        ref to ophth for yearly checkup
    Follow-Up:
        3 months.
        ***** Graphic *****
      Date Created: 04/26/2003
      Date of Service: 04/28/2003
      Patient Number: 31 Chart ID: 12
        Last Modified: 11/22/2006

Patient: Adams, Patti G 06/29/42   **Page 1 of 1**

Sample 12   History & Physical Report

History and Physical
Patient: Sykes, Chris J 05/22/01
Date of Service: 11/27/2006
Chief Complaint:
Acute Diarrhea.
Present Illness:
Pt c/o watery diarrhea which began 2 days ago. Notes the diarrhea is moderate.
Comes on suddenly. - Pt denies nausea, vomiting, pain. - Pt has not noted stools
floating or food particles within stool. - History of sick contacts, antibiotic use,
foreign travel, bad food exposure. Past Hx of similar episodes: Negative. Family Hx
of similar episodes: Negative.
Allergies:
Penicillin
pollen
Current Medications:
Allegra 30mg i po q am
Nasacort AQ 55mcg ii puffs each nostril q am
Children's aspirin, benedryl
Past Medical History:
Chickenpox
Family Medical History:
HTN, Mother, father and sister have had consistent problems with allergies.
Social History:
Review Of Systems:
GENERAL: + - no weight change, fever, chills, night sweats, generalized
weakness Gastrointestinal: + -Appetite is normal. No dysphagia, dyspepsia, abd.
pain, heartburn, nausea, vomiting, vomiting blood or coffee ground material,
jaundice, constipation, melena, blood in or on stools, hemorrhoids.
Examination:
Vitals: Temp: 98.6 Wt: 42.0 Ht: 41.0
GENERAL: + - Well developed. Well nourished. In no distress / evident discomfort /
Appears ill. ABDOMEN: + - Bowel sounds present and normal. - No evidence of
scarring or past surgical procedures. - Flat, soft, nontender, without rebound or
guarding. No fluid wave elicited. - No evidence of masses, organomegaly or
abdominal aneurysm. - Normal to percussion. RECTAL: + - No abnormality. No
masses, hemorrhoids, no fissures. - Hemoccult: Negative.
Impression:
Diarrhea, Acute 787.91
Plan:
Flagyl 500mg i po bid #10 rf x0
Discussed keeping up hydration and eating crackers until diarrhea remits. Once
better add complex carbohydrates to diet (cereals, rice, potatoes, bread). Avoid
fatty foods until well. Watch for lactose intolerance. Pt Instr: Diarrhea given

Suburban Medical Group
H&P for Pt: Sykes, Chris J 05/22/01   Page 1 of 2

Sample 13   Routing Slip

Suburban Medical Group
101 Elm Street
Sherman, TX 77521
(214) 674-2000   Fax (214) 674-2100

Adams, Patti G 06/29/42
198 Elm St
Sherman, TX 77521
Home #: (214) 766-7676
Work #:
Pager:
EMail: mom5645566@aol.com
SS#: 876-45-6676
Sex: F
Employer: Home Engineer

Home Fax:
Work Fax:
Mobile #: (214) 777-7987

Marital Status: Married
Pt ID #: 31

Date of Service: 04/28/2003
Doctor: John O. Smith, M. D.
   E&M Code Recommended: 99214
Diagnosis:
   HTN 401.9
   DM, Adult Onset,NID, Controlled 250.00
   Hypercholesterolemia 272.0
Tests:
   CBC 85025
   SMAC 80054
   Lipid Panel   80061
   HGBA1C 83036
Other Procedures:
   Ear Irrigation 69210
ref to ophth for yearly checkup
Followup:
   3 months.

Patient Insurance Info
Group Name: Retired Teachers Association
Group/Policy No: 78329
Guarantor: Adams, Patti G 06/29/42
Certif No: 876456676
Insured
CoPay: 10.0

Insurance Company: United Healthcare
Mail Claim To: Claims
Attention:
Address: 19900 Molson Dr.
City: San Antonio
State: TX
Zip: 77890
Phone: 8008880404
Details:
EMail:
URL:

Prepared by
SpringChartsEMR

appendix B

Source Documents for Single-User Computers

Sample 1   **Patient Information Sheet**

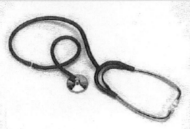

Suburban Medical Group

101 Elm Street
Sherman, TX 77521

PH: (214) 674-2000
FX: (214) 674-2100

APPOINTMENT: TIME: _10:00 AM_   DATE: _____

PATIENT INFORMATION SHEET

Patient Name: _____HILL_____, __CHLOE ELIZABETH_____
Last, First, Middle

Previous and/or Maiden Name(s): _____N/A._____

Date of Birth: ___10/8/89_____   SS #: ___048-69-4281___

Street Address: __78 RICHARDS ST._____

City/State/Zip: __LOGANLEA___, __MO___ __65807_____

Phone Numbers: Home: _417-881-3968_   Cell: _____

Email address (if applicable): ___ceh89@hotmail.com_____

Sex: (Circle one): Male, (Female)

Marital Status (Circle one): Married, Widowed, Divorced, (Single,) or Separated

Patient's Employer: ___LOGAN CITY_____

Work Phone: _417-969-4123_ Fax Phone: _417-969-7821_

Signature of Patient or Patient/Guardian:

_____CEHill_____.

Sample 2   Primary Insurance Card Information

Physician Visit & Hospital Program

Office Visit:
Deposit
$35

CHLOE ELIZABETH HILL
Member Number 041020102
Group Number 76022

Galaxy Health
Network
National Provider Network

Members: *In an Emergency Seek Medical Attention First.*

For questions or to locate a provider visit www.iabbenefits.com
or call 800-275-1171.
Before seeking hospital services you must register for CAP benefits.
To register call 800-975-3322.
Members Are Responsible For Network Contracted Rates Incurred.
Members are required to register for referral authorization before
seeking hospital services.

PROVIDERS:
Send bills to: IAB; PO Box 224767; Dallas, TX 75222
For questions call: 866-404-5970

For lab work use Quest Diagnostics or call 800-975-3322.
In Emergency please admit the patient and call 800-975-3322 by the next business day.
All members have limited inpatient and outpatient benefits.
Underwritten by various insurance companies.
This program is administered by IAB
701 Highlander Blvd., Ste 500, Arlington, TX 76015

Sample 3   Patient Intake Sheet

Suburban Medical Group

101 Elm Street
Sherman, TX 77521

PH: (214) 674-2000
FX: (214) 674-2100

Patient Name: _HILL, CHLOE ELIZABETH_
Last, First, Middle

Date of Birth: _10/8/89_   SS #: _048-69-4281_

FAMILY HISTORY

	Age	State of Health	Occupation	IF DECEASED Cause of Death	Age of Death
Father	50	GOOD	CONSTRUCTION		
Mother				BREAST CANCER	45
Brothers	24	ASTHMA			
	12	GOOD			
Sisters					

Have YOU OR ANY OF YOUR BLOOD RELATED FAMILY MEMBERS had

	YES	NO	RELATIONSHIP
Cancer (List type)	✓		MOTHER - BST CNCR
High blood pressure	✓		AUNT - MOTHERS SISTR
Bleeding disorder		✓	
Tuberculosis		✓	
Diabetes		✓	
Kidney disease		✓	
Heart disease	✓		UNCLE - FATHER'S BROTHR
Arthritis		✓	
Gastrointestinal disorder		✓	
History of drug/alcohol abuse		✓	

PERSONAL HISTORY: QUESTIONS RELATED TO YOUR PAST HEALTH HISTORY.

PROBLEM LIST: Comment on positive answers in space below or on additional sheet.

HAVE YOU HAD?	YES	NO	ALLERGIES:	YES	NO		YES	NO		YES	NO
			Drugs/Medication: Please list	✓		Recurrent colds or chronic cough	✓		Disease or injury of bones or joints		✓
Measles		✓	CODEINE			Shortness of Breath		✓	Back problems	✓	
German Measles		✓				Asthma and/or hay fever	✓		Weakness, Paralysis		✓
Mumps		✓				Pain/Pressure in Chest		✓	Dizziness, fainting		✓
Chicken Pox	✓		Foods: Please list			Heart murmur		✓	Frequent Urination		✓
Malaria		✓	PEANUTS			Rheumatic fever		✓	Kidney disease		✓
Gum or Tooth Problem			SHELLFISH CAUSES RASH			High or Low Blood Pressure		✓	S. T. Ds.		✓
Sinusitis			Head injury/ unconsciousness or concuss ion			Recurrent diarrhea or constipation or both		✓	Chronic skin disease eczema or psoriasis		✓
Eye Problem	✓		Seizure disorder/Epilepsy		✓	Jaundice or Hepatitis		✓	Tumor, cancer, cyst		✓
Ear, Nose, Throat Problems TONSILLITIS	✓		Recurrent or severe headache, migraine headache	✓		Gallbladder disease or gallstones		✓	FEMALES ONLY		
Surgery List			Asthmatic/Bronchitis		✓	Eating disorder		✓	Excessive flow		✓
APPENDECTOMY			Insomnia		✓				Irregular Periods		✓
			Frequent Anxiety	✓		Hernia, rupture		✓	Severe Cramps	✓	

	YES	NO
A. Has your physical activity been restricted during the past five years? (give reasons and duration)		✓
B. Have you ever had radiation treatments to the head or neck?		✓
C. Have you received treatment or counseling for a nervous condition.	✓	
D Have you had any illness or injury or been hospitalized, other than already noted? (Give details)		✓
E. Have you been rejected for or discharged from military service because of physical, emotional, or other reasons?		✓
F Have you lived or traveled outside of the U.S.A.?	✓	

ROUTINE MEDICATIONS. List medications you take regularly including non-prescription & herbals.
ALEVE - 275 mg   CLARITIN D-24
CALCIUM SUPPLEMENTS
MULTI-VITAMIN

Name/address/phone of your primary care physician.
DR JON CLARK
1200 E. WOODHURST
WATERFORD, MO 65804 (417) 890-6777

Social History:
1. Tobacco Use: ☐Yes, ☒No, ☐Mild, ☐Moderate, ☐Heavy, ☐Smokeless Tobacco, Packs Per Day? _____   2. Alcohol Use: ☐Non Drinker, ☒Social Drinker, ☐Heavy Drinker
3. Caffeine Use: ☒Yes, ☐No, Cups Per Day _3_ 4. Illicit Drug Use: List _____ N/A _____   5. Sexually Active: ☐Yes, ☒No, Age Started? _____
6. Education: ☐ Elementary, ☐High School, ☒College, ☐Post-Graduate 7. Occupation: _STUDENT_

Additional Information:
Hospital Preference - _ST. JOHNS_
Lab Preference - _LAB CORP_

HIPAA Notice of Privacy Practices Acknowledgement

✓   I agree to receive **Suburban Medical Group's** Notice of Privacy Practices electronically that can be reviewed and printed at www.smg.com or.

____   I acknowledge receipt of this Notice and that updates will be made available at this website.

Please check one of the above and sign the document _____CEHill_____   _____
(Patient/Legal Guardian)   (Date)

Rev B-2S-2008

Sample 4   Default Pharmacy Information

Walgreens

Crn Campell Ave. & Battlefield St.   Office:(417) 887-8546
Loganlea, MO 68504   Fax:(417) 887-5623

Category: Pharmacy

Sample 5   Immunization Record Card

VACCINE ADMINISTRATION RECORD
FOR CHILDREN & TEENS
LOGANLEA, MO 65801
(417) 889-2222   Fax

Immunizations for Hill, Chloe E 10/08/89
HFlu 02/05/1990
MMR 04/10/1990
Varicella 04/10/1990
IPV 08/15/1990
HepatitisA 10/15/1990
IPV 04/15/1991
DaPT 10/05/1991
IPV 04/15/1994
DPT 04/15/1994
DPT 10/15/2001
MMR 10/15/2001
HepatitisB 06/02/2002
Meningococcus 08/19/2005
HFlu 05/05/2007
date printed: 08/28/07

Sample 6   Office Visit Notes

	COMPLAINT AND TREATMENT (Diagnosis, when possible) (Underline every new diagnosis)	
Date		L. Smith. Physician

Name CHLOE HILL   Soc. Sec. # 048-64-4281

Address see intake sheet.

Address

CC	Allergies, congestion, cough, runny nose.
PI	Pt reports sys began gradually 5 days ago. Cough - onset 3 days ago No fever. Nature of cough is dry. Has tried to treat w/ OTC meds. Seems worse in evenings. Ass. sys include itchy eyes. Overall getting worse
ROS	Normals: No weight change, fever, chills, no sweats or generalized weakness
VITALS	Temp: 99° Resp: 25 Pulse: 75 BP: 121/62 Ht. 62 in Wt: 115
EXAM	General: Well developed, well nourished. Alert. Oriented to person, place + time. In no apparent distress Abnormals: Nose: congested with boggy Turbinates, copious bilateral discharge EYES: dark circles under both eyes. swollen conjunctiva w/ bilateral tearing
DX:	Allergic Rhinitis (477.9)
RX:	Allegra 30 mcg i po q am #30 rf xprn Nasacort AQ 55 mcg ii puff each nostril q am #16.5 gm bott. rf xprn Serevent inhaler 21 mcg ii puff bid #13g canister rf xprn.
Tests:	Strep Screen
Proc.	Nebulizer c̄ Albuterol. (0.5 cc in 2cc NS)
Other	Customary discussion of prescribed medication. Pt instruction sheet given: Allergies.
F/u	RTC prn or 1 year F/u.
	10:20 AM J. Smith MD

HS-

Sample 7 Patient Excuse Note

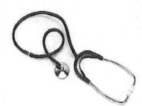

Suburban Medical Group

101 Elm Street
Sherman, TX 77521

PH: (214) 674-2000
FX: (214) 674-2100

EXPLAINED ABSENCE

DATE: _____

TO: *Spfld Community College*

Please excuse this ~~students~~/employees absence today due to our office visit from

_10:00 AM_ to _12:00_ am/~~pm~~

John O. Smith M.D.

By: _____

Sample 8   Letter to Primary Care Physician

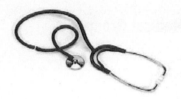

Suburban Medical Group

101 Elm Street
Sherman, TX 77521

PH: (214) 674-2000
FX: (214) 674-2100

Jon D. Clark
Clark Family Medicine
1200 E. Woodhurst St.
Waterford, MO 65804

Re: Chloa E. Hill   10/8/89

Dear Dr. Clark:

Thank you for allowing me to participate in this pt's care. If you have any questions or observations for me, please do not hesitate to call.

Below please find a copy of the recent examination

Sincerely,

J.D. Smith MD

Sample 9   Letter to Patient

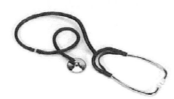

Suburban Medical Group

101 Elm Street
Sherman, TX 77521

PH: (214) 674-2000
FX: (214) 674-2100

Chloe E. Hill
78 Richards St
Loganlea, MO 65807.

RE: Lab Results from Recent Visit

Dear Ms. Hill:

Please find enclosed lab results from our recent visit. Included is a basic explanation of the lab results.

If you have any questions regarding these results, please call the office + schedule an appointment to meet with me.

Thank you for allowing me to be your physician. Stay well.

Sincerely,

John D. Smith, MD.

Sample 10   Patient Lab Results

TEST PERFORMED AT:
Lab Corp
4380 Federal Dr. Suite 100
Marsdon, MO 65803

PATIENT:
Hill, Chloe Elizabeth
DOB: 10/08/1989
Gender: F

Ordering Physician: John O. Smith MD
  Accnt No: 444051
Lab Specimen: No N321850003

Test Name	In Range	Out Of Range	Reference Range
Strep Screen	Normal		Normal

Test Date: 08/05/2003

Exercises for the Networked Computer Environment

The following exercises (designated with N) correspond to the exercises within the chapters but are intended for use in a networked computer environment. Please use these exercises if you are using SpringCharts in a networked computer environment.

CHAPTER 3 INTRODUCTION AND SETUP

Exercise 3.1(N) Setting Your User Preferences (LO 3.3)

1. Double-click on the SpringCharts icon on your desktop. **Note:** This is the only time you will double-click while using Spring-Charts. Once the program is opened, all functions are activated by a single click of the mouse.
2. SpringCharts is designed to give each user the ability to change certain functions of the program. These preferences will adjust when the user logs on. Select the *File* menu on the main window and choose *Preferences>User Preferences*. Set up your preferences based on the items selected in the *Set User Preferences* window shown at the right.
3. In a **network version** of SpringCharts you have already been assigned a password to log on to the program. Select the *Password* tab and change your password, verify it, and click on the [Change Password] button. Record your new password below.
4. Once again click on the first preferences tab and save all the changes.
5. Submit your new password to your instructor.

New Password: _____

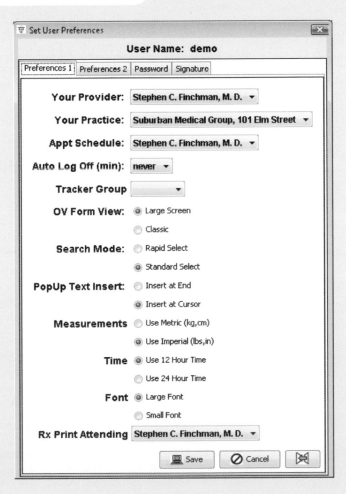

Exercise 3.2(N) Adding a New Address ^(LO 3.4)

1. In the *New* menu of the main screen select *New Address.*
2. Enter the name and demographics of your primary care physician. If you do not have one, please make up a fictitious doctor and demographics. In the *Category* field you will select *Physician.* Choose the medical specialty in the *Specialty* field. The *Account #* field is for internal use only; it could be used to reference the entry in another software program. Save the information.
3. Enter your neighbor's name and demographics as a clinic employee. You will not fill in the *Company* and *Specialty* fields. Although SpringCharts users are set up as *Users* in the *Administration Panel* of SpringCharts Server, they need also to be entered in the *Address Book* as employees in order to capture the address and other information. Save the information.
4. Set up a pharmacy of your choice. You will start by entering information in the *Company* field. (You will not need to fill out the *name* information.) In this entry you will not fill out the *Specialty* field. Save the information.
5. Set up a Testing Facility. This could be a lab company. As with the pharmacy, you will not fill out the *name* information or choose a *Specialty* field. Be sure to use *Testing Facility* in the *Category* field so the program can display this entry in the appropriate place in SpringCharts. Add the other demographic details. Save the information.
6. Locate each address that you recorded by searching by the *Name* or *Category* field in the *Address* window. Open the address by highlighting it on the list.
7. Print out each of your addresses by selecting the [Print Card] button. Write your name on each sheet and submit to your instructor.

Exercise 3.3(N) Adding a New Patient ^(LO 3.5)

1. Select the *New* menu on the main screen. Select the *New Patient* submenu and enter yourself as a patient. Note the first name is filled out first. Save the information.

> Note: The date of birth can be entered by using the mmddyyyy format (without the punctuation) in the *Date of Birth* field. The punctuation will occur automatically after you tab off the field. Another method of selecting the patient's date of birth is by using popup calendar to the right.

2. Once again, open a *New Patient* window and record a patient's first name, middle initial, and date of birth. Click the [Copy Patient] button and type: *adams* in the rapid select *Choose Patient* window. Select *Patti Adams.* Note the family information that is copied from an existing patient. Complete the remaining information. The *Home Phone* will need to remain the same in order for these two patients to be linked in the same household list. Save the information.
3. Select the main *Edit* menu and then choose the *Patients* submenu. Select *Zip Code* as the *Search* criterion and type: 77521 in the *Search* field and click the [Search] button. You will be provided a list of all the

patients in the database having this specific zip code. Select *Patti Adams* and add a *Work Phone* to her demographics. Click the [Save] button.

4. Click the [Export] button and select *Export List*. Choose the [Open in Word Processor] option and SpringCharts will recreate the list of patients with a zip code of 77521 into your computer's default word processing program. In most cases this will be Notepad™. From here the list can be printed out and saved. You will notice that the date of birth is in the yyyymmdd format. Notepad defaults to the font size that was last used on the computer. If your text size appears abnormal, change the font under the *Format* menu in Notepad to 10 points.

5. Print out your list and submit to your instructor.

Exercise 3.4(N) Adding a New Insurance (LO 3.6)

1. Click on the *Edit* menu on the main menu. Select the *Insurance* submenu. Click the [New Insurance Company] button and add a new insurance company to SpringCharts. If you have your own insurance card you may want to record this information. If not, you can make up an insurance company and the demographics. Save the new insurance company.

2. Highlight the newly added insurance company and select the *Universal Export* button in the lower right corner. Select the [Open in Word Processor] button.

3. In the word processing program, type your name at the top of the insurance information.

4. Print the document and submit to your instructor.

CHAPTER 4 THE CLINIC ADMINISTRATION

Exercise 4.1(N) Working the Patient Scheduler (LO 4.2)

Note: Your instructor will assign you a day on the calendar into which you will schedule your patient for an office visit.

1. With your mouse in hand, left click on an [OPEN] icon on your designated appointment schedule day. Assign a patient to this appointment slot by clicking on the [Choose Patient] button. With the *Choose Patient* window open, type in the first few letters of your last name. Select your name then type a reason for your visit in the *Note* field. Add your initials after the note. Click the [Done] button.

2. Choose any free hour on the day that you scheduled your patient and block out time from the schedule for a staff meeting. Click on the *OPEN* time slot and type *Staff Meeting* in the *Note* field. Click on the [Block this Time] button in the *Edit Appointment* window. Do this exercise three more times until the entire hour is blocked.

3. Click on another *OPEN* slot on that particular appointment schedule. Type a new patient's name in the *Patient* field then type in a reason for the visit in the *Note* field. Add your initials after the note. Click the [Done] button.

4. Add the established patients, Sally Dalton and Robert Underhagen, to the day that you have open. Add the reason note "UTI" (urinary tract infection) to Sally and the reason note "Lab" to Robert. Remember to add your initials after the note for each patient that you add to the schedule.

5. Add two new patients to the same appointment schedule along with appropriate reason notes.

6. Print the schedule that you have open and submit to your instructor. Circle your name on the schedule.

7. Chart yourself as a No Show. Save the No Show documentation under the *Encounter* tab. The program will indicate the charting of the No Show. Click on the [Get Chart] button in the *Edit Appointment* window. Click on the "+" sign to the left of the *Encounter* tab in the upper right panel of the patient's chart to view the No Show entry. Clicking on the No Show entry will display the details in the lower window. The *No Show* note can be further modified by clicking on the [Edit] button.

Exercise 4.2(N) Working the Patient Tracker (LO 4.3)

1. Add yourself to the patient tracker by clicking one time on your patient's name in the office schedule and selecting the [Track Pt] button. You will notice the program automatically selects *Waiting Room* as the default location. Immediately click [Done]. You will also notice the program stamps the time that your patient entered into the patient tracker.

2. Let us assume we are working for a clinic that has allocated the color flags as:

   a. Blue—A patient visit for Dr. Finchman
   b. Yellow—A patient visit for a nurse check only
   c. Green—A self-pay patient
   d. Red—A patient visit for lab work only
   e. Black—A patient visit for a specific office procedure
   f. Fuchsia—A Medicaid patient

   Click on your name in the patient tracker and use the color flags along the top of the *Edit Tracker* window to indicate that the patient is coming in for a nurse check and has Medicaid as her primary insurance. Assign your patient a *Ready* status and click the [Done] button.

3. Click on your patient in the waiting room and move the patient to one of the exam rooms. Give the patient a status of *Nurse Check* and save him/her back into the patient tracker.

4. Assume your employment is in the clinical area of office. You will want to make the patient tracker into the main screen on your computer. Do this by accessing the *Actions Menu* on the main screen.

5. A walk-in patient has arrived at the clinic. The patient is not on the schedule. This is an established patient. Click one time on the patient tracker header bar and type just one letter for the patient's last name in the *Rapid Select* window. Select a patient from the list and click [Done] in the *Edit Tracker* window.

6. Now that you have finished the nurse check on your patient (your name), click one time on your patient's name in the tracker and now click on the final [CheckOut] button in the *Edit Tracker* window. You will notice the program changes the location to *Done* and the status to *Done* and removes the color flags from the patient.

7. Go to the *Tracker Archive* window in the *Edit* menu. The *Edit Tracker Archive* window will display the patients who were processed through the patient tracker today. Click on your patient and notice the *Time In* and *Time Out* stamp on the right-side panel. (LO 4.6)

8. Click on the [Export] button and export the list of names to *Open in Word Processor*.

9. Print out the list of patients, circle your name, and submit to your instructor. Close the *Edit Patient Tracker* window.

Exercise 4.3(N)   Working with the ToDo List (LO 4.4)

1. You will now function as an office manager. Click on the *ToDo List* header bar. In the *New ToDo/Reminder* window, type *Plan Staff Meeting* in the empty item field. Click on the [Send] button. You will notice the new ToDo item added to your *ToDo List* with a green bar. Sometime throughout the day you will work on this task. Click the *Plan Staff Meeting* ToDo item. The program adds a checked box to the item. The next time you log onto SpringCharts this item will have been removed.

2. Again, click on the *ToDo List* header bar. In the *New ToDo/Reminder* window select *Call Pt* and *Check Lab* from the pop-up text panel. Click the [Link to a Patient] button. In the *Choose Patient* window, type in "under," and conduct a search. Highlight Robert Underhagen and select the [Send] button. You will notice the new ToDo item added to your list of tasks. This item will have a blue color bar indicating it is linked to a patient. At some point during the day you will process this task. Click on the Robert Underhagen item. You will notice Robert's chart opens, enabling you to access the patient's phone number and other important information. Close the patient's chart and notice the red checked box added to this ToDo item.

3. Open a *New ToDo/Reminder* window. From the pop-up text select *Order Supplies*. In the ToDo field also type "*bandages*." In the *ToDo* drop-down list, select *Jan*. Select the [Send Later] button and choose any date next month. Click the [Send] button. This ToDo item will appear in Jan's *ToDo List* on that specific date.

4. Create a new ToDo/Reminder for yourself. Type or select some pop-up text. Link it to the patient Rusty Day. Send it to yourself in the future. Go to the main *Edit* menu and select *My ToDo List*. Find the item that you scheduled for yourself in the future. Click on the Red X in the upper right corner to exit this window.

Exercise 4.4(N) Working the Messages Center (LO 4.5)

1. Once again you will function in the role of the office manager. Click one time in the *Message* header in the lower right quadrant. Click [No] to the question: *Does this message concern a Patient?* In the subject line (RE:), type the subject: *Staff Meeting.* In the body of the message invite the staff to the meeting, giving the time and location. Click in the [MultiSend] button in the middle of the *New Message* window. Check several of the staff including yourself. Click on the [Send] button. You will notice the new message appears in you own message center at the top of the list displaying the subject, date, and time that the message was sent.

2. As the office manager, you would like to save this message so you can send it out again next month. Click on the staff meeting message in your message center. Click on the [Save] button in the middle panel of the *Message* window. The program will remove the message from the message center and indicate that the message has been archived. In the main *Edit* menu select the *Message Archive* option. The *Message Archive* window will display any archived message. Next month you will want to click on the *Staff Meeting* message then select the [Re-Activate Message] button to send the message back into your message center, from where it can be sent out again to coworkers. Close the *Message Archives* window by clicking on the 'X' in the upper right corner.

3. Print out the archived message and submit to your instructor.

4. Once again, click one time in the *Message* header. Click [Yes] to the question: *Does this message concern a Patient?* In the *Choose Patient* window, type your last name and select yourself as the patient. You will notice the program adds the patient's demographics to the left side of the *New Message* window and the patient's name in the subject field. Let us now assume you are employed in the doctor's office as a front office receptionist. You have received a phone call from the patient asking for a prescription refill of Lipitor. No clinic staff workers are available so you will need to send the doctor a message. You will notice that there is no pop-up text in the right panel regarding a patient calling requesting a refill. You will want to add it so you don't have to type this item each time.

   Click on the pop-up text edit icon. In the *Edit PopUp Text* window, type: *Patient called requesting refill.* on an empty line. Click the [Done] button to save the new pop-up text item. You will now see the line of text that you added into the *Edit PopUp Text* window. Click in that new pop-up text and it will be placed in the body of the new message.

   Now you will need to select the medication that your patient is requesting as a refill. Click on the *Rx* icon in the lower section of the message pad. This will open a window displaying the patient's routine medications and the patient's previous prescriptions that have been prescribed by the clinic. Because your patient is new to the clinic, there are no medications on file. Search for and select a Lipitor medication from the *Find* field, then click the [Save] button. The program adds the medication in question to the message note.

Your patient has asked that her prescription be sent to the *Walshop Pharmacy*. Click on the [Pharm List] button and select the appropriate pharmacy. The program will ask you if you want to update the patient's chart to reflect this as the patient's default pharmacy. Click on "No." The selected pharmacy is added to the body of the message note. Find your logon name in the drop-down list and send the message to yourself.

5. Let us now assume we are a doctor and we have received the message that you just created. At some point during the day we will check our electronic messages. You will notice the recently sent message regarding your patient in the *Messages* center. Click on the message. The doctor will most likely want to check the patient's chart and review lab results and medication history. Click on the [Get Chart] button. Close the patient's chart. Dr. Finchman wants to refill the prescription without authorizing any more refills and would like to set up an appointment with the patient to conduct another lipid panel. Click on the medication in the lower portion of the *Message* window. Change the *Refills* field to 0 and click the [Save] button. Click on the Edit pencil icon and edit Dr. Finchman's pop-up text and add the following sentences on three separate lines: *OK to refill. Call patient when prescription is called in. Schedule an appointment with patient ASAP to conduct further tests.* Click the [Done] button. The updated text will be refreshed in the window. Click in the body of the message and hit your enter key to start a new paragraph. Select the three new sentences just added to your pop-up text. Again, hit your enter key to start a new line of text. Click once on the time and initial stamp buttons in the lower right corner of the *Message* window.
    Click the [Send Back] button.

6. In the *Messages* center, open the message sent to you from Dr. Finchman. Once you have completed the assigned task you will want to print out the prescription and save this message into the patient's chart. Click on the printer icon located just below the *Rx* button on the message pad. Let's add the doctor's license and DEA number to the script.

7. Click the [Print Rxs] button to print a copy of the prescription and submit to your instructor.

8. Edit your pop-up text. In the *Message Body* section, add two lines of type: *Called in the meds below.* and *Called and arrange an appt with Dr. Finchman for ___.* Save your work. In the open message window, select the two new sentences from your pop-up text selection and complete the last sentence. Using the time and initial buttons, stamp your initials and the time below your selected sentences.

9. Select the [Chart It] button in the middle of the *Message* window. You will be presented with an option to save the message as an encounter or place the note in another area of the chart. Save it as an encounter. Click the [Save] button.

10. Open your patient's chart by clicking on the patient's name either in the office calendar or in the patient tracker. Click on the [Get Chart] button. Click the "+" sign in the care tree in the upper right panel of the chart. Click on the message that you recently saved. The details of the message can be seen in the lower right corner of the patient's

chart. You will also notice the medication added to the *Prescription Hx* panel in the face sheet of the chart.

11. Print out the message using the [Print] button below and submit to your instructor.

12. Close the chart.

CHAPTER 5 THE PATIENT'S CHART

Exercise 5.1(N) Building Category Preferences (LO 5.3)

1. Open your own chart by selecting the *Open a Chart* icon (see margin reference) on the main menu. Type in the first few letters of your last name in the rapid select window. Select your name. Your chart will be empty except for your demographic information.

2. Within your chart, click on the "*Show chart/face sheet*" icon (see margin reference) to open your face sheet edit window.

3. Click on the [Social Hx] navigation button on the left-hand side and locate the list of *Preferences* beginning with "Tobacco Use:" in the lower right panel. This list of *social history preferences* was created on SpringCharts Server and will provide the user with a rapid way to enter data into the patient's face sheet. Copy this list into the appropriate table below. This activity is similar to how the administrator of SpringCharts created this list on the Server. Because the list will appear as category headings in the *Face Sheet* window, you can place a colon (:) after each group heading.

4. Similarly, locate the *Preferences* list under the [PMHX] and [FMHX] navigation buttons of the face sheet and record the lists in the respective columns below.

Social Hx	Past Hx	Family Hx

Exercise 5.2(N) Building a Patient's Face Sheet (LO 5.3)

1. Open your own chart by selecting the *Open a Chart* icon (see margin reference) on the main menu. Type in the first few letters of your last name in the window. Select your name. Your chart will be empty except for your demographic information.
2. Within your chart, click on the "*Show chart/face sheet*" icon (see margin reference) to open your face sheet edit window.
3. The window opens to the *Allergies* section. In the *Allergy* field, type "Peni" and press the search button. Select "Penicillins" from the list. The program adds this drug to your allergy list. Repeat the activity by adding the drug "Codeine" and "Peanut Containing Prod." In the *Other Sensitivities* window type the medication "erythromycin," then select "causes nausea" from the *Allergy Notes* pop-up text.
4. Click on the *Social Hx* navigation button (see margin reference). In the *Preferences* window select the "Tobacco Use:" category. (This list is being pulled from the *Administration Category Preferences* setup window on SpringCharts Server.) Now select the appropriate pop-up text from the *Social Hx* category in the upper window, for example, *Tobacco Use: Non Smoker.* Also select *Alcohol Use* and *Living Arrangements* categories and add the necessary pop-up text to further define the category.

Note: You will need to place your cursor after the *Preferences* category item that you selected in the left panel and then click on the pop-up text item. The placement of the cursor determines where the pop-up text is inserted.

5. Select the next navigation button—*PMHX* (see margin reference). (Once again you will notice the *Preferences* window displaying up to 30 past medical items that were customized in the *Category Preferences* window of the *Administration* menu on SpringCharts Server.) Select several items from the *Preferences* list. If a patient indicates a medical condition that is not in the rapid-select list, search for the diagnosis by code or description in the *Dx* field in the upper right. Type "HTN" for hypertension, hit the search icon and select the diagnosis.
6. Select the *FMHX* navigation button (see margin reference). Choose several medical conditions that may be appropriate for family medical history. Select "Father Died At Age:," place your cursor at the end of this phrase in the *Other FMHX* window and then type an age. Press your [Enter] key to place your cursor on the next line. Select "Cause of Death:" in the *Preferences* list; place your cursor at the end of this phrase and select a medical condition from the list. Repeat this activity with other family members.
7. Select the *Referred By* section (see margin reference) and type "Hart" in the *Address* field. Click the search button and select Dr. Harry Hart as the referring physician.
8. Select the *Chart Note* navigation button (see margin reference). It contains data about the patient that the medical staff do not want buried in various encounters. Select "Prefers Hospital" and

"Religion," then place your cursor at the end of these selections and type in the completed information.

9. Select the *Routine Meds* section (see margin reference). In the upper right *Drug* quadrant, search and select the following *Routine Meds:* Diovan, Glucophage, and Lipitor. In the *Routine Medications* window edit Diovan and Glucophage by clicking on each of the medications and removing the strength, directions, quantity, and refills. (Many times a new patient will not know these details; therefore it is important not to have this information in the face sheet if the patient has not supplied these details.) Save the edited medications. Click 'Yes' to the alert question: *Are you sure you want to leave the Strength blank?* Select several OTC (over the counter) items from the *Routine Meds* pop-up text in the lower right quadrant.

10. The *Problem List* (see margin reference) contains all the current medical conditions of the patient. It may be different from the PMHX list because some of the past medical history may no longer be current problems. Select several ailments from the *Problem List* pop-up text. Remember all pop-up text in SpringCharts can be customized for each user.

11. Place your [Caps Lock] on and type "DELINQUENT ACCOUNT" in the *Chart Alert* window (see margin reference). Additional text can be chosen from the *Chart Alert* pop-up text.

12. Click on the [Back to Chart] button. You will notice that all the data selected is now positioned in the various face sheet categories within your chart.

13. Click on the Insurance category section in the face sheet of your chart. Enter your group name, policy number, and other details. Select an insurance company from the provided list. Save the information. Your face sheet is now complete. Save the information.

14. Once again, click on the "*Show chart/face sheet*" icon (see open face sheet icon in margin reference) to open your face sheet edit window. Click on the [Print FS] button in the bottom left portion of the screen. This will print out your patient's face sheet report.

15. Submit your face sheet report to your instructor.

Exercise 5.3(N) Ordering an Imaging Test (LO 5.7)

1. Open your patient's chart. Dr. Finchman has recommended a magnetic resonance imaging of your patient's head.
2. Under the *Actions* tab select the *Imaging* submenu. Order an *Imaging Test*, an MRI of the Brain – With & Without contrast. Click the [Done] button.

Exercise 5.4(N) Recording and Viewing Vitals (LO 5.8)

1. Open your chart. Under the *New* menu select *New Vitals Only*.
2. Record your vitals. Under the *Actions* tab select the *Imaging* submenu. Order verbiage from the pop-up text. Click the [Done] button and *Save and Skip Billing*.

3. Close and reopen your chart by selecting your name from the *Recent Charts* menu on the Main menu bar.
4. Open the *Actions* menu within the patient's chart. Select *Graph Vital Signs* and view the various graphed vitals.
5. Open the Body Mass Index graph and print a copy.
6. Write your name on the sheet and submit to your instructor.

Exercise 5.5(N) Creating a Letter About a Patient (LO 5.8)

1. Open your chart. Under the *New* menu select *New Letter ABOUT Pt.*
2. Select the referring physician, Dr. Harry Hart, from the [Get Address Book] button.
3. Choose the pop-up text that begins with: "Thank you for allowing me to participate . . . ."
4. Click on the edit pop-up text icon (see margin reference).
5. Add the following sentence on an empty line: *Below please find a copy of the patient's recent lab results.* Click on the [Done] button.
6. Place the cursor in the letter body on a new line and select the newly added pop-up text sentence. Also, click on the sentence: *I will update you on this patient's progress after our next appointment.*
7. Click on the [Add Chart Notes] button and select the lipid panel results from the *Chart Entry* window. The lab test results will be added to the body of the letter.
8. Select the signature icon to the right of the *Close* field (see margin reference) and select your user name.
9. Print the letter, allow for the printing of your letterhead, and submit to your instructor.
10. Click on the [Done] button and select *Letters* as the category to which the letter will be stored in the patient's care tree.
11. In your chart, click on the "+" expand symbol beside the *Letter* category in the care tree to see the saved copy of the letter.

Exercise 5.6(N) Creating a Test Report for a Patient (LO 5.8)

1. Open your chart. Under the *New* menu select *New Test Report to Pt.*
2. Highlight the lipid panel in the *Select Text* window. You will notice that the program automatically adds the test description to the bottom of the test results.
3. Place your cursor in the body of the report under the section heading *Problems*. Select *Elevated Cholesterol* from the pop-up text in the lower right panel.
4. Click on the down arrow in the pop-up text category window to reveal the list of pop-up text categories. Select *Report-Recs*. Place your

cursor under the section heading *Recommendations*. Now select the following pop-up text line items: *Low cholesterol diet. Regular exercise program. Please make an appointment to see the doctor as soon as possible.*

5. Print the test report and submit to your instructor.
6. Click on the [Done] button and store a copy of the report under the *Reports to Patient* category in the care tree. You will notice a "+" expand symbol has been placed beside the *Reports to Patients* header in the care tree. Click the "+" symbol to see the saved report.

CHAPTER 6 **THE OFFICE VISIT**

Exercise 6.1(N) Building an Office Visit Note [LO 6.2]

1. Open your own patient chart. On the chart menu select *New>New OV*. In the *Office Visit* screen notice the face sheet information on the right-hand side of the window.
2. Add another past medical history item to your face sheet by right-clicking in the PMHX section of the face sheet panel on the left side and selecting *Edit*. In the face sheet window choose another medical item either from the list of *Preferences* in the lower left or search for a new diagnosis in the upper right. Click the [Back to Chart] button in the lower left.

Note: The OV screen will be positioned behind the patient's chart window. To bring it to the foreground simply click on the top edge of the OV window. **Do not close the patient's chart.**

3. Let us assume you are visiting the doctor because of a flare-up with seasonal allergies. Click on the [CC] navigation button in the upper left of the *Office Visit* screen. Notice the *S Panel* of pop-up text that appears in the right-hand panel. You do not have all the appropriate pop-up text that you need to document the chief complaints of seasonal allergies. Click on the edit pencil to the right of the pop-up text category to open the *Edit PopUp Text* window. Locate the *S Panel* category on the left column. In the empty space, type *Allergies, Runny nose, Itchy eyes* all on separate lines. (Place a comma after each symptom.) Using the arrows to the left, move your new text items up one by one and position them under the word *Congestion* in the list. (As the word moves up the list you will need to click the corresponding arrow on that line to continue to move the word.) Click the [Done] button to return to the *Office Visit* screen. The added words will now appear in your list. In the pop-up text list select: *Allergies, Runny nose, Itchy eyes, Congestion.* The words will be added to the lower left quadrant.
4. Select the yellow [PI] navigation button. In the *S Panel* pop-up text, select the sentence: *Cough. Onset . . . days ago. No fever. Etc.* Place

your cursor after the word *Onset* in the lower left quadrant and type *3-5*. Place your cursor after: *Nature of cough is* and type *productive*. Place your cursor after: *Has tried to treat with* and type *OTC meds*. Highlight and delete the phrase: *during the day* (Be sure to use the [Delete] key on your key pad, **not** the [Delete] button in the *Office Visit* screen. The [Delete] button in the *Office Visit* screen will delete the entire OV.) Add the word: *night*. Place your cursor after the phrase: *Associate symptoms include,* then select *HA* from the popup text. (HA is an abbreviation for headache.) Place your cursor after: *Overall is getting* and type *worse*. As you can see, the more pop-up text you have available, the less typing needs to done in SpringCharts.

5. Select the [ROS] navigation button. Notice that the text chosen under *CC* and *PI* is placed into the upper *SOAP* format. A new category of pop-up text opens up for you. Select *ROS-Normal:* from the pop-up text. Click in the text box in the lower left corner and hit the [Enter] key to place your cursor on the next line. Select: *GENERAL:* and *No weight change, fever, chills, night sweats . . .* from the pop-up text. Once again click in the text box and hit the [Enter] key to start a new line. Select: *CV:* and *No chest pain, arrhythmia, syncope, dyspnea, exertional dyspnea . . .* from the pop-up text.

6. Click on the drop-down arrow in the pop-up text category field and select the *ROS: HEENT* category. Click on the pop-up text edit icon. In the *Edit PopUp Text* window select the *ROS: HEENT* category. Replace the word: *Tic.* with the word: *No* (You will need to scroll down to locate the word). Click the [Done] button. Refresh the *PopUp Text* window in the *Office Visit* screen. Place your cursor on a new line in the text box. From the new pop-up text list select: *EYES:* and *No* and *Blurred vision* and "+" and *Excessive tearing*. Your new sentence should look like: *EYES: No Blurred vision. + Excessive tearing*. Place your cursor on a new line in the text box and create the following note from the pop-up text: *EARS: No Ear pain. No Discharge*. (Scroll down the list to see these other items.) Start a new line in the text box and select the following pop-up text: *NOSE: Rhinorrhea*. On a new line in the text box add: *THROAT: Sore throat*.

7. Select the [Vitals] navigation button. All previously created text is now added to the *SOAP* format. Fill out some vital information on yourself. Remember you do not have an abnormal temperature. *HC* stands for head circumference and is used by pediatricians to record head measurements for developing infants. BMI (body mass index) is grayed out because the program will calculate this item from the height and weight measurements.

8. Select the [Exam] navigation button. You will notice the vitals were added to the O (Objective) portion of the *SOAP* note. You are now presented with a new category of pop-up text. Select: *GENERAL: Well developed. Well nourished. Alert . . .* place your cursor on a new line in the text box. Add the following note: *HEAD: Normocephalic. Atraumatic*. Click on the drop down arrow in the pop-up text category field and select the new category: *PE-ENT*. On a new line in the text box add the following text: *Nose: _ Clear discharge _ Mucosal thickening*. This is all we will do of the physical exam notation in this exercise. You now have an idea of how a provider will move from one pop-up text category to another to select text appropriate to the exam.

9. Select the [Dx] navigation button. In the diagnosis field in the upper right, type: *alle* and press the *Search* icon. From the list of provided diagnoses select: *Allergic Rhinitis 477.9*.

10. Select the [Rx] navigation button. You will notice the allergies in red in the upper right window. In the *Prescription* search field type: *alle* and press the search icon. In the *Prescription* field search for and select *Allegra 180mg* and *Flonase 50mcg*. Click on the *Print Prescription* icon in the lower left corner of your OV screen. In the *Prescription Printing Options* window select the license and DEA number to print on the prescription form.

11. Print the prescription and submit to your instructor.

12. Select the [Other Tx] navigation button. In the supplied pop-up text select: *Discussed that daily vacuuming with a HEPA filtered vacuum cleaner, eliminating danderous indoor pets . . .*

13. Select the [F/U-Rem] navigation button. In the *f/u Panel* pop-up text select *1 month* for the follow-up. Place your cursor in the text box and hit the [Enter] key to start a new line. In the pop-up text select: *Pt urged to see Allergist promptly for _*. Place the cursor after the word *for* and type: *chronic allergies*.

14. Click on the "*create a reminder*" icon to the left of the text box see margin reference). You will notice that the *New ToDo/Reminder* window is already linked to the patient. Write a note to the front desk to schedule an appointment in 1 month. While you're in this window go ahead and add *Schedule appointment* to the list of pop-up text items. Remember to select the appropriate pop-up text category *ToDo-Reminder* when you're in the *Edit PopUp Text* window. Now you will not have to type this phrase again. Send the *ToDo/Reminder* note to Jan.

15. Click on the [Done] button in the OV screen. Click the [Save and Skip Billing] button. We will come back later and create a routing slip for this office visit. The OV note has been added to the list of encounters in the care tree of your patient's chart. Close the chart.

Exercise 6.4(N)   Activating a New Diagnosis (LO 6.3)

1. Open your chart. This may be done by clicking on the *Open Chart* icon (see margin reference). Select your chart by typing in your last name. Click the "+" sign next to the *Encounters* in the care tree. Highlight the office visit that you recently created. In the lower right quadrant of the patient chart select the [Edit] bottom to open the *Office Visit* screen.

2. Let's assume that the physician wants to select another diagnosis that has not been activated into the SpringCharts' list. Click on the [Dx] navigation button. The provider is searching for the diagnosis: *Pulmonary congestion*. In the diagnosis search field type: *pulm* and click the search icon. Pulmonary congestion is not yet activated.

3. Click on *Database* on the menu bar and select *New Diagnosis*. In the *New Diagnosis* window click on the [Lookup] button. In the search field type: *pulmonary* and search the database. You will notice a large number of diagnoses listed in the diagnoses database. Highlight any

diagnosis to add it to the *New Diagnosis* window. The physician will use the same description as supplied by the database so check the *Use ICD name for Brief name* box. Save the newly activated code.
4. Back in the *Office Visit* screen, search for the new diagnosis by typing: *pulm* in the diagnosis search field. Select a new ICD-9 code. It will be added to the patient's diagnosis for this office visit.

Exercise 6.5(N) Activating a New Medication (LO 6.4)

1. The provider needs to add another medication that is not yet activated to the SpringCharts list. Click on the [Rx] navigation button. In the prescription field type: *deconsal*. It is not in the list. Once again, select *Database* on the OV menu bar, then *New Drug*. The provider has the option to fill out the details of the new drug or click the [Lookup] button and search for Deconsal in the drug database. Click on the [Lookup] button. In the *LookUp Drug* window, type: *deconsal* *and* search and select any of the medications. In the *New Drug* window, type: *1-2 cap PO q12h* in the *directions* field and *30* in the *Quantity* field. Put 0 in the *Refills* field. Save the new medication.
2. In the prescription search field of the OV screen search for Deconsal again. Select the newly activated drug.
3. Click the [Done] button in the OV screen and *Save and Skip Billing* of the office visit. Close the patient's chart.

Exercise 6.6(N) Creating an Examination Report (LO 6.7)

1. Open your patient's chart. Highlight the recent office visit note. Click on the [Report] button at the bottom of the patient's chart screen. The program will automatically open the OV window and display the examination report on the screen.
2. Print the report by clicking on the [Print] button in the report window and submit to your instructor. You will notice that SpringCharts automatically places the letterhead, patient's name and address, the greeting, and introduction in the report letter. Close the report window.

Exercise 6.7(N) Creating an H&P Report (LO 6.7)

1. In the OV window, click on the *Tools* menu and select *H&P*. The *History & Physical Report* is speedily created. You can see that an H&P contains relevant information from the current physical exam as well as documentation from the patient's face sheet.
2. Print the report and submit to your instructor.
3. Click the [Done] button and save the H&P under the *H&P* category in the care tree.

Exercise 6.8(N) Creating an OV Note Report (LO 6.7)

1. With your office visit window still open, click on the [Print] button and print the entire office visit note. As you will see, the OV note is not preaddressed to any entity and may be used to send to a referring physician or other consultant.
2. Submit the OV note to your instructor. You have already seen that office visit notes, among other things, can be added to the body of a letter and printed, faxed, or e-mailed to the patient or other concerned entities. Close the OV window.
3. In the patient's chart you will notice the *Report to Patient* and the *Office Visit* saved as *Encounters* in the care tree and *H&P* saved under that category in the care tree. Click on the "+" sign beside the *H&P* category and highlight the recently created H&P report. The report will be seen in the lower right quadrant, where it can be edited and printed. Close the patient's chart.

Exercise 6.9(N) Creating an Excuse Note (LO 6.10)

1. Open your patient's chart. Open the recent office visit note. Click on the *Tools* menu and select *New Excuse/Note/Order* then *New Excuse/ Note*. In the *Note* window select pop-up text to excuse the student's absence from college for the time period that you were at the doctor's office. Add your signature to the note.
2. Print the excuse note and submit the OV note to your instructor.
3. Click the [Done] button in the OV screen. Click on the "+" sign to the left of the *ExcusesNotes* category in the care tree and see the saved note. The note is displayed in the lower right window.

Exercise 6.10(N) Creating a Routing Slip (LO 6.11)

1. Open your patient's chart. Open the recent office visit note. Click on the *Tools* menu and select *Resend Routing Slip/Transaction*. You will see in the *Routing Slip* window the diagnoses and follow-up information recorded from the OV note. The *E&M Coder* in the middle section is recommending the E&M code of 99202. Click on the [Details] button in the bottom area of the *Routing Slip* window and read about the body systems and areas that were reviewed during the office visit. Click [OK] and use the recommended code by clicking on the [Use Code] button.
2. Print the *Routing Slip* by clicking the [Print] button and submit to your instructor. Click on the [Send] button. Close the OV window and the patient's chart.
3. In the main *Practice View* screen, select the *Edit* menu and choose the *Routing Slips* option. In the *View Routing Slip* window you will see the routing slip you just created. This is where the billing person

will come to retrieve the routing slips for each day in order to bill the insurance companies or other responsible parties. In a linked environment to a PMS program, this routing slip code information will have been sent to the PMS interface.

CHAPTER 7 CLINICAL TOOLS

Exercise 7.1(N) Creating and Conducting a Chart Evaluation (LO 7.1)

1. Because you cannot access SpringCharts Server from your computer, we will go through the exercise of setting up a chart evaluation item and recording the information below. Typically, in a network environment in a medical office this information would be placed on the server. Open your web browser and proceed to the website: http://www .guideline.gov. Once on the National Guideline Clearinghouse™ website, type in *pap smear* in the *Search* field and conduct a search. Locate the title for *Cervical screening recommendations and rationale*. Read through a portion of the article and note down the appropriate age that Pap smears should begin and end, who should get them, and how frequently they should be conducted. Close the web browser and record the information in the illustration below. Fill in the appropriate radio buttons and information. In the *Should have* field write Pap smear 88150. Make sure you translate the recurring time frame into weeks. We will not link a Pap smear to any specific diagnosis on the *Only If* section of the chart evaluation item window.

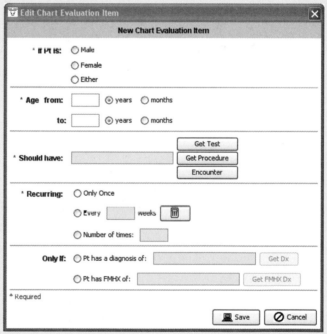

2. Open your patient's chart. Locate the *Chart Evaluation* icon on the toolbar and conduct a chart evaluation. Let's assume we recommend all the displayed criteria to the patient, so we will check the *Mark this Completed* radio buttons. Record the patient's response. Perhaps the patient is declining the DT shot and will schedule on the next visit. If the Pap smear screening is displayed, go ahead and indicate the patient has agreed to have it done today. Click the [Done] button.
3. Click on the "+" sign to the left of the *Encounter* category in the care tree and notice the addition of the chart evaluation screenings. The details will be seen below in the lower right window.

Exercise 7.2(N) Ordering a Test in an Office Visit (LO 7.2)

1. Let's go ahead and order the Pap smear screening. Open a new office visit in your patient's chart. In the OV screen, select the *Routine Well Visit* pop-up text under the [CC] navigation button.
2. Record some routine well vitals under the [Vitals] navigation button.
3. Select the diagnosis code for a *Well Woman* under the [Dx] Navigation button.
4. Now let's order the Pap smear test. Choose the appropriate navigation panel button for tests and type *pap* in the search field. Selecting the test will place it in the lower window. Click the [Order Selected test] button at the bottom and the test is added to the OV note.
5. To print the order for the test, click on the printer icon *below* the [TEST] button in the lower left text panel. You will notice the diagnosis added to the *Orders* window from the OV note. Add the patient's insurance information to the Order Form by clicking the [Add Pt Ins] button.
6. Print the order note and electronically sign it. Submit the printed Order Form to your instructor.
7. Click the [Done] button inside the *Orders* window and chart the order form under the *Encounters* category in the care tree.
8. Record a 3-year follow-up for the patient from the [F/U-Rem] navigation panel. If you do not have *3 years* in your pop-up text then you need to add it by clicking on the edit pencil icon. Remember to choose the appropriate category in the *Edit PopUp Text* window, add the new text, and then move it up to the most suitable position. Return to the OV screen.
9. Send a *New ToDo/Reminder* to the front desk to *Schedule appointment in 3 years*.
10. Close the office visit and create a routing slip. Choose the recommended E&M code in the *Routing Slip* window.
11. Print the *Routing Slip* and submit to your instructor.
12. Click the [Send] button to send the *Routing Slip*. Close the patient's chart.

Exercise 7.3(N) Adding Items to the Superbill (LO 7.4)

The screen shot displayed below is a copy of the Superbill setup window on SpringCharts Server. Because we cannot access the server we will complete the form below.

1. In the *Section Titles* field below print: *Preventive E&M Codes.* In the two columns below print the following list of new patient (NP) and established patient (EP) **codes** in the first column and the description in the next column.

99381	NP < 1 yr old
99382	NP 1–4 yrs old
99383	NP 5–11 yrs old

99384   NP 12–17 yrs old
99385   NP 18–39 yrs old
99386   NP 40–64 yrs old
99387   NP 65+ yrs old
99391   EP < 1 yr old
99392   EP 1–4 yrs old
99393   EP 5–11 yrs old
99394   EP 12–17 yrs old
99395   EP 18–39 yrs old
99396   EP 40–64 yrs old
99397   EP 65+ yrs old

Under the *Supplies* heading, type the following codes and descriptions:
A4550   Surgical Tray
D5982   Surgical Stent
D5988   Surgical Splint

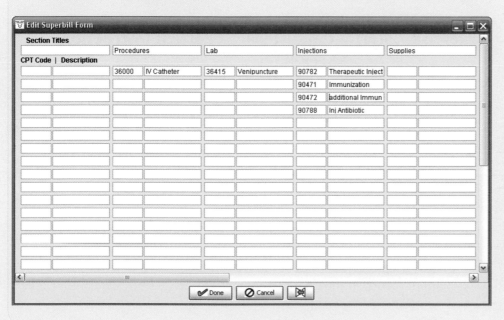

Exercise 7.4(N) Creating a New Patient Information Sheet (LO 7.5)

1. Click on the *New* menu in the main *Practice View* screen and select the *New Patient Instruction*. Click [OK] in the information window and select the [Write your own] button.
2. Open your Web browser and type in the URL address: www.familydoctor.org.
3. In the *Women* section click on any topic to locate an instruction sheet. You may also select the *More* link to locate many more instructional sheets for women.
4. Select *Printer friendly version*. To highlight this information, place your cursor at the beginning of the article's name, and with your left

mouse button depressed, drag the cursor to the end of the instruction page. Right-click on any highlighted area and choose *copy.* Close the Web page and return to the SpringCharts program. Click in the *Patient Instruction* window. Using your key pad, press the [Ctrl]+[V] keys. Highlight the bottom section of the instruction that begins with *Reviewed/Updated* and delete this section. At the bottom of the instruction sheet type: *For more information contact our office at (214) 674–2000.*

5. Change the *Patient Instruction Name* to the topic of your selected information sheet and click the [Save] button.
6. To view all the patient instructions in the program select the *Edit* menu and choose *Patient Instructions.* You will notice your instruction sheet listed here. In this window instruction sheets can be modified, exported, and deleted, and new ones can be created. Close the window.

Exercise 7.5(N) Administering a Patient Instruction Sheet (LO 7.5)

1. Open your patient's chart. Locate the office visit note in the *Encounter* category of the care tree that dealt with the well woman visit. Highlight the OV note and click [Edit] in the lower window.
2. In the OV screen select the *Tools* menu and choose the *Patient Instructions* option. Click on the instruction sheet you recently added in the *Choose Patient Instruction* window.
3. Print the instruction sheet. Write your name on it and submit it to your instructor.
4. Close the OV note and skip billing. View the bottom on the OV note in lower right window of the patient chart. Notice the phrase: *Pt Instr: ____ given* recorded in the OV note. This now becomes a permanent record in the patient's chart.

Exercise 7.6(N) Adding a Patient's Care Plan (LO 7.6)

1. Let's add a care plan to a patient's chart. Open your patient chart. Select the OV note in the care tree that dealt with the allergy symptoms. Edit the OV note.
2. In the OV screen select the *Tools* menu and choose *Care Plan.* In the *Care Plan/Guideline* window, click on the [NGC] button. (Care plans can be attached from a location stored on the computer or a computer on the network or downloaded from the *National Guidelines Clearinghouse.*)
3. On the NGC website type: enter *seasonal allergies* in the search field and search for the care plan. Locate and open the *Allergic Rhinitis* plan. Highlight just the recommendations information, copy the information, and close the web browser. Paste the material into the *Care Plan/Guideline* window by using the [Ctrl]+[V] keys. Take out any unnecessary spaces below headings in the text. Click the [Done] button, close the OV screen, and skip billing.

4. You will notice the care plan added to the bottom of the OV note in the lower right corner on the patient's chart.
5. Print the OV Note by clicking on the [Print] button in the lower right. Submit the document to your instructor.
6. Close the patient chart.

Exercise 7.7(N) Operating the Drug and Allergy Checking Feature (LO 7.7)

1. Let us check for any drug allergies in a medication that we have prescribed. Open your patient chart. Locate the OV note for allergies. Open the OV window.
2. Select the [Rx] navigation button in the OV window. You will see the medications prescribed in the lower central window: Allegra, Flonase, and Deconsal.
3. If the *Drug Allergy/Interaction Checking* button (pill bottle) to the left of the prescription window is not grayed out, it indicates that you have Internet connection. If you have connection, you may click on this icon and the Pharmacy Web Service will check for any known allergic reactions between the medicine you are prescribing and your listed allergies and your current medications. It appears that there are no allergies. If you were successful logging into this data, you may now close this window. This information cannot be printed out; it is for the provider's eyes only. Close the OV note.

Exercise 7.8(N) Importing A Document (LO 7.9)

1. Open your patient's chart and select *Import Items* from the *New* menu. Select the *Import File Cabinet Document* option.
2. Let's import a patient's insurance card. It will be helpful to have a copy in the chart. Fill out the document name in the *File Cabinet Document* window. Select the chart tab: *Insurance Card.* In the description box type: *Galaxy Health Network—Primary Ins.*
3. Click the [Sign] button to add your initials only.
4. Click on the [Attach] button and choose the *Existing* option (because your computer is not attached to a scanner).
5. Maneuver in the *Open* dialogue box to find your *EHR Material* folder. Your instructor will inform you where the *EHR Material* folder is located. Open the folder and select the *Ins Card* file. Make sure the file name shows in the *File name* field. Click the [Open] button to attach the file. If you were successful the file will be shown in blue in the *File Cabinet Document* window.
6. Click the [Done] button. The newly imported file will show up under the Insurance Card tab in the care tree.
7. Click on the [Doc] button in the lower right of your patient's chart to view the document. You may have to expand the window to see the entire image.
8. Print the document. Write your name on it and submit it to your instructor.

CHAPTER 8 **TEMPLATES AND POP-UP TEXT**

Exercise 8.1(N) Creating an Office Visit Template (LO 8.2)

1. Open your patient chart. Open the office visit note that you created dealing with the *allergies, runny nose, itchy eyes, and congestion* complaints. Select the *Database* menu and choose *Copy OV To Template*. Name the new template: *Adult Allergies (User name)*. For example, Adult Allergies User 25. Save the template. Close the *Office Visit* screen, skip billing, and close your patient chart.
2. Click on the main *Edit* menu and select *Templates*. Locate your *Adult Allergies* template under the office visit templates list. Click on the *CC* navigation tab on the right. Remove all the chief complaints: allergies, runny nose, etc. Remove the verbiage in the *F/U-Rem* segment dealing with the patient returning to the clinic as needed. Save the edited template.

Exercise 8.2(N) Activating an Office Visit Template (LO 8.2)

1. Open your patient's chart. Open a new OV note screen from the *new* menu.
2. Click on the *CC* navigation button. Your patient mentions that she has a runny nose and congestion. She believes she has allergies again. You notice in the lower right-hand window that the patient was in your office on a prior date with the same complaints. With your mouse highlight *Allergies, runny nose, congestion.* (Do not highlight the date.) Click on the *copy highlighted text to note* button and the previous chief complaints are added into the new OV note.
3. Enter some vitals in for your patient. Remember the patient doesn't have an elevated temperature.
4. Knowing that you have a template for adult allergies, click on the [Template] button at the bottom of the window and choose the *Adult Allergies* template that you created. The template will be added into the OV note augmenting the chief complaints and vitals that you have already added.
5. Your patient mentions that her cough started about 7 days ago and she tells you she does not have a headache. Click on the [PI] navigation button. This brings the PI text to the lower center text box where it can be edited. Change the cough onset time to 7 days. **Remember to use the [Delete] key on your keyboard, not the [Delete] button in the OV screen.**
6. Perhaps you decide not to give her Flonase, which is in the template. Click on the [Rx] navigation button and highlight *Flonase* in the lower center window and delete the medication.
7. Print the prescription and submit to your instructor.
8. Save the office visit and edit the routing slip. Use the recommended E&M code and [Send] the routing slip. See how the introduction of a template into the OV notes greatly enhances the speed of documentation. You will see the completed OV note saved under the *Encounter* category in the care tree of your patient's chart. Close the chart.

Exercise 8.3(N) Creating and Using a Letter Template (LO 8.4)

1. Create a new letter template by accessing the *New* menu in the *Practice View* screen and choosing *New Template>New Letter Template*. In the *Letter Template* window type the subject (*Re*): *Welcome*. In the body of the letter *(Text)* type a letter dealing with welcoming a new patient to the clinic and giving the names and phone numbers of key personnel. You may want to start the letter like this: *Thank you for your recent visit to our clinic. I want to welcome you and give you the names of a few key contact people here at the clinic.* (This letter will be sent out to all new patients coming into the clinic.) The program will automatically add a 'close' to the letter.
2. Give the letter template the name: *New Patient Letter + (User name)* and click the [Save] button.
3. Open your patient chart. Click on the *New* menu and select *New Letter to Pt.* You will notice that the letter is already addressed to the patient and is complete with greetings and closure. Click on the [Template] button at the bottom of the screen and locate your *New Patient Letter.* Highlighting the item will add it into the body of the letter.
4. To add the signature to the bottom of the letter, click the *signature* icon at the bottom of the letter and select a signature line. You will be given the option of your default doctor (this was set up initially under *User Preferences*) or your name.
5. If you used your proper e-mail address when setting up this patient, the letter can be e-mailed to the patient by clicking on the [Email Letter] button to the right or the letter may be printed or faxed by selecting the [Print] button at the bottom.
6. **Print the letter.** Add the letterhead and electronically sign the letter when prompted. **Submit the letter to your instructor.**
7. Click the [Done] button and saved the letter under the *Letters* category in the care tree. Save the letter as: *New Patient Letter.* You will notice the letter displayed in the lower right window and stored under the *Letter* category.

Exercise 8.4(N) Adding Pop-up Text (LO 8.5)

1. Let's add some pop-up text that will enable us to more thoroughly document the recent office visit of your patient for the regular Pap smear. Click on the *File* menu in the *Practice View* screen and select *Preferences>PopUp Text*.
2. Choose the *S Panel* and scroll down until you find an empty line. Type: *Routine Pap smear exam.* Using the arrows to the left, move the text up until it is placed under the line *Follow-Up*.
3. Because this will be text that is used for a wellness exam, we want to make sure we have appropriate text in the *ROS – Normals* panel. Locate this category. Scroll down in this panel and find an empty line. Type: *Patient denies abdominal pains.* and *Patient states she is*

not pregnant. on two separate line items. Using the arrows to the left, move the text up and position it in the *GU/GYN (female):* area under the line beginning: *No urgency, dysuria, nocturia, . . .* Click on the [Done] button.

Exercise 8.5(N) Using Pop-up Text (LO 8.5)

1. Open up your patient chart. Locate the office visit note regarding the Pap smear exam and open the OV note. Click on the [CC] navigation button and select the text: *Routine Pap smear exam* from the *S Panel* pop-up text.

> Note: When a user selects a series of pop-up text, the text wraps by default. If the user wants to have each new category of text on a new line, he/she will have to click at the end of the previous line of text in the lower center window and hit the *Enter* key. This will place the cursor on the next line. When selecting new pop-up text it will go to where the cursor is positioned.

2. Click on the [ROS] navigation button. Start each new section on a new line by placing the cursor on a new line in the lower central text box. Select all the *ROS-Normals* text starting with *GENERAL:* down through *GU/GYN (female):*
3. Click on the [Exam] button. Start each new section on a new line and be sure to use the heading names. Again, select all the *O (Normals)* text starting with *GENERAL:* down through *GU/GYN (female): . . .* Your text in the lower center window should finish with: *Pap smear performed.*
4. While performing the physical exam, the physician notices several benign lesions on the skin. Start a new line in the lower center text box then drop down the pop-up text category list and choose *O (Abnormals).* Locate the *Skin* heading and select *SKIN: _maculopapular lesions* to be added into the text box.
5. Notice the enormous amount of text that was effortlessly compiled detailing the patient's review of systems and the physician's exam. Click the [Done] button and the [Save and Edit Routing Slip] button. Notice in the *Routing Slip* window that the E&M code recommendation is now 99215. Even though your diagnosis code and text code remained the same, a great volume of documentation was added to the OV note indicate the thoroughness of the exam. This is now indicated by pressing the [Details] button.
6. Let us assume this patient is a Medicaid recipient. Rather than choose the recommended E&M code, you will choose a preventive E&M code that we listed in the superbill earlier. Highlight the *EP 18–39 yrs old* for an established patient wellness visit.
7. **Print the routing slip and submit it to your instructor.**
8. [Send] the routing slip and close your patient chart.

CHAPTER 9 TESTS, PROCEDURES, AND DIAGNOSIS CODES

Exercise 9.1(N) Ordering a Lab Test and an Imaging Test (LO 9.1)

1. Open your patient's chart. In the *Actions* menu of the chart select: *Lab>Order New Lab.*
2. Order a CBC (complete blood count) for the patient.
3. Again in the *Actions* menu of the chart select: *Imaging>Order Imaging Item.*
4. Order an MRI of the head, without contrast.
5. Access the *Edit* menu on the *Practice View* screen and locate the CBC test and the MRI under the *Pending Tests* option.
6. Close the *Pending Tests* window.

Exercise 9.2(N) Processing a Reference Lab Result (LO 9.2)

1. Under the *Edit* menu on the *Practice View* screen, locate the *Reference Lab* option.
2. Open the *Imported Reference Lab Tests* window and locate the complete blood count lab for Patti Adams. Highlight the test to open the *Imported Lab Data* window. The imported lab shows the patient's results both in range and out of range.
3. In a networked environment of a medical facility, typically a medical technician would select the [Match] button of this imported lab and match it to a pending test that was ordered for this patient. The data would be placed into the pending test automatically and the test saved into the patient's chart. Because we are all working with the same test we will not be able to do this. Instead we will input the data manually.
4. Leave the *Imported Lab Data* window for Patti Adams open and open the pending CBC test that you ordered for your patient in the *pending test* item of the *Edit* menu. With your mouse maneuver the two windows so that you see them side by side. Now begin copying the lab results from the imported lab into the pending lab. You will notice that you have more analytes on the imported test than are listed on the pending test. Click on the [Ignore] button to ignore the additional items on the imported lab.
5. Click the [Tech Sign] button and select the appropriate testing facility from the address list.
6. Click the [ToDo] button and send a *ToDo/Reminder* to the physician alerting him or her to the completed test that is now available. Use your pop-up text. You will notice that the ToDo item is already linked to your patient.
7. Click on the *Complete* radio button and then the [Done] button. Close the reference lab windows.

8. The physician will now open the *Completed Tests* window under the *Edit* menu. In the *Completed Tests* window locate the CBC test for your patient. Notice the analytes that are out of range. The physician will now click the *Dr Viewed* radio button and then the [Done] button to send the completed test into the patient's chart.
9. Open your chart. Locate the newly added lab in the care tree.
10. **Print out the lab and submit to your instructor.**

Exercise 9.3(N) Ordering and Processing a Lab Test (LO 9.3)

1. Open your chart and order a new lab from the *Action* menu within the chart. In the order test window, type "lip" and search with the icon (see margin reference). Select "Lipid Panel," then click the [Done] button.
2. Select "Pending Tests" from the main *Edit* menu. Highlight the "Lipid Panel" just ordered for your chart.
3. Enter in some lab results in the various fields. Check the normal ranges to the right. Place some results in range and some out of range. Click on the [Tech Sign] button and then select an appropriate [Testing facility]. Enter an ID number for the incoming lab.
4. Send a *To/Do* to Dr. S. Finchman indicating that a lab result is ready to be looked at. Select "Check Lab" from the available pop-up text. Send the *ToDo*.
5. Click the "Complete" radio button then click the [Done] button. Close the *Pending Test* window.
6. Let us now assume you are Dr. Finchman. Under the *Edit* menu open the *Completed Test* window.
7. Select the "Lipid Panel" test that was just completed for your chart. Notice the lab items that are outside the normal ranges. Open the patient's chart by clicking the [Get Chart] button (see margin reference). Look in the **Routine Meds** section of the face sheet and note that the patient is on the cholesterol-lowering drug Lipitor.
8. Close the chart and send a message (see margin reference) to Jan requesting that she call the patient and schedule an appointment ASAP. Place your cursor in the body of the message and start a new line by pressing the [Enter] key. Now choose the appropriate pop-up text. Initial the message by clicking the [init] button. Send the message to Jan.
9. Check the *Dr. Viewed* radio button in the completed lipid panel test and click the [Done] button. Close the *Completed Test* window.
10. Open your chart and notice the "+" expand sign added to the *Lab* category of the care tree. Click on the expand sign and you will see the recently completed lab panel. Highlight the lipid panel and the results can be viewed in the lower right quadrant of the patient's chart.
11. **Click on the [Print] button at the bottom and submit a copy of the completed test to your instructor.**

Exercise 9.4(N) Processing a Lab Manually ^(LO 9.3)

1. Locate your pending test for a Pap smear for your patient in the *Pending Tests* list of the *Edit* menu in the *Practice View* screen. Highlight the pending test.
2. In the results window, type *Normal* in the upper left window. Click the [Tech Sign] button indicating the inputting clinician. Click the [Testing Facility] button and choose a facility. Click the *Complete* radio button then the [Done] button. The pending test is now removed from the list.
3. Open the same test in the *Completed Tests* area of the *Edit* menu. You will notice it is stamped "Normal." Remember that only those logged on as physicians have the *Dr Viewed* radio button available in this window. The physician has multiple choices for administration in this window including getting the patient's chart. Check the *Dr Viewed* button and then click the [Done] button. The test is removed from the completed list and sent into the patient's chart. Close the *Completed Tests* window.
4. Open your patient chart. Click on the "+" sign beside the lab category in the care tree. Notice the addition of the Pap test.
5. **Print out the lab and submit to your instructor.**

Exercise 9.5(N) Creating a Test Report ^(LO 9.4)

1. Inside your patient chart open a *New Test Report to Pt* under the *New* menu.
2. Select the Pap lab test in the upper right panel. Because this is a "normal" result, we can delete the *Problems* and *Recommendations* headings in the report.
3. Print out the report and submit to your instructor.

Exercise 9.6(N) Creating a New Lab Test ^(LO 9.6)

1. Open the *Tests* option in the *Edit* menu of the *Practice View* screen. Click on the [List Lab Tests] button and see if you can locate a complete metabolic panel (CMP) test.
2. Because a CMP is not set up for this medical practice we will need to create a new lab test so the clinic can order the test and so that we can match the results to the pending test. Click on the [New Lab Test] button and fill in the test name and the CPT code. The test name will be CMP + your user name, for example, CMPUser35. The CPT code is 80052.
3. Next we will need to build the analytes that make up the panel. They are listed in alphabetical order in the left side window. When you highlight an analyte it will be added into the right side window.

Below is a list of lab components that you will need to select from the list of analytes to make up the CMP panel:

Glucose, BUN, Creatinine, Sodium, Potassium, Chloride, Bicarbonate (see no. 4 below), Calcium, Total Protein, Albumin, AST, ALT, Alkaline Phosphotase, Total Bilirubin, Globulin, and A:G Ratio (see no. 4 below).

4. When you cannot find a specific lab item in the left window you will need to create it. Click on the [New Lab Item] button and select one of the four options for the layout of the analyte. Based on the following lab item details below, create the new analyte. Once created, it will be added into the resource list in the *Create a New Lab Test* window. It then can be selected for the lab panel that you are building.

    Bicarbonate – a Number, Code – 99999, Low Range – 22, High Range – 32, UOM (Units of Measure) – MMOL/L
    A:G Ratio – a Number, Code – 99999, Low Range – 1.0, High Range – 2.3, UOM – Ratio

5. Now that the CMP panel has been built, click [Done] to save the test. You can now find the CMP listed in the *List Lab Test* window.

Exercise 9.7(N) Creating a New Imaging Test (LO 9.6)

1. Open the *Tests* window in the main *Edit* menu. Click on the [List Imaging Tests] button. Examine the list of imaging tests that are in the SpringCharts system. See if we have activated a test for an x-ray of the larynx with contrast. Close this window.

2. In order to add this imaging test, click on the [New Imaging Test] button. You will notice the [Lookup] button. This will access the CPT dictionary database of SpringCharts. Press *Lookup*.

3. In the *Lookup CPT Code* window, type the code 70373 and hit the search icon. When the new code has been located, highlight it. The description and code are added to the *New Imaging Test* window. Delete the term *Laryngography* and replace it with *Xray Larynx*. Click [Save] and the new code will be added to the list of activated imaging tests. Click on the [List Imaging Tests] button again to view the new test.

Exercise 9.8(N) Creating a New Procedure Code (LO 9.7)

1. Let's create a new procedure code. We need the procedure: Destruction of Benign Lesion – 17111. First of all, we need to check to be sure the code is not already activated. Open the *Edit* menu in the *Practice View* screen and select *Procedures*.

2. In the *Edit Procedure* window select *CPT Code* as the search mode and type 17111 in the search field. Click the [Search] button.

3. A new procedure code can be activated in the *New* menu of the *Practice View* screen; however, because we have the *Edit Procedure* window open we can activate a new code from here. Click the [New] button on the right side. You can either type the procedure name or code in the upper fields or look up the code in the CPT dictionary database.

4. To access the CPT database click the [Lookup] button. In the *Search Procedure Master List* window, select *CPT Code* as the search mode in the first drop down list and type 17111 in the search field. Click the [Search] button. When the code has been located, click the [Select] button.

5. The new code and description is added to the *Edit Procedure* window. Now we have to categorize it. Drop down the *Category* list and choose *Surgery*.

6. There is text that we need to add to this procedure that will be consistent each time the procedure is conducted. Click the [PopUp Text] button. In the *PopUp Text Composer* window select the paragraph that begins with: *Pt was advised of the purpose, benefits . . . .* and click the [OK] button. The text is now added to the *Detail* window and will be associated with this code. Save the new procedure code and close the window.

Exercise 9.9(N) Using Diagnosis and Procedure Codes (LO 9.7)

1. Open your patient chart and launch a new office visit.

2. Under the [CC] navigation button select the pop-up text *Follow-Up*. Because maculopapular skin lesions were discovered during a previous wellness check, this will be a follow-up visit that was scheduled to conduct the removal procedure.

3. Add several normal vitals.

4. Under the [Exam] navigation button, choose the *(O Abnormals)* as the pop-up text category. Scroll down and select the text: *SKIN: +maculopapular lesions*.

5. In the [Dx] navigation area, search for any diagnosis starting with *lesion*. Type in *lesion*. The pigmented lesion is not the one we want to use, so we will need to activate another diagnosis code. In the *Database* menu of the OV screen select *New Diagnosis*. To access the ICD dictionary database click the [Lookup] button. In the *Lookup Dx Code* window, search for the main 102 code. From the list select: *Yaws; Other Early Skin Lesions*. The diagnosis description and code is placed in the *New Diagnosis* window. Perhaps the physician does not commonly refer to the diagnosis by this name; rather than select the *Use ICD name for Brief name* box, the physician will enter *maculopapular lesions* in the *Dx Brief Name* field and add your user name. For example, Maculopapular Lesion User35. Save the newly activated diagnosis.

6. In the diagnosis field of the OV screen, type *mac* and search for the code you just activated. From the presenting list select the new code.

7. Under the [Proc] navigation button click the drop-down list of procedure categories. Select *Surgery* and choose the newly activated CPT code—destruction of benign lesion.

8. Click on the [F/U-Rem] navigation button. You will notice all the text that was associated with this procedure during its creation is now added into the body of the *SOAP* note. Choose a follow-up in 1 week.

9. Click on the *create a reminder* icon and send a ToDo/reminder to Jan at the front desk to schedule an appointment on 1 week. Use the appropriate pop-up text and send the ToDo item. Click the [Done] button and create a routing slip.

10. In the *Routing Slip* window bill for the surgical tray that you find itemized in the *Superbill Form* in the right panel, you will **not** need to choose an E&M code because this visit will not be billed as an office visit, but rather a procedure.

11. **Print the routing slip and submit to your instructor.** Send the routing slip and close your patient chart.

CHAPTER 10 PRODUCTIVITY CENTER AND UTILITIES

Exercise 10.1(N) Creating a New Bulletin Post (LO 10.1)

1. Click on the bulletin board icon on the tool bar of the *Practice View* screen. Click on the [New] button to open a new bulletin.

2. Highlight the phrase: *New Bulletin* and replace it with the name of a bulletin you would like to post. Remember the purpose of the bulletin board is to place items for general viewing. If a message or directive needs to be sent to another coworker, the message center or the ToDo/reminder sections of the program would be used for that purpose. Bulletins could be information and directions about an office gathering, parties, things for sale, and so on.

3. On the next lines of your new bulletin type the details of your message. Complete your bulletin by adding your name and user log on. You can color your bulletin by accessing the color options under the [Color] button. Now click the [Save] button.

4. **Print a copy of your original bulletin and submit to your instructor.**

Exercise 10.2(N) Faxing a Prescription Electronically (LO 10.2)

1. In the *Productivity Center* menu open the *Address Book* option. Change the search criterion on the right side to *Category*. In the *Find* field, type *pharmacy* and conduct the search.

2. Select the *Walshop Pharm*. If there is no fax number in the *Address* window, add a fax number to the *Work Fax* field and click the [Save] button. Close the *address* window.

3. Open your patient chart. Select the office visit note under the *Encounter* category of the care tree that deals with the adult allergy symptoms. Click on the [Edit] button to open the OV screen.

4. In the OV screen, click on the [Rx] navigation button to display the three prescriptions that were ordered. Click on the printer icon in the lower center section of the screen.

5. In the *Prescription Printing Options* window select *Use Digital Signature* and *Print License No on Rx*. Click on the [Fax] button.

6. In the *Fax* window conduct a search for a pharmacy by clicking on the search icon. In the *Fax Number Lookup* window choose *Category* as the search criterion. In the search field type: *phar* and click the [Search] button. In the list of displayed pharmacies select the Walshop Pharmacy. On the right side, the fax number will be displayed that you typed in earlier. Click the radio button beside the fax number and click the [Select] button.

7. Back in the *Fax* window type in the *Subject* field: *Prescription*. Check the box to *Send InterFax Header* and click the [Send] button. The fax will now be transmitted to the pharmacy.

Exercise 10.3(N) Processing an Inbound Electronic Fax (LO 10.2)

1. Access the *Inbound Fax List* option in the *Production Center* menu. If the medical facility had an account set up with InterFax, any inbound faxes would be listed here. Because we are not currently interfaced with this web service, we will retrieve our fax from the *EHR Material* folder on the desktop. Within this folder, locate the document regarding an MRI evaluation and open it.

2. With the left-click of your mouse held down, highlight the document. Right-click inside the highlighted area and select *Copy*. Close the fax image and close the *EHR Material* folder *window*.

3. Open the *Pending Tests* window under the *Edit* menu, locate and open the MRI of brain test for your patient. Click in the *Results* text box and press [Ctrl]+[V] on your keyboard. The MRI evaluation will be pasted into the pending test.

4. Click the [Tech Sign] button to add your initials and choose the appropriate testing facility. Add the ID number from the MRI evaluation. Select the interpreting physician.

5. Send a *ToDo* to Dr. Finchman (scfmd) notifying him of the completed MRI test that he will need to look at. Select the pop-up text: *Check XRay*. You will notice it is already linked to the patient and descriptive text is already applied. Send the item. Click in the *Complete* radio button and click the [Done] button. Close the *Pending Tests* window.

6. Now, as Dr. Finchman, open the *Completed Tests* window in the *Edit* menu. Select the MRI test for your patient. Send a *Message* to Jan to have her call the patient and schedule an appointment. Click on the *Dr. Viewed* radio button and the [Done] button.

7. Open your patient's chart and view the MRI test under the *Imaging* category in the care tree.
8. Click on the MRI item and select the [Print] button in the bottom right window.
9. **Print the MRI report and submit to your instructor.** Close the patient's chart.

Exercise 10.4(N) Working with the Time Clock (LO 10.3)

1. If the *Time Clock* submenu is not visible in the *Productivity Center* menu you will need to activate the feature in SpringCharts.
2. Click on the *Administration* menu on the main screen and select the *Time Clock Setup* submenu.
3. Check the *Enable time clock* box and select *demo* as the administrator. Click the [Done] button.
4. You will now need to close down the SpringCharts program and reboot it for this feature to be activated.
5. Access the *Productivity Center* menu and select *Time Clock*. In the *Time Clock* window click the *In* box and then confirm the click-in. Your time-in is stamped into the window.
6. You have clocked in after the hour. Let's say that you were actually in the clinic but had forgotten to clock in. Click the [Request Change] button and edit your existing time. Highlight your time and the *Edit Time Clock Item* window will open.
7. On the right-hand side, change the time back to the top of the hour. In the *Request Reason* text box state the reason why you clocked in so late and click the [Send] button.
8. The program has now sent your request to the office administrator as an item in the administrator's ToDo list, marking it with an orange bar. The administrator is able to open the item and either approve or deny the request. If the administrator approves the request, the user's time clock will be adjusted to reflect the newly requested time. Close the *Time Clock* window.

Exercise 10.5(N) Adding a New My Website Link (LO 10.4)

1. Under the *Productivity Center* open the *My Websites* option. In the *My Websites* window, click on the [Edit] button.
2. Enter the phrase *Patient Instructions* in the first blank space on the left. Move your cursor to the far left. In the right side field place the cursor to the far left of the field and, following the same format as the other links, type in the web address: http://www.familydoctor .org. Save your website addition.
3. In the *My Websites* window click on the newly added *Patient Instructions* link. The Internet browser will be activated and you will access the website directly from SpringCharts. This website has a wealth of

patient instructional sheets that can the copied into SpringCharts as patient instructions or printed directly from the website.

4. Close the Internet browser and the *My Websites* windows.

Exercise 10.6(N) Calculating an Estimated Delivery Date (LO 10.5)

1. Open the pregnancy calculator under the *Utility* menu.
2. Let us assume your last menstrual period was 6 weeks ago (sorry guys!). Select that date from the calendar. The date will be automatically entered into the LMP field and the estimated age of your baby calculated along with the estimated date of delivery. Congratulations!

Exercise 10.7(N) Searching the Medical Database (LO 10.6, 10.7)

1. Under the *Utilities* menu select the *Search Database* option. Click [Yes] to "Search all patient records now" and "Yes" in the next window.
2. Select the [Drug] button as the criterion to search by. Type *Lipitor* in the *Select Drug* window and conduct a search. The program will display all strengths of the drug Lipitor; click on all of the medications one by one to add them to the *Selected Drug* window. Click the [Done] button and the program will begin searching the patient database for patients who have been prescribed with the medication Lipitor.
3. Click the [Form Letter] button. In the *Form Letter* window type in the subject: *Drug Recall*. In the text field type the body of the letter informing the patients about the drug recall and the need to contact the doctor's office to schedule a visit. When completed click the [Done] button.
4. In the *Choose Action* window select the [Print Letters] button. Choose "Yes" to chart the letters, "Yes" to print the letterhead, and "Yes" to sign the letters electronically. Print the letters.
5. Open Russell Dean's chart. Under the *Encounters* category in the care tree you will find a copy of your letter saved in the patient's chart. Close the chart.
6. **Submit your patient letter to your instructor.**

Exercise 10.8(N) Archiving a Patient's Record (LO 10.8)

1. Select the *Patients* option in the *Edit* menu of the *Practice View* screen. In the *Edit Patient* window locate and highlight your patient.
2. Archive your patient by pressing the [Archive] button in the lower right. You will see your patient's name disappear from the patient list.
3. Try to search for your patient again. Close the *Edit Patient* window.
4. Open the *Edit* menu once again and select *Patient Archives*. In the *Patient Archives* window, search for your patient. Highlight the

patient in the list and select the [View Chart] button in the *Archive Patient* window. The *Archive Patient* window will also enable you to reactivate the patient into the active lists in SpringCharts if necessary. Close the *Patient Archives* window.

5. Let's reactivate your patient. In the *Edit* menu open the *Patient Archives* window. Locate the archived patient. This time select the [Reactivate Patient] button. You will be shown a progress bar indicating the patient is being placed back into the active list of patients in SpringCharts.

CHAPTER 11 APPLYING YOUR KNOWLEDGE
A. Practice View Screen
1. Office Schedule

Exercise 11.1(N)

1. Let's set up a new male patient: Use the name of your cousin for your new patient.

   Address: 6021 Hodges Place
   Mansfield, TX 76063
   DOB: 10/5/83
   SS#: 456-78-2371
   Home Phone: (817) 473-0328
   Work Phone: (817) 966-2484
   Cell Phone: (817) 504-0903
   E-mail: mycousin@nofencedland.net
   Employer: No Fenced Land Company
   Your cousin is married and has two children.
   He carries insurance on the family. His assigned doctor is
   Dr. Finchman, the family's primary care physician.

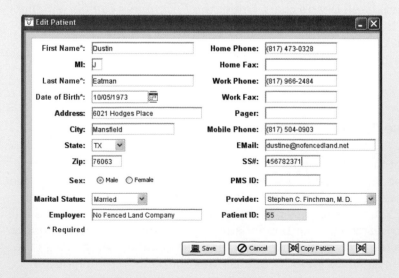

2. Let's set up your cousin's son. Remember, to add family members of the same household you can use the [Copy Patient] button in a *New Patient* window. Locate your cousin; his address and home phone will be copied into the new patient record. Add your cousin's son's name; he was born on October 16, 2005. He does not have an e-mail address. His Social Security number is 456-67-9451.

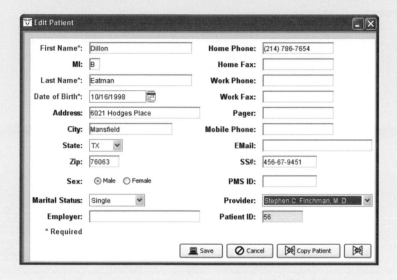

Exercise 11.2(N)

1. Place your cousin on an open spot on today's or tomorrow's schedule. He is presenting for a routine well visit.
2. Choose a future day and block out 1 hour of the day for a staff meeting.

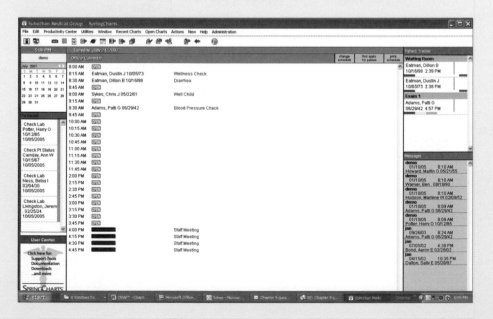

3. Your cousin indicates on the sign-in sheet that his cell phone number has changed to (214) 766-8271. Update the patient's record under the *Edit* menu.

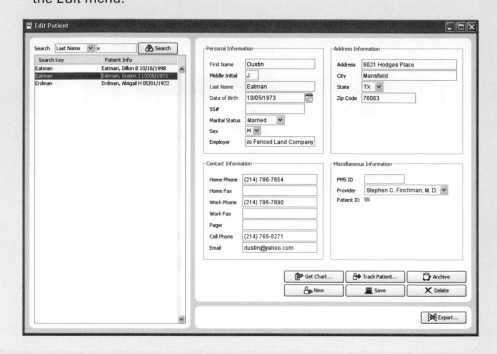

2. Patient Tracker

Exercise 11.3(N)

1. Add your cousin to the *Waiting Room* in the patient tracker by clicking on his name in the schedule.
2. The clinic has assigned the following *Patient Tracker* colors and their associative usage:

Blue—Dr. Finchman
Yellow—Dr. Smith
Green—Self Pay
Red—Lab Work
Black—Procedures
Fuchsia—Commercial Insurance
Assign your cousin the appropriate colors.

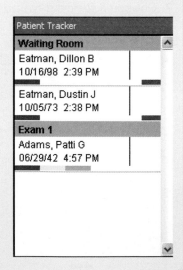

Exercise 11.4(N)

1. Add the insurance information to the program and the patients' charts.

Insurance Company: Prudential Financial Group + your user name. For example, Prudential Financial Group User35
Mail Claim To: NFL Group Claims
Address: PO Box 18974
City: Plano
State: TX
Zip: 56781
Phone: (800) 281-9823

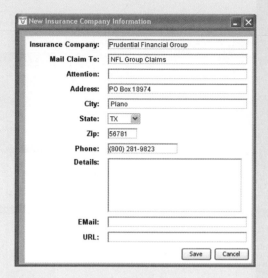

Group Name: NFL Claims
Group Number: 10978NFL
OV Co-Pay: $25
Guarantor: the father

Make a note in the *Details* box of your cousin's son's *Edit Patient Insurance* window: *Insurance Confirmed.*

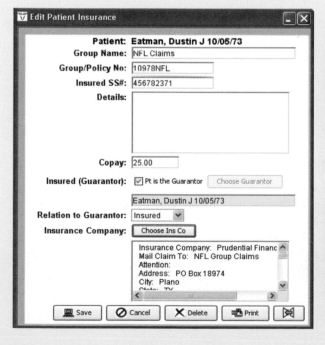
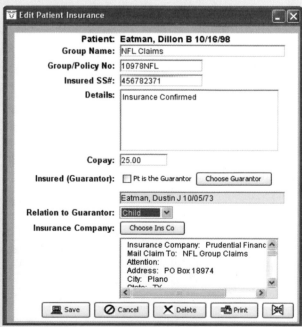

Exercise 11.5(N)

1. Set up the patient tracker as the main view.

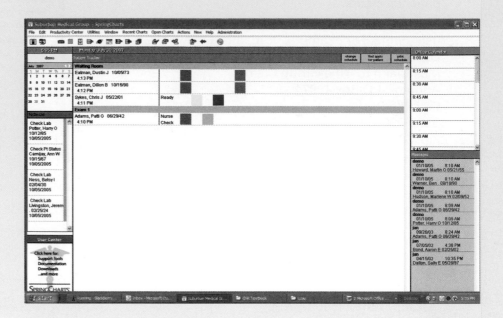

2. Move your cousin into an open exam room and give him a status to *Nurse Check*.
3. Place your cousin's son into the waiting room. Although your cousin is not on the schedule you can add him to the tracker by clicking one time on the *Patient Tracker* title bar.
4. Assign your cousin's son the status of *Ready* and appropriate colors.

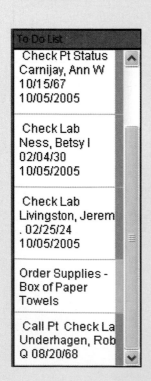

3. To Do List

Exercise 11.6(N)

1. Send yourself a *ToDo* message to *Order Supplies – Box of Paper Towels*. Use both pop-up text and typing.
2. Send yourself a *ToDo* message to call a patient and check the patient's lab. Use exiting pop-up text and link to the patient: Robert Underhagen.

Exercise 11.7(N)

1. Open the *Edit PopUp Text* window and add the sentence: "Remind *patient about scheduled labs*" in the *ToDo/Reminders* category.

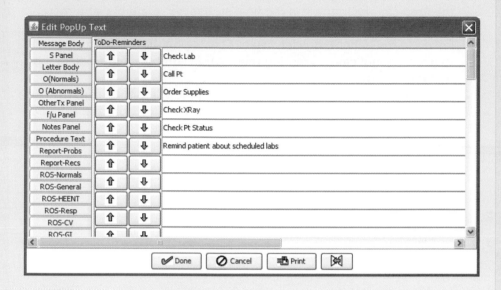

2. Send yourself a *ToDo* message to call a patient and remind the patient about scheduled labs. Select any patient and send the *ToDo* item to yourself in 2 weeks. Check *My ToDo List* and find the future item in the *Edit ToDo* window.

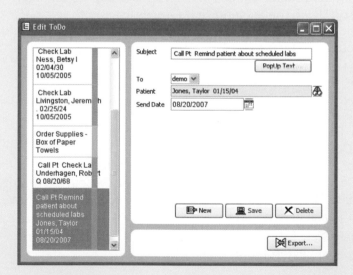

4. Message

Exercise 11.8(N)

1. Mr. Dean has called the doctor's office to request some samples of the medication Lipitor. The medical staff is not available so a message is created at the front desk. Open a *New Message* window linked to the patient: Russell Dean. Create pop-up text that indicates that the patient called wanting medication samples. Now select the text for the note.
2. Mr. Dean had requested some drug samples of Lipitor. From the [Rx] button in the *New Message* window, select Lipitor from the *Previous Prescription* list. Save the medication to the note.
4. Send the message to Dr. Finchman.

B. Patient Chart Screen

1. Face Sheet

Exercise 11.11(N)

1. Open your cousin's chart. Open the face sheet window of the chart. Build the following entries into the face sheet.

   Allergies: Mold extracts and latex. In the *Other Sensitivities* window type: *Cat hair,* then select: *causes hives* from the pop-up text list.

   Social History: Using the existing *Preferences* list and the *Social Hx* PopUp Text, create the following social history. You will need to add only the occupation by free typing.

   Tobacco Use: Nonsmoker.

   Alcohol Use: Social Drinker.

   Caffeine Use: Yes. Cups Per Day: 4.

   Marital Status: Married.

   Occupation: Sales.

   Education: College.

   Past Medical History: Choose asthma and bronchitis from the *Preferences* list. Search for *Fracture of Rib* in the upper *Dx* search window.

   Family Medical History: Using the *Preferences* list build the following family medical history data:

   Brother: Heart Disease

   Mother: Hypercholesterolemia

   Father Died At Age: 59

   Cause of Death: Heart Disease

   Referred By: This patient was referred by Dr. Able Body.

Chart Note: Click on the edit icon for the pop-up text. In the *Edit PopUp Text* window select the *Chart Note* category and add the following hospitals: *St. Johns Hospital, Cox Medical Centers,* and *Physicians Hospital*—indent each line three spaces. Using the up and down arrows, position the new text under the *Prefers Hospital* line. Now move an empty line between the list of hospitals and the line *Religion*. Click the space bar to add an invisible character on the empty line. This will create a space between the text lines. Save the material in the *Edit PopUp Text* window.

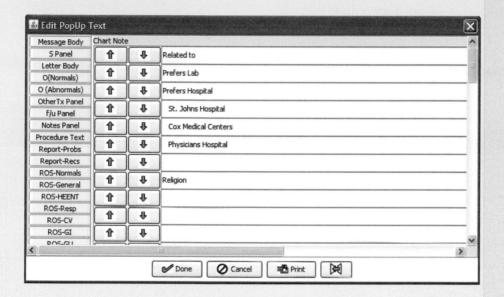

In the face sheet window check your results with the figure below.

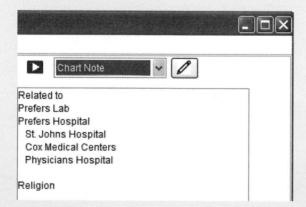

Select the text: Prefers hospital

St. Johns Hospital

Routine Meds: Select the following medications:

Aleve – 275 mg

Lipitor – 20 mg

Aspirin – 81 mg

Edit the Lipitor entry and change the number of refills to 0.

In the *Notes and OTC Meds* window select: *Omega-3*

Problem List: Select *Allergic Rhinitis 477.9* and *Bronchitis 466.0* from the pop-up text list. In the upper *Dx* search area, search for and select *Abdominal Pain.*

Chart Alert: In the *Edit PopUp Text* window select the *Chart Alert* category and add the following sentence: *Insurance approval needed for elective surgery.* Save and select the new text.

Click on the [Back to Chart] button and check your work with the figure below.

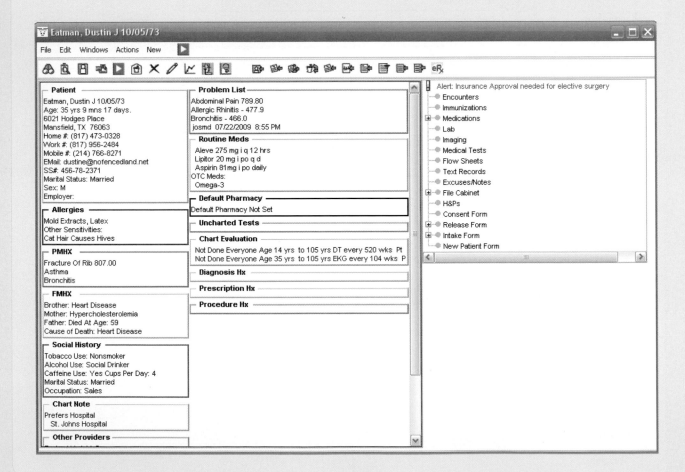

2. Patient Chart Activities

Exercise 11.12(N)

Run a Chart Evaluation of your cousin's chart by accessing the *Evaluate Chart* feature. Record the patient's response that he will get a DT shot today. Mark the recommendation as "Completed" and then save the evaluation. Check your results in the patient's chart under the *Encounter* tab in the Care Tree.

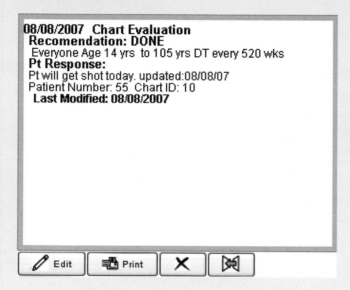

08/08/2007 Chart Evaluation
  Recomendation: DONE
   Everyone Age 14 yrs to 105 yrs DT every 520 wks
  Pt Response:
  Pt will get shot today. updated:08/08/07
  Patient Number: 55 Chart ID: 10
   Last Modified: 08/08/2007

Edit | Print | X | ▶◀

Exercise 11.13(N)

Check the *Household List* located in the *File* menu of the father's chart. This list will provide access to the other patient charts of the same household.

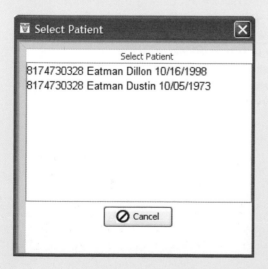

Select Patient

Select Patient
8174730328 Eatman Dillon 10/16/1998
8174730328 Eatman Dustin 10/05/1973

Cancel

Exercise 11.14(N)

The following pharmacy supplied by the father will need to be added to the SpringCharts address book. Because you are working in a network environment you will need to create a unique address for the pharmacy below. **Be sure to add the street name in parentheses after the company's name so that you can distinguish it on the list**

Walgreens (_____)
Crn _____ Av. & _____ St.
_____, TX 76063
Ph: (817) ____-_____
Fx: (817) ____-_____

Under the *Edit* menu in the father's chart, add this new pharmacy as the patient default pharmacy. The patient's preferred pharmacy will be displayed in the *Prescription Hx* portion of the face sheet.

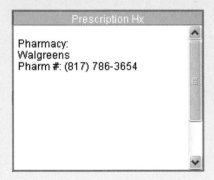

Prescription Hx

Pharmacy:
Walgreens
Pharm #: (817) 786-3654

Exercise 11.15(N)

1. Add your cousin's photo to his chart by accessing the *Pt Photo* feature under the *Edit* menu. By selecting the [Edit] button direct your search in the *Open* dialogue window through the "*Desktop*" access to locate your cousin's photo in the *EHR Material* folder saved to your desktop. It the folder was not previously downloaded from the Online Learning Center at www.mhhe.com/HamiltonEHR2e, you will need to do so now.

2. Click on the *Pt Photo* category in the patient's care tree to view the father's photo below.

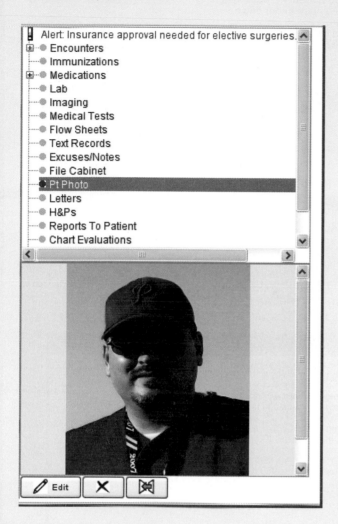

Exercise 11.16(N)

1. Your patient (who goes by your name) has called on the telephone and is requesting a list of medication that has been prescribed for him/her at your office. By using both pop-up text and typing, record the details of the conversation by accessing the *New TC Note* under the *New* menu in your patient's chart. Initial- and time-stamp the note by using the [Sign] button. Save the telephone note and skip billing.

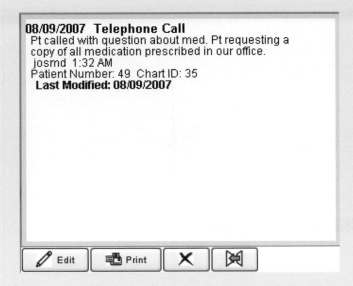

08/09/2007 Telephone Call
Pt called with question about med. Pt requesting a
copy of all medication prescribed in our office.
 josmd 1:32 AM
Patient Number: 49 Chart ID: 35
 Last Modified: 08/09/2007

2. In your patient's chart print out the list of all medications prescribed to him by accessing the *Medications List* under the *Actions* menu.

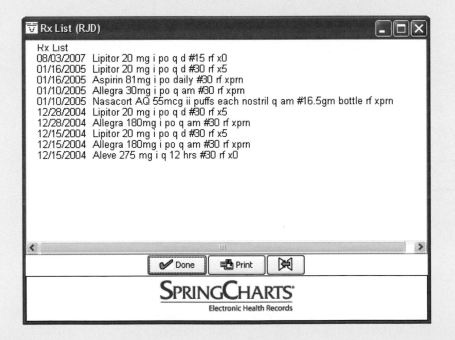

Rx List (RJD)

Rx List
08/03/2007 Lipitor 20 mg i po q d #15 rf x0
01/16/2005 Lipitor 20 mg i po q d #30 rf x5
01/16/2005 Aspirin 81mg i po daily #30 rf xprn
01/10/2005 Allegra 30mg i po q am #30 rf xprn
01/10/2005 Nasacort AQ 55mcg ii puffs each nostril q am #16.5gm bottle rf xprn
12/28/2004 Lipitor 20 mg i po q d #30 rf x5
12/28/2004 Allegra 180mg i po q am #30 rf xprn
12/15/2004 Lipitor 20 mg i po q d #30 rf x5
12/15/2004 Allegra 180mg i po q am #30 rf xprn
12/15/2004 Aleve 275 mg i q 12 hrs #30 rf x0

SPRINGCHARTS®
Electronic Health Records

Exercise 11.17(N)

1. Open a *New Nurse Note* under the *New* menu of your cousin's chart. Choose a *Well Adult* diagnosis and record the inoculation of a DT shot. You will need to select the *Immunization* category under the

Choose Procedure window to locate the DT procedure. Once selected, click on the DT procedure and change the procedure detail to lot number 2695A. Add your initials and time by selecting the [Sign] button. Save the nurse note under the *Encounters* tab and send a routing slip.

2. In the *Routing Slip* window select *Immunization 90471* from the *Superbill Form* for the administration of the injection. Send the routing slip. Check the details of the *Nurse Note* in the patient's chart.

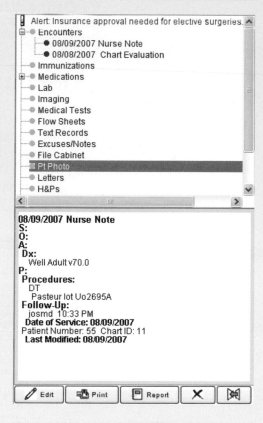

Exercise 11.18(N)

Open your patient's chart. Your patient is diabetic and comes into the clinic on a regular basis to have his/her vitals taken. Under the *New* menu in the chart complete a *Vitals Only* panel. The patient is 5 ft 4 in, and weighs 156 pounds. You can complete the other vitals yourself. Remember BMI is calculated automatically from the height and weight. Head circumference (HC) is only used in a pediatric situation for head growth of infants. By using pop-up text found under the *Notes* tab indicate that the patient's blood pressure was taken on his/her right arm. Save the new vitals under the *Encounter* tab and skip billing.

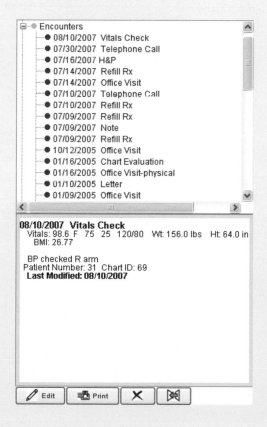

C. Office Visit Screen

1. Office Visit Note

Exercise 11.19(N)

1. In your cousin's chart open a *New OV* window under the *New* menu. The patient has come to the doctor's office for his annual well checkup. Under the chief complaint (CC) navigation button select: *Routine Well Visit*. Using the time and initial icon buttons in the lower middle of the OV screen, stamp the chief complaint note with the time and initial stamp.
2. Under the [Vitals] button complete the well vitals for the patient.
3. Save the office visit under the encounter tab and skip billing. Close the patient's chart and update the patient's status on the Patient tracker to "Doctor Ready."

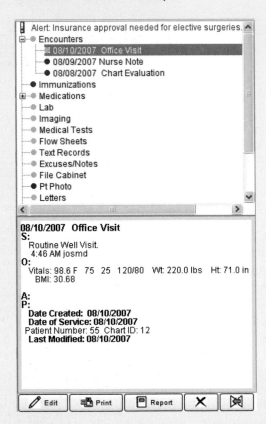

Exercise 11.20(N)

1. Reopen the patient's chart and highlight the partially completed office visit note. Click on the [Edit] button to open the *Office Visit* screen.

2. Under the review of systems (ROS) navigation button select the following:

ROS-Normal:

GENERAL: No weight change, fever, chills, night sweats, generalized weakness.

HEENT: No headache, dizziness, lightheadedness, diplopia, tearing, eye pain, blind spots, excessive blinking, tinnitus, ear pain or discharge, nose bleeding, nasal obstruction, nasal discharge, gingival bleeding, dental problem, sore throat, hoarseness, difficulty swallowing, neck stiffness, neck pain.

PULMONARY: No wheezing, cough, congestion, hemoptysis, respiratory infections, tuberculosis, chest wall pain.

CV: No chest pain, arrhythmia, syncope, dyspnea, exertional dyspnea, orthopnea, paroxysmal nocturnal dyspnea, intermittent claudication, dependent edema, varicose vein, phlebitis, heart murmur, hypertension.

GI: No change in appetite, difficulty swallowing, indigestion, heartburn, belching, nausea, vomiting, hematemesis, hematochezia, abdomen pain, flatulence, changes in bowel habits, constipation, diarrhea, abnormal stools, incontinence, hemorrhoids, jaundice.

3. Under the [Exam] button select the following pop-up text:

GENERAL: Well developed. Well nourished. Alert. Oriented to person, place, and time. In no apparent distress.

HEAD: Normocephalic. Atraumatic.

EYES: Eyes and lids appear symmetrical. No exudate. Sclera clear. PERRLA, EOMI. Discs sharp.

EARS: External auditory canals and TMs normal. Hearing normal as tested by whisper and Rinne/Weber.

MOUTH/THROAT: Dentition good. Normal mucosa, tongue, gingiva, and oropharynx. Palate elevates in midline. No thrush, erythema, or exudate.

CV: RRR, normal S1 S2, no S3/S4, murmur, gallop, rub, arrhythmia, or heave. PMI normal in location and character.

ABDOMEN: Bowel sounds are normal. No evidence of scarring or past surgical procedures. Abdomen is flat, soft, and nontender, without rebound or guarding. No evidence of masses, organomegaly, or abdominal aneurysm. Normal to percussion.

MUSCULOSKELETAL: Posture normal. Pulses normal and symmetrical. Motor strength normal. Sensory normal and symmetrical to soft touch and pin prick. Joints show normal range of motion and are without erythema or effusions. Nails: Normal capillary filling and appearance w/o clubbing or pitting. No masses or dependent edema noted.

RECTAL: No mass palpable. Prostate normal in size, shape, and consistency for age. Guaiac negative.

4. Select the [Dx] button and choose the *Well Adult* code from the *Previous Diagnosis* window.

5. Order a CBC and a SMAC under the [Test] button. Because these tests will be conducted at an outside testing facility you will want to print a physician's order form and save a copy in the patient's chart under the *Notes* category in the care tree. Add the patient's primary insurance to the order form.

6. **Print the order form and compare with the figure below. Submit to your instructor.**

Suburban Medical Group
101 Elm Street
Sherman, TX 77521
(214) 674-2000   Fax (214) 674-2100

Date: 08/10/07
Pt: Eatman, Dustin J 10/05/73
Address: 6021 Hodges Place   Mansfield, TX 76063

Physician Order

Orders:
CBC 85025
SMAC 80054

Diagnosis:
Well Adult v70.0

_____

Patient Insurance Info
Group Name: NFL Claims
Group/Policy No: 10978NFL
Guarantor: Eatman, Dustin J 10/05/73
Certif No: 456782371
Insured
CoPay: 25.0

Insurance Company: Prudential Financial Group
Mail Claim To: NFL Group Claims
Attention:
Address: PO Box 18974
City: Plano
State: TX
Zip: 56781
Phone: 8002819823
Details:
EMail:
URL:

Prepared by
SpringChartsEMR   **Suburban Medical Group**

---

7. The doctor decides to give the patient a flu shot during the office visit because of the upcoming flu season. Under the procedure button type *flu,* then search for and select flu shot. Highlight the flu shot procedure

and change the Aventis Pasteur number to UO701BA and the vaccine date to today's date, for example, 30JUNE08. Date-, time-, and initial-stamp the procedure note.

8. Under the [OtherTx] button select the counseling notes: *Discussed weight loss strategies. Encouraged Pt to exercise 30 minutes 5 times a week.*

9. Plan a follow-up for 1 year. Select the *Create a Reminder* icon and send a *ToDo/Reminder* note to Jan to call the patient and check the lab work (use pop-up text). Send it to her so that she will receive it in 3 business days.

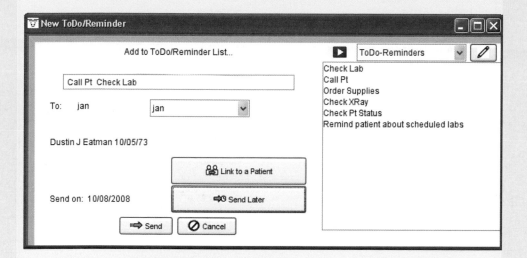

10. Save the office visit note and create a routing slip. From the Superbill form, select the venipuncture procedure because of the blood draw and the CPT code 90472 because of the additional inoculation that was done. (These additional codes are added to the routing slip at this time rather than in the OV note because they are essential for billing purposes, even though they are not critical to the note.) Depending of whether you did Exercise 11.17 (the nurse note) on the same day or a different day from this exercise, the E&M coder will recommend either a new or established patient visit E&M code. Let us assume this office visit note was created on the same day as the nurse note. If the E&M coder recommendation is not for a new patient you will need to choose the appropriate E&M code for a new patient from the drop-down list at the bottom of the routing slip. Send the routing slip.

11. Under the main *Edit* menu locate the routing slip just generated.

12. Print the routing slip. Compare your results with the figure below. Submit to your instructor.

Suburban Medical Group
101 Elm Street
Sherman, TX 77521
(214) 674-2000   Fax (214) 674-2100

Eatman, Dustin J 10/05/73
6021 Hodges Place
Mansfield, TX 76063
Home #: (817) 473-0328
Work #: (817) 966-2484
Pager:
EMail: dustine@nofencedland.net
SS#: 456-78-2371
Sex: M
Employer: No Fenced Land Company

Home Fax:
Work Fax:
Mobile #: (214) 766-8271

Marital Status: Married
Pt ID #: 55

Date of Service: 08/10/2007
Doctor: Stephen C. Finchman, M. D.
    99205 NP-Comprehensive
Diagnosis:
    Well Adult v70.0
Tests:
    CBC 85025
    SMAC 80054
Other Procedures:
    Immunization 90471
    additional Immunization 90472
    Venipuncture 36415

    Flu Shot 90658
Discussed weight loss strategies. Encouraged
pt to exercise 30 minutes 5 times a week.
    Followup:
    1 year

Patient Insurance Info
Group Name: NFL Claims
Group/Policy No: 10978NFL
Guarantor: Eatman, Dustin J 10/05/73
Certif No: 456782371
Insured
CoPay: 25.0

Insurance Company: Prudential Financial Group
Mail Claim To: NFL Group Claims
Attention:
Address: PO Box 18974
City: Plano
State: TX
Zip: 56781
Phone: 8002819823
Details:
EMail:
URL:

epared by
gChartsEMR

2. Office Visit Activities

Exercise 11.21(N)

In your cousin's chart print a copy of the recent office visit note. Submit to your instructor.

Suburban Medical Group
101 Elm Street Sherman, TX 77521
(214) 674-2000

08/10/2007 Office Visit
S:
    CC:Routine Well Visit.
    4:46 AM josmd
    PI: Routine Well Visit.
    ROS: ROS-Normal:
    GENERAL: No weight change, fever, chills, night sweats, generalized weakness.
    HEENT: No headache, dizziness, lightheadedness, diplopia, tearing, eye pain, blind spots, excessive blinking, tinnitus, ear pain or discharge, nose bleeding, nasal obstruction, nasal discharge, gingival bleeding, dental problem, sore throat, hoarseness, difficulty swallowing, neck stiffness, neck pain.
    PULMONARY: No wheezing, cough, congestion, hemoptysis, respiratory infections, tuberculosis, chest wall pain.
    CV: No chest pain, arrhythmia, syncope, dyspnea, exertional dyspnea, orthopnea, paroxysmal nocturnal dyspnea, intermittent claudication, dependent edema, varicose vein, phlebitis, heart murmur, hypertension.
    GI: No change in appetite, difficulty swallowing, indigestion, heartburn, belching, nausea, vomiting, hematemesis, hematochezia, abdomen pain, flatulence, changes in bowel habits, constipation, diarrhea, abnormal stools, incontinence, hemorrhoids, jaundice.
O:
    Vitals: 98.6 F 75 25 120/80 Wt: 220.0 lbs Ht: 71.0 in
    BMI: 30.68

    GENERAL: Well developed. Well nourished. Alert. Oriented to person, place, and time. In no apparent distress.
    HEAD: Normocephalic Atraumatic.
    EYES: Eyes and lids appear symmetrical. No exudate. Sclera clear. PERRLA, EOMI. Discs sharp.
    EARS: External auditory canals and TMs normal. Hearing normal as tested by whisper and Rinne/Weber.
    MOUTH/THROAT: Dentition good. Normal mucosa, tongue, gingiva, and oropharynx. Palate elevates in midline. No thrush, erythema, or exudate.
    CV: RRR, normal S1 S2, no S3/S4, murmur, gallop, rub, arrhythmia, or heave. PMI normal in location and character.
    ABDOMEN: Bowel sounds are normal. No evidence of scarring or past surgical procedures. Abdomen is flat, soft, and nontender, without rebound or guarding. No evidence of masses, organomegaly or abdominal aneurysm. Normal to percussion.
    MUSCULOSKELETAL: Posture normal. Pulses normal and symmetrical. Motor strength normal. Sensory normal and symmetrical to soft touch and pin prick. Joints show normal range of motion and are without erythema or effusions. Nails: Normal capillary filling and appearance w/o clubbing or pitting. No masses or dependent edema noted.
    GU (male): RECTAL: No mass palpable. Prostate normal in size, shape, and consistency for age. Guiaic negative.
A:
    Dx:
        Well Adult v70.0
    P:

Patient: Eatman, Dustin J 10/05/73
Prepared by
SpringChartsEMR

Page 1 of 2
Suburban Medical Group

Tests:
    CBC
    SMAC
Procedures:
    Flu Shot
        Aventis Pasteur UO701BA x 30JUNE08 Fluzone
        0.5 IM
        08/10/2007 5:38 AM josmd
Other Tx:
    Discussed weight loss strategies. Encouraged pt to exercise 30 minutes 5 times a week.
Follow-Up:
    1 year
    Date Created: 08/10/2007
    Date of Service: 08/10/2007
Patient Number: no Patient reference Chart ID: not Charted
    Last Modified: 08/10/2007

Patient: Eatman, Dustin J 10/05/73
Prepared by
SpringChartsEMR

Page 2 of 2
Suburban Medical Group

Exercise 11.22(N)

1. The father is requesting a history and physical report of his medical encounter to take with him. Open the current office visit note and select the H&P report from the *Tools* menu.
2. Print **the report. Submit to your instructor.**
3. Save the H&P report under the *H&Ps* category in the care tree. Close the *Office Visit* screen.

History and Physical
Patient: Eatman, Dustin J 10/05/73
Date of Service: 08/10/2007
Chief Complaint:
 Routine Well Visit. 4:46 AM josmd
Present Illness:
 Routine Well Visit.
Allergies:
 Mold Extracts, Latex
 Cat Hair causes hives
Current Medications:
 Aleve 275 mg i q 12 hrs
 Lipitor 20 mg i po q d
 Aspirin 81mg i po daily
 Omega-3
Past Medical History:
 Fracture Of Rib
 Asthma Bronchitis
Family Medical History:
 Brother: Heart Disease Mother: Hypercholesterolemia Father Died At Age: 59
 Cause Of Death: Heart Disease
Social History:
 Tobacco Use: Nonsmoker. Alcohol Use: Social Drinker. Caffeine Use: Yes. Cups
 Per Day: 4 Marital Status: Married. Occupation: Sales Education: College.
Review Of Systems:
 ROS-Normal: GENERAL: No weight change, fever, chills, night sweats,
 generalized weakness. HEENT: No headache, dizziness, lightheadedness,
 diplopia, tearing, eye pain, blind spots, excessive blinking, tinnitus, ear pain or
 discharge, nose bleeding, nasal obstruction, nasal discharge, gingival bleeding,
 dental problem, sore throat, hoarseness, difficulty swallowing, neck stiffness, neck
 pain. PULMONARY: No wheezing, cough, congestion, hemoptysis, respiratory
 infections, tuberculosis, chest wall pain. CV: No chest pain, arrhythmia, syncope,
 dyspnea, exertional dyspnea, orthopnea, paroxysmal nocturnal dyspnea,
 intermittent claudication, dependent edema, varicose vein, phlebitis, heart
 murmur, hypertension. GI: No change in appetite, difficulty swallowing, indigestion,
 heartburn, belching, nausea, vomiting, hematemesis, hematochezia, abdomen
 pain, flatulence, changes in bowel habits, constipation, diarrhea, abnormal stools,
 incontinence, hemorrhoids, jaundice.
Examination:
 Vitals: Temp: 98.6 Pulse: 75 Resp: 25 BP: 120/60 Wt: 220.0 Ht: 71.0
 GENERAL: Well developed. Well nourished. Alert. Oriented to person, place, and
 time. In no apparent distress. HEAD: Normocephalic. Atraumatic. EYES: Eyes and
 lids appear symmetrical. No exudate. Sclera clear. PERRLA, EOMI. Discs sharp.
 EARS: External auditory canals and TMs normal. Hearing normal as tested by

Suburban Medical Group
H&P for Pt: Eatman, Dustin J 10/05/73   Page 1 of 2

whisper and Rinne/Weber. MOUTH/THROAT: Dentition good. Normal mucosa,
tongue, gingiva, and oropharynx. Palate elevates in midline. No thrush, erythema,
or exudate. CV: RRR, normal S1 S2, no S3/S4, murmur, gallop, rub, arrhythmia, or
heave. PMI normal in location and character. ABDOMEN: Bowel sounds are
normal. No evidence of scarring or past surgical procedures. Abdomen is flat, soft,
and nontender, without rebound or guarding. No evidence of masses,
organomegaly or abdominal aneurysm. Normal to percussion.
MUSCULOSKELETAL: Posture normal. Pulses normal and symmetrical. Motor
strength normal. Sensory normal and symmetrical to soft touch and pin prick.
Joints show normal range of motion and are without erythema or effusions. Nails:
Normal capillary filling and appearance w/o clubbing or pitting. No masses or
dependent edema noted. GU (male): RECTAL: No mass palpable. Prostate
normal in size, shape, and consistency for age. Guiaic negative.
Tests:
CBC pending
SMAC pending
Flu Shot
Aventis Pasteur UO701BA x 30JUNE08 Fluzone 0.5 IM 08/10/2007 5:38 AM josmd
Impression:
Well Adult v70.0
Plan:
Discussed weight loss strategies. Encouraged pt to exercise 30 minutes 5 times
a week.
1 year

John O. Smith, M. D.

Suburban Medical Group
H&P for Pt: Eatman, Dustin J 10/05/73   Page 2 of 2

4. Close the patient's chart. Update the patient tracker to reflect the father being sent to the *Checkout Desk* with a status of *Ready.* Save the *Edit Tracker* window. Reopen it and click on the [CheckOut] button. The patient tracker will show the patient in the "Done" section with the *Routing Slip* stamp.

Done

Eatman, Dustin J 10/05/73
6:58 AM   √ *Routing Slip*   Done

CHAPTER 12 **ELECTRONIC RECORDING**

Exercise 12.1(N)

1. Using *Source Document 1—Patient Information Sheet (see Appendix D, page 346)*, complete a *New Patient* profile.
2. **Using the universal export button, open the patient information in the word processor, print, record your name on the document, and submit to your instructor.**

Exercise 12.2(N)

1. Using *Source Document 2—Primary Insurance Card Information (see Appendix D, page 347)*, set up a new insurance company in SpringCharts. Save the insurance information.
2. **Using the universal export button, open the insurance information in the word processor, print, record your name on the document, and submit to your instructor.**

Exercise 12.3(N)

1. Using *Source Document 2—Primary Insurance Card Information (see Appendix D, page 347)*, add the primary insurance details to the patient's face sheet.
2. **Using the [print] button, print the patient and insurance information, record your name on the document, and submit to your instructor.**

Exercise 12.4(N)

1. Using *Source Document 3—Patient Intake Sheet (see Appendix D, page 348)*, add the PCP (primary care physician) to SpringCharts address book.
2. **Using the [print] button, print the patient and insurance information, record your name on the document, and submit to your instructor.**

Exercise 12.5(N)

1. Using *Source Document 3—Patient Intake Sheet (see Appendix D, page 348)*, complete the face sheet of the patient's chart.
2. **Print the face sheet. Record your name on the document and submit to your instructor.**

Exercise 12.6(N)

1. Using *Source Document 4—Default Pharmacy Information (see Appendix D, page 349),* add a new address entry to the Address Book in SpringCharts.
2. **Using the [Print Card] button, print the insurance card information. Record your name on the document and submit to your instructor.**

Exercise 12.7(N)

Using *Source Document 4—Default Pharmacy Information (see Appendix D, page 349),* set up the patient's default pharmacy.

Exercise 12.8(N)

1. Import the patient's photo into the chart. Access the *EHR Material* folder on your "Desktop." Locate Chloe Hill's patient picture file and import into the patient's chart.
2. Open the patient's chart to display the imported picture. Also move the scroll bar in the *Prescription Hx* window to display the default pharmacy.
3. **Using the [Print Screen] button on your keyboard, copy the patient chart screen and paste into a word document. You may have to resize the picture to fit the page. Record your name on the document and submit to your instructor.**

Exercise 12.9(N)

1. Using *Source Document 5—Immunization Record Card (see Appendix D, page 349),* update the patient's immunization archive in the patient's chart.
2. **View the immunization and print the list. Record your name on the document and submit to your instructor.**

Exercise 12.10(N)

1. In the patient's chart perform a Chart Evaluation and record the patient's agreement to have the indicated items conducted.
2. Print the chart evaluation. Record your name on the document and submit to your instructor.

Exercise 12.11(N)

1. Using *Source Document 6—Office Visit Notes (see Appendix D, page 350,* record the notation into a *New OV* window in the patient's chart. Complete Exercises 12.12 and 12.13 from within the OV note. Create a Routing Slip.
2. **Using the [Print] button, print the OV Note. Record your name on the document and submit to your instructor.**

Exercise 12.12(N)

1. Create a *Prescription Form* from within the OV note for the medication prescribed to the patient.
2. **Print the prescription form. Record your name on the document and submit to your instructor.**

Exercise 12.13(N)

1. Create an *Order Form* from within the OV note for the tests that are ordered. Add the patient's primary insurance.
2. **Print the order form. Record your name on the document and submit to your instructor.**

Exercise 12.14(N)

1. Using *Source Document 7—Patient Excuse Note (see Appendix D, page 351),* create an excuse note for the patient within the patient's chart.
2. **Print the excuse note. Record your name on the document and submit to your instructor.**

Exercise 12.15(N)

1. Using *Source Document 8—Letter to Primary Care Physician (see Appendix D, page 352),* create a letter about the patient in the patient's chart. Save it under the *Letter* category.
2. **Print the letter. Record your name on the document and submit to your instructor.**

Exercise 12.16(N)

1. Using *Source Document 9—Letter to Patient (see Appendix D, page 353),* create a letter to the patient in the patient's chart. Save it under the *Letter* category.
2. **Print the letter. Record your name on the document and submit to your instructor.**

Exercise 12.17(N)

Using *Source Document 10—Patient Lab Results (see Appendix D, page 354),* record the lab results into the patient's *Pending Test.* Process the *Pending Test* into the *Completed Tests* area from where you will save it into the patient's chart.

Exercise 12.18(N)

1. Create a *New Test Report* from within the patient's chart. Remove the *Problems* and *Recommendations* headings from the report.
2. **Print the report. Record your name on the document and submit to your instructor.**

appendix D

Source Documents for Network Version

Sample 1   Patient Information Sheet

Suburban Medical Group

101 Elm Street
Sherman, TX 77521

PH: (214) 674-2000
FX: (214) 674-2100

APPOINTMENT: TIME: _10:00 AM_   DATE: _____

PATIENT INFORMATION SHEET

Patient Name: _____ Create a Patient's Name _____
Last, First, Middle

Previous and/or Maiden Name(s): _____N/A._____

Date of Birth: _10/8/89_   SS #: _048-69-4281_

Street Address: _78 RICHARDS ST._

City/State/Zip: _LOGANLEA, MO 65807_

Phone Numbers: Home: _417-881-3968_ Cell: _____

Email address (if applicable): _ceh89@hotmail.com_

Sex: (Circle one): Male, (Female)

Marital Status (Circle one): Married, Widowed, Divorced, (Single,) or Separated

Patient's Employer: _LOGAN CITY_

Work Phone: _417-969-4123_ Fax Phone: _417-969-7821_

Signature of Patient or Patient/Guardian:
CEHill

Sample 2   Primary Insurance Card Information

Physician Visit & Hospital Program

Office Visit:
Deposit
$35

Member Number 041020102
Group Number 76022

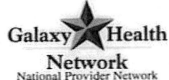

Galaxy Health
Network
National Provider Network

Members: *In an Emergency Seek Medical Attention First.*

For questions or to locate a provider visit www.iabbenefits.com
or call 800-275-1171.

Before seeking hospital services you must register for CAP benefits.
To register call 800-975-3322.

Members Are Responsible For Network Contracted Rates Incurred.

Members are required to register for referral authorization before
seeking hospital services.

PROVIDERS:
Send bills to: IAB; PO Supply No. ; Dallas, TX 75222
For questions call: 866-404- Supply last four digits.

For lab work use Quest Diagnostics or call 800-975-3322.

In Emergency please admit the patient and call 800-975-3322 by the next business day.
All members have limited inpatient and outpatient benefits.
Underwritten by various insurance companies.
This program is administered by IAB
701 Highlander Blvd., Ste 500, Arlington, TX 76015

Sample 3 Patient Intake Sheet

Suburban Medical Group

101 Elm Street
Sherman, TX 77521

PH: (214) 674-2000
FX: (214) 674-2100

Patient Name: _____ , *Add your new patient's name here*
Last, First, Middle

Date of Birth: _10/8/89_____ SS #: _048-69-4281_

FAMILY HISTORY

	Age	State of Health	Occupation	IF DECEASED Cause of Death	Age of Death
Father	50	GOOD	CONSTRUCTION		
Mother				BREAST CANCER	45
Brothers	24	ASTHMA			
	12	GOOD			
Sisters					

Have YOU OR ANY OF YOUR BLOOD RELATED FAMILY MEMBERS had

	YES	NO	RELATIONSHIP
Cancer (List type)	✓		MOTHER - BST CNCR
High blood pressure	✓		AUNT - MOTHERS SISTR
Bleeding disorder		✓	
Tuberculosis		✓	
Diabetes		✓	
Kidney disease		✓	
Heart disease	✓	✓	UNCLE-FATHER'S BROTHR
Arthritis		✓	
Gastrointestinal disorder		✓	
History of drug/alcohol abuse		✓	

PERSONAL HISTORY: QUESTIONS RELATED TO YOUR PAST HEALTH HISTORY.

PROBLEM LIST: Comment on *positive* answers in space below or on *additional sheet.*

HAVE YOU HAD?	YES	NO	ALLERGIES:	YES	NO		YES	NO		YES	NO
			Drugs/Medication: Please list	✓		Recurrent colds or chronic cough	✓		Disease or Injury of bones or joints		✓
Measles		✓	CODEINE			Shortness of Breath		✓	Back problems	✓	
German Measles		✓				Asthma and/or hay fever	✓		Weakness, Paralysis		✓
Mumps		✓				Pain/Pressure in Chest		✓	Dizziness, fainting		✓
Chicken Pox	✓		Foods: Please list			Heart murmur		✓	Frequent Urination		✓
Malaria		✓	PEANUTS			Rheumatic fever		✓	Kidney disease		✓
Gum or Tooth Problem		✓	SHELLFISH CAUSES RASH			High or Low Blood Pressure		✓	S. T. Ds.		✓
Sinusitis	✓		Head injury/ unconsciousness or concuss ion		✓	Recurrent diarrhea or constipation or both		✓	Chronic skin disease eczema or psoriasis		✓
Eye Problem		✓	Seizure disorder/Epilepsy		✓	Jaundice or Hepatitis		✓	Tumor, cancer, cyst		✓
Ear, Nose, Throat Problems TONSILLITIS	✓		Recurrent or severe headache, migraine headache	✓		Gallbladder disease or gallstones		✓	FEMALES ONLY		
Surgery List APPENDECTOMY			Asthmatic/Bronchitis	✓		Eating disorder		✓	Excessive flow		✓
			Insomnia		✓				Irregular Periods		✓
			Frequent Anxiety	✓		Hernia, rupture		✓	Severe Cramps	✓	

		YES	NO	
A. Has your physical activity been restricted during the past five years? (give reasons and duration)			✓	
B. Have you ever had radiation treatments to the head or neck?			✓	
C. Have you received treatment or counseling for a nervous condition,		✓		
D. Have you had any illness or injury or been hospitalized, other than already noted? (Give details)			✓	
E. Have you been rejected for or discharged from military service because of physical, emotional, or other reasons?			✓	
F. Have you lived or traveled outside of the U.S.A.?		✓		

ROUTINE MEDICATIONS. List medications you take regularly including non-prescription & herbals.

ALEVE - 275 mg   CLARITIN D-24
CALCIUM SUPPLEMENTS
MULTI-VITAMIN

Name/address/phone of your primary care physician.
DR JON *Add docor's last name.*
1200 E. WOODHURST
WATERFORD, MO 65804 (417) 890-6777

Social History:

1. Tobacco Use: ☐Yes, ☒No, ☐Mild, ☐Moderate, ☐Heavy, ☐Smokeless Tobacco, Packs Per Day? _____ 2. Alcohol Use: ☐Non Drinker, ☒Social Drinker, ☐Heavy Drinker
3. Caffeine Use: ☒Yes, ☐No, Cups Per Day _3_ 4. Illicit Drug Use: List _N/A_ 5. Sexually Active: ☐Yes, ☒No, Age Started? _____
6. Education: ☐ Elementary, ☐High School, ☒College, ☐Post-Graduate 7. Occupation: _STUDENT_

Additional Information:
Hospital Preference - _ST. JOHNS_
Lab Preference - _LAB CORP_

HIPAA Notice of Privacy Practices Acknowledgement

✓ I agree to receive **Suburban Medical Group**'s Notice of Privacy Practices electronically that can be reviewed and printed at www.smg.com or,

_____ I acknowledge receipt of this Notice and that updates will be made available at this website.

Please check one of the above and sign the document _____CEHill_____   _____

(Patient/Legal Guardian)   (Date)

Rev B-2S-2008

Sample 4   Default Pharmacy Information

Walgreens (Place Locate Here)

(Add Your Own Address)   Office:(417) 887-8546
Loganlea, MO 65804   Fax:(417) 887-5623

Category: Pharmacy

Sample 5   Immunization Record Card

VACCINE ADMINISTRATION RECORD
FOR CHILDREN & TEENS
LOGANLEA, MO 65801
(417) 889-2222   Fax

Immunizations for : Your Patient's Name
HFlu 02/05/1990
MMR 04/10/1990
Varicella 04/10/1990
IPV 08/15/1990
HepatitisA 10/15/1990
IPV 04/15/1991
DaPT 10/05/1991
IPV 04/15/1994
DPT 04/15/1994
DPT 10/15/2001
MMR 10/15/2001
HepatitisB 06/02/2002
Meningococcus 08/19/2005
HFlu 05/05/2007
date printed: 08/28/07

Sample 6   Office Visit Notes

	COMPLAINT AND TREATMENT (Diagnosis, when possible) (Underline every new diagnosis)	
Date		*J. Smith* ___ Physician
Name	Your Patient's Name	
Address	see intake sheet.	Soc. Sec. # 048-64-4281
Address		

CC Allergies, congestion, cough, runny nose.

PI Pt reports sys began gradually 5 days ago. Cough - onset 3 days ago. No fever. Nature of cough is dry. Has tried to treat w/ OTC meds. Seems worse in evenings. Ass. sys include itchy eyes. Overall getting worse.

ROS Normals: No weight change, fever, chills no sweats or generalized weakness.

VITALS Temp: 99° Resp: 25 Pulse: 75 BP: 121/62 Ht. 62in Wt. 115

EXAM General: Well developed, well nourished. Alert. Oriented to person, place + time. In no apparent distress.
Abnormals: Nose: congested with boggy turbinates, copious bilateral discharge
EYES: dark circles under both eyes. swollen conjunctivae w/ bilateral tearing

DX: Allergic Rhinitis (477.9)

RX: Allegra 30 mcg i po q am #30 rf xprn
Nasacort AQ 55 mcg ii puffs each nostril q am #16.5 gm bottle rf xprn
Serevent inhaler 21 mcg ii puffs bid #13g canister rf xprn.

Test: Strep Screen

Proc. Nebulizer c Albuterol. (0.5 cc in 2cc NS)

Other Customary discussion of prescribed medication.
Pt instruction sheet given: Allergies.

F/u RTC prn or 1 year F/u.

10:20 AM   J. Smith MD

H5-

Sample 7   Patient Excuse Note

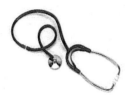

Suburban Medical Group

101 Elm Street
Sherman, TX 77521

PH: (214) 674-2000
FX: (214) 674-2100

EXPLAINED ABSENCE

DATE: _____

TO: *Spfld Community College*

Please excuse this ~~students~~/employees absence today due to our office visit from

10:00 AM to *12:00* ___ am/pm

John O. Smith M.D.

By: _____

Sample 8   Letter to Primary Care Physician

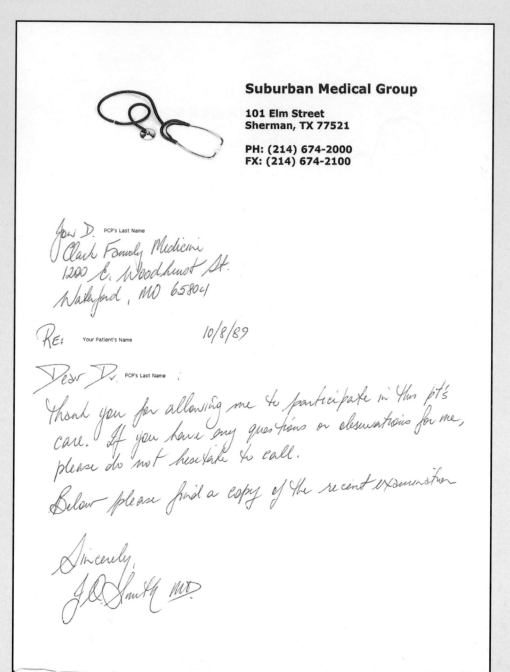

Suburban Medical Group

101 Elm Street
Sherman, TX 77521

PH: (214) 674-2000
FX: (214) 674-2100

Your D.   PCP's Last Name
Clark Family Medicine
1200 E. Woodhurst St.
Waterford, MO 65804

RE: Your Patient's Name   10/8/89

Dear Dr.   PCP's Last Name   :

Thank you for allowing me to participate in this pt's care. If you have any questions or observations for me, please do not hesitate to call.

Below please find a copy of the recent examination

Sincerely,

J.D. Smith MD

Sample 9   Letter to Patient

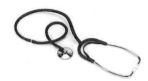

Suburban Medical Group

101 Elm Street
Sherman, TX 77521

PH: (214) 674-2000
FX: (214) 674-2100

Your Patient's Name

78 Richards St
Loganlea, MD 65807.

RE: Lab Results from Recent Visit

Dear Ms. Patient's Last Name :

Please find enclosed lab results from our recent visit. Included is a basic explanation of the lab results.

If you have any questions regarding these results, please call the office + schedule an appointment to meet with me.

Thank you for allowing me to be your physician Stay well.

Sincerely,

John D. Smith, MD

Sample 10   Patient Lab Results

TEST PERFORMED AT:
Lab Corp
4380 Federal Dr. Suite 100
Marsdon, MO 65803

PATIENT:
Your Patient's Name
DOB: 10/08/1989
Gender: F

Ordering Physician: John O. Smith MD
  Accnt No: 444051
Lab Specimen: No N321850003

Test Name	In Range	Out Of Range	Reference Range
Strep Screen	Normal		Normal

Test Date: 08/05/2003

glossary

A

Addendum An addendum is a medical note added subsequent to the original note that will supplement the clinical information.

AMA AMA is the acronym for the *American Medical Association*, which was founded in 1847. Its purpose is to promote the art and science of medicine in order to improve professional and public health concerns in America's health-care system.

Ambulatory EHR The word *ambulatory* indicates the ability to walk from one place to another. When referring to EHR programs it indicates those used in physicians' offices as contrasted with EHR programs used in inpatient settings.

Analyte See *Lab Analyte*

Appointment Schedule The appointment schedule displays past, current, and future appointments for patients. Multiple appointment schedules can be created in one program to display patient appointments for several medical providers and other resources. Appointment schedules can show a variety of appointment length slots.

ARRA The American Recovery and Reinvestment Act of 2009, commonly known as the stimulus package, was passed by Congress to stimulate the economy through investments in infrastructure, unemployment benefits, transportation, education, and health care.

ASP Application Server Provider enables a doctor's office to access an EHR via the Internet; the EHR software and database are housed and maintained by a separate company in a remote location.

B

Body Mass Index BMI is the measurement of choice for studying obesity. BMI is calculated by a mathematical formula that divides a person's weight by height in meters squared (BMI = kg/m^2).

C

Care Plans Care plans or practice guidelines are specific documents that provide a "road map" to guide all who are involved with a patient's care, outlining the appropriate treatment to ensure the optimal outcome. A caregiver unfamiliar with the patient should be able to find all the information needed to care for this person in the care plan.

Care Tree The dynamic care tree in the patient's electronic chart lists categories that hold encounters (progress notes), tests, excuse notes, letters, reports, and other current records.

Category Preferences The category preference table on SpringCharts Server enables the clinic administrator to create customized predetermined lists of medical data. The lists are displayed in SpringCharts on each computer and enable the rapid selection of items from these checklists to build the face sheet and other areas of the program.

CCHIT Certification Commission for Healthcare Information Technology is an independent non-government organization that seeks to accelerate the adoption of EHRs with a credible certification program.

CCR Continuity of Care Record is a core set of provider-oriented health data reflecting the most relevant and timely facts about a patient's health care. It is vendor and technology neutral, enabling the access of patient information between health-care providers.

Chart Alert The chart alert allows for the inclusion of important text that will appear in red above the *Encounters* category on the chart's care tree.

Chart Evaluation The chart evaluation feature is used to define criteria to search patient charts for health screening needs.

CHI Consolidated Health Informatics is a federal government initiative that seeks to provide adoption of health information interoperability standards for health vocabulary and messaging.

CMS Centers for Medicare and Medicaid Services, formerly known as the Health Care Financing Administration (HCFA). It is the federal agency responsible for administering Medicare, Medicaid, HIPAA, CLIA, and several other health-related programs.

Connectivity   The ability to make and maintain a connection between two or more points in a tele-communications system. It allows for the viewing and/or transfer of data from one computer system to another.

CPT Codes   CPT codes stands for *Current Procedural Terminology*. The CPT five-digit codes were developed by the American Medical Association (AMA) and have been adopted by insurance carriers and managed care companies as the means to identify common medical procedures, e.g., "82270 – Fecal occult blood test."

D

DICOM   The Digital Imaging and Communications in Medicine standard was created to aid in the distribution and viewing of medical images, such as CT scans, MRIs, ultrasound, and x-rays.

Drug Formularies   Drug formularies are databases of approved medications in drug therapy categories and include information on recipe for the preparation, safety, effectiveness, and cost.

Drug Monographs   Drug monographs are highly detailed and thoroughly documented studies on drugs. They provide such information as the composition, description, method of preparation, dosage, adverse effects, overdose, warnings, and research.

E

E&M Code   Evaluation and Management codes are five-digit Current Procedural Terminology (CPT) codes used by a physician to report evaluation and management services with a patient. The E&M encounter may include documenting a patient's medical history, a physical examination, and medical decision making. An E&M encounter may be with an inpatient, an outpatient, or a consultation and may occur in any number of medical settings.

E&M Coder   The E&M coder stands for *The Evaluation & Management Coder*, which is a built-in function of SpringCharts that recommends the appropriate evaluation and management code for office visits. The coder looks for keywords used within the review of systems and exam of body areas, organs, and systems in the office visit note. The E&M coder then

uses this information along with the number of diagnoses chosen and whether the encounter is an initial or subsequent visit to determine the E&M code for billing.

EHR   Electronic Health Records is the most commonly accepted term for software with a full range of functionalities to store, access, and use patient medical information.

Electronic Chart   The electronic chart is the repository for patient medical data through computer automation in the medical office/clinic. Similar to the traditional paper chart, it holds such static information as the patient's medical history and medical problems as well as the dynamic information including office visit notes, tests, letters, and reports concerning the patient.

EMR   Electronic Medical Records is the term for software that lacks a full range of higher-end functionalities to store, access, and use patient medical information.

Encounters   The encounters tab in the electronic care tree stores many of the documents that are created from encounters with the patient.

Encrypted   When computer data is changed from its original form to be transmitted securely so as to be unintelligible to unauthorized parties and then decrypted back into its original form for use.

E-Prescribing   Electronic prescribing is the use of computerized tools, usually embedded in an EHR program, that create and sign prescriptions for medicines. E-prescriptions replace the handwritten prescriptions and are sent to pharmacies over the Internet via clearinghouses.

Export Chart   Export chart enables you to export any portion of the chart as a text file by selecting items from a list of chart entries. The text file can be e-mailed and opened in a Word Processor program by the recipient.

F

Face Sheet   The face sheet contains more consistent patient information such as demographics, allergies, problem list, past medical history (PMHX), family medical history (FMHX), social history, and so on. It is initially set up for a new patient.

FMHX   A family medical history is a record of health information about a person's close relatives. Because families have many factors in common, including their genes and lifestyles, medical information from three generations of relatives can give clues to a patient's increased risk of developing a particular condition.

G

Graphic User Interface   Software program screen that can display icons, subwindows, text fields, and menus designed to standardize and simplify the use of the computer program by typing in fields and by using a mouse to manipulate text and images.

H

Healthcare Common Procedure Coding System (HCPCS) codes   Codes used by CMS (Medicare & Medicaid) to indicate medical supplies such as durable medical equipment and other medical procedure codes; coding supplies ensures uniformity for billing and financial reimbursement.

HIPAA   Health Insurance Portability and Accountability Act of 1996 enforces standards for electronic patient health, administrative, and financial data.

History & Physical Report   A History & Physical report is often referred to as an H&P. It is the documentation of the patient's medical history combined with the physical exam.

HITECH   The Health Information Technology for Economic and Clinical Health (HITECH) Act was passed as part of ARRA in 2009 and governs finance and development within the health-care industry, including expansion of HIPAA's coverage to business associates of HIPAA covered entities.

HL7   Healthy Level 7.5 is an international computer language by which various health-care systems can communicate. HL7 is currently the selected standard for the interfacing of clinical data between software programs in most institutions.

I

ICD-9 Codes   ICD-9 Codes stands for the *International Classification of Diseases, Ninth Revision.* The ICD has become the international standard diagnostic classification for all medical data dealing with the incidence and prevalence of disease in large populations and for other health management purposes, e.g., "474.00 – Tonsillitis (chronic)."

Imaging Tests   Imaging tests consist of x-rays, CT scans, MRIs, and so on.

Imperial Units   Having to do with weights and measures that conform to the standards legally established in Great Britain. This measurement system is still widely used in the United States.

Interoperability   Interoperability is the ability of a software program to accept, send, or communicate data from its database to other software programs from multiple vendors to communicate.

Intranet Technologies   Intranet technology is a privately maintained computer network that provides secure accessibility to authorized persons, especially members or employees of an organization enabling the sharing of software, database, and files.

IOM   Institute of Medicine gives advice and information about government policies that affect human health.

L

Lab Analyte   A lab analyte is a blood test compound that is the subject to its own specific chemical analysis. A lab panel is composed of multiple analytes that will undergo analysis.

LAN   Local Area Network is a wired or wireless connection of computers on a single campus or facility.

M

Medicare Part B   That part of the Medicare insurance program that covers physicians' supervision, outpatient hospital care, diagnostic tests, ambulance services, and other ambulatory services. Part A of Medicare covers hospitals, skilled nursing facilities, home health agencies, and other non-ambulatory services.

Message Archive   The message archive is a storage area for saved messages for each user. A sent or received message that is not regarding a patient can be saved as an archived message from where it can be reactivated. Messages regarding patients are saved into the patient's chart.

Metric Units   Having to do with weights and measures relating to the metric system, which is mandatory in a large number of countries; also known as the International System of Units.

MIPPA The Medicare Improvements for Patients and Providers Act of 2008. The act re-establishes Medicare reimbursement for providers, reduces racial and ethnic disparities among Medicare recipients, and reins in certain rapidly growing Medicare supplemental insurance policies.

N

No Show is a term used to indicate a patient missed a scheduled appointment without calling in advance to inform the clinic of their intentions and/ or to reschedule.

O

Office Visit An office visit is defined in SpringCharts as an encounter with a medical provider in which the patient's chief complaints, body systems, vitals, physical exam, diagnoses, and medications, among other things, are reviewed and documented.

P

Patient Status The patient status allows the clinical staff to know in *general terms* what is currently happening with the patient or what needs to be done next. The *Status* is chosen from a drop-down list that is customized by the clinic.

Patient Tracker The patient tracker enables all users across the network to see at a glance the current location and the status of all patients in the clinic. It records the time each patient entered and left the clinic.

Pending Tests The pending tests window displays all the ordered tests (lab, imaging, and medical tests) that are awaiting incoming results.

PHI Protected Health Information regulated under HIPAA covers the protection of any past, present, or future medical and mental health condition whether in oral or recorded form or other medium.

PHR Personal Health Records allows the patient access via the Internet to store and update personal medical information and make inquiries to their doctor about prescriptions, appointments, or concerns.

PMHX The Past Medical History of a patient is information gained by clinicians regarding the patient's past major illnesses, previous surgeries/ operations, and current ongoing illnesses. This information is used to help in formulating a diagnosis and providing medical care.

PMS Acronym for Practice Management System, a software program that manages, among other things, financial transactions, both charges and payments, and the billing of insurance claims and patient statements.

Point of Care Point of care is the time and place of care being given to the patient from the health-care provider.

PopUp Text Large groups of text in SpringCharts enabling the clinic and clerical staff rapid selection of predefined text to complete office visits, letters, reports, messages, and so on. It consists of 34 static categories and 20 categories that can be customized to suit the need of each user. Each category has the capacity to hold 60 lines of customized type.

R

Reference Labs Reference labs are specific lab companies that transmit electronic data to SpringCharts using HL7 language and protocols. Some of the many reference lab companies are LabCorp, Quest, Spectrum, Carilion, WestCliff, and Antek.

ROI Return On Investment is the measure, expressed as a percentage, of the amount that is earned on a company's total purchase or investment calculated by dividing the total capital into earnings or financial benefits.

Routine Meds Routine meds is an abbreviation for the patient's current routine medications. They are listed in the patient's electronic chart.

Routing Slip A routing slip is a form that contains the medical office's most common procedure and diagnosis codes and descriptions. It also contains the patient's name, demographics, and billing information and may or may not include pricing. In a paper environment the physician usually indicates on the routing slip which procedures and diagnoses were used in the office visit. With an EHR only the codes and description that were selected in the office visit will print on the routing slip. Some other names for a routing slip are superbill, encounter form, and fee ticket.

S

SOAP The letters S-O-A-P is an acronym for SUBJECTIVE, OBJECTIVE, ASSESSMENT, and PLAN. The SOAP note is convenient way for health-care providers to lay out the documentation of an office visit exam and to improve communication among medical staff members.

SpringLabs SpringLabs is a SpringCharts feature that provides the capability of automatically receiving lab test results directly from the reference lab by using Electronic Data Interchange (EDI) standards and protocols over a secure Internet connection.

Superbill A superbill typically contains the medical office's most common procedure and diagnosis codes and descriptions for the purposes of recording the physician's selection and billing. However, in SpringCharts the superbill is designed to display codes and items that are often overlooked in the OV exam and can be billed.

SureScripts SureScripts is the national clearinghouse for e-prescribing. The clearinghouse connects a network of thousands of physicians, pharmacists, and payers nationwide, enabling them to exchange health information and prescribe medication without paper.

T

Tablet PC A Tablet PC is a portable, handheld personal computer, with the ability to document directly on the screen with a stylus pen.

Telehealth The use of electronic and communication technology to deliver medical information and services over large and small distances through a standard telephone line.

Template A template is an electronic file that is predesigned with a set format and structure. It serves as a model for a letters, faxes, and reports that need to be filled in to be completed.

TemplateWare A SpringCharts add-on feature that provides pre-built office visits notes, orders and letters, as well as popup text for specific specialists.

Toolbar The toolbar offers a lineup of icons that give the user shortcut access to the most commonly used functions of the program.

Tracker Archive The tracker archive provides a record of all patients that have been entered in to the patient tracker. The tracker archive groups patients by date and tracks such information as the time that the patient entered and left the clinic.

U

Urgent Message An urgent message is the means by which an instant message can be sent to another coworker on the network. The urgent message is not stored with the other messages in the system; rather it is displayed as a popup window in SpringCharts.

User Preferences Setup window in Spring-Charts that enables each user to preset the default practice name, physician name, schedule, and various other features that will be displayed when the user logs into the program.

W

Wellness Screenings Wellness screenings are periodic medical checkups to test for or inoculate against significant diseases. They are preventive services given before the onset of chief complaints.

notes

Chapter 1 An Introduction to Electronic Health Records

1. Andrew H. Melczer, Ph.D., et al., "Background on Electronic Health Records for Small Practices," Illinois State Medical Society, January 2005.
2. Tyler Chin, *Growth in Electronic Medical Record. AMNews.* www.amednews.com, February 9, 2004.
3. *Bush Proposes Update to Patient Records,* Associated Press, April 27, 2004
4. *Transcript: Obama's Speech to Congress,* CBS, February 24, 2009.
5. Agency for Healthcare Research and Quality (AHRQ) at www.ahrq.gov/clinic/
6. Andrew H. Melczer, Ph.D., et al., "Background on Electronic Health Records for Small Practices," Illinois State Medical Society, January 2005.
7. J. Tim Scott, Ph.D., Thomas G. Rundall, Ph.D., Thomas M. Vogt, M.D., M.P.H., et al., *Kaiser Permanente's Experience of Implementing an Electronic Medical Record: A Qualitative Study,* vol. 1, February 24, 2006. http://www.commonwealthfund.org
8. L. Stammer, 2001. Chart pulling brought to its knees. *Healthcare Informatics,* 18:107–108.
9. D. Dassenko and T. Slowinski, 1995. Using the CPR to benefit a business office. *Healthcare Financial Management,* 49:68–70, 72–73.
10. J. Mildon and T. Cohen, 2001. Drivers in the electronics medical records market. *Health Management Technology,* 22:14–6, 18.
11. Andrew H. Melczer, Ph.D et al., "Background on Electronic Health Records for Small Practices," Illinois State Medical Society, January 2005.
12. *The American Recovery and Reinvestment Act of 2009 Summary of Key Health Information Technology Provisions.* March 5, 2009. http://www.himss.org/content/files/HIMSSSummaryOfARRA.pdf

Chapter 2 Standards for Electronic Health Records

1. *Certification Commission for Healthcare Information Technology* Home Page. www.cchit.org/
2. Ibid.
3. United States Department of Health and Human Services, news release. July 18, 2006. www.hhs.gov/news/press/2006pres/20060718.html
4. Incentive Program Made Simple. *http://www.cms.hhs.gov/EPrescribing*

index

Healthcare Information and Management Systems Society (HIMSS), 23

Help, for *Productivity Center,* 227

High Security, 36

HIMSS (Healthcare Information and Management Systems Society), 23

HIPAA (*see* Health Insurance Portability and Accountability Act of 1996)

History:
  in chart notes, 80
  of diagnosis, 81–82
  in EHRs, 2–11
  in EMRs, 2
  on face sheets, 79
  outbound fax history, 213–214
  PMHX, 79
  of prescriptions, 81–82
  of procedures, 81–82
  social, 79
  of standards, 17

History & Physical (H&P) reports, 111
  in networked computer environments, 302
  and office visits, 128
  sample, 275
  and *Tools* menu, 132

HIT (Health Information Technology), 24

HITECH, 19

HL7 (Health Level Seven), 20

Household List, 87

H&P reports (*see* History & Physical reports)

Human Gene Nomenclature (HUGN), 21

I

ICD codes, 18, 205–206

ICD-9 Codes (International Classification of Diseases, Ninth Revision), 122–123, 183

Identify Patient, 187

Illinois Medical Society, 8

Imaging tests, 90–91, 93, 200–201
  creating new, 200–201, 314
  ordering, 90–91, 93, 296
  storage of, 194

Immunization records, 92, 267–268, 281

Imperial units, 34

Import File Cabinet Documents, 157–163

Import items, 102–103, 177

Import Items, 102–103

Inbound fax lists, 214–216, 317–318

Initial Only, 119

Institute of Electrical and Electronic Engineers 1073 (IEEE), 20

Institute of Medicine (IOM), 17, 22–23
  Committee on Data Standards for Patient Safety, 22
  and EHRs, 7

Insurance information:
  adding, to SpringCharts, 43–44
  on face sheets, 82
  malpractice, 10
  primary, 82, 279

Insurance window, 43, 44

InterFax™, 64, 212–213

Internal messages, 61–65
  concerning patients, 63–65
  non-patient messages, 61–63

International Classification of Diseases, Volume 9 (*see* ICD-9 Codes)

Internet technology, 3

Interoperability, 4, 23, 32

Intranet technologies, 3

IOM (*see* Institute of Medicine)

K

Kaiser Permanente, 9

L

Lab analytes (lab items), 188, 198, 199

Lab test(s), 197–200, 311–314
  creating new, 197–200, 313–314
  ordering, 90–91, 195–196, 312
  storage of, 194

Lab test name, 185–187

Lab test results, 183–189, 193, 270
  processing, 187–190, 311–312
  sample, 270, 286

Laboratory Logical Observation Identifier Name Codes (LOINC), 20

Labs, reference, 185

LAN (Local Area Network), 2–3

Large Screen view, 33

Last menstrual period (LMP), 220

Legislation, 7

Letter templates, 168, 172–175, 309

Letters (*see* Messages)

LMP (Last menstrual period), 220

Local Area Network (LAN), 2–3

Location allocations, 54–55

Lock Chart feature, 88

Locking, of notes, 97, 99

LOINC (Laboratory Logical Observation Identifier Name Codes), 20

Lookup/Search icon, 213

Low Security, 36

Lytec™, 31, 33

M

MacExchange, 31

Macintosh computers, 191

MacPractice™, 31

Malpractice insurance, 10

Match, 187

Match Test, 188

Match Test Analyte, 188

Mayo Clinic (Rochester, Minnesota), 2

Measurements, 34

Medicaid, 11

Medical Center Hospital of Vermont, 2

Medical Database, 224, 319

Medical decision support, 22

Medical tests, 200
  creating new, 200
  ordering, 90–91
  storage of, 194

Medicare, 11

Medicare Improvements for Patients and Providers Act of 2008 (MIPPA), 25–26

Medicare Part B, 26

Medications:
  discontinued, 125–126
  on face sheets, 80–81
  in Networked computer environments, 301
  in office visits, 123–126
  over the counter, 80
  routine, 80–81, 114

Medications list, 91

Medisoft™, 31, 33

Message archives, 62–63

Messages, 61–67
  concerning patients, 63–65, 237–239, 269, 297, 326
  e-mails, 68–69
  form letters, 222–223
  internal, 61–65
  in networked computer environments, 292–294
  non-patient, 61–63
  to patient, 268, 285
  to primary care physician, 284
  urgent, 68

Metric units, 34

MIPPA (Medicare Improvements for Patients and Providers Act of 2008), 25–26

My ToDo List, 60, 61

My Websites feature, 219–220, 318

N

National Alliance for Health Information Technology (NAHIT), 23

National Council on Prescription Drug Programs (NCDCP), 20

National Guideline Clearinghouse (NGC), 142, 153

National Provider Identification (NPI)
number, 96
NCDCP (National Council on
Prescription Drug Programs),
20, 26
NDCHealth, Inc., 31
Negative test results, 191
Networked computer environments,
287–354
applying your knowledge in,
320–344
clinic administration in, 289–294
clinical tools in, 303–307
electronic recording exercises, 341–354
office visits in, 298–303
patients charts in, 294–298
productivity center and utilities for,
316–320
source documents for, 345–354
templates and pop-up text in,
308–310
tests, procedures, and diagnosis
codes in, 311–316
New Address window, 38–40, 288
New Drug window, 124, 301
New Excuse, 102, 132
New Form, 101
New Insurance Company button,
43, 289
New Letter ABOUT Pt, 99–101,
104–105
New Letter to Pt, 99
New menu, 93–103
New Note, 93–94, 102, 132
New Nurse Note, 94
New Order, 102, 132
New OV, 93, 109
New Patient feature, 41, 288–289
New Rx Refill, 94–97
New TC note, 97–98
New Test Report, 101, 105
New ToDo/Reminder, 59–61
New Vitals Only, 98–99, 112
NewCrop™, 116, 124
NGC (*see National Guideline*
Clearinghouse)
"No Show," 51
Notes:
to appointments, 50
chart notes, 80
creating new, 93–94, 96, 102, 132
excuse notes, 271, 283, 302
follow-up, 118
locking, 97, 99
nurse notes, 94
TC notes, 97–98
(*See also* Office visit notes)
NPI (National Provider Identification)
number, 96
Nurse note, 94

O

Obama, Barack, 7
Objective component (SOAP), 110
Office visit (OV), 33, 109–138,
253–256
Actions menu, 131
addendums to, 137–138
adding data to, 167
building, 110–122
creating, 167–169
discontinued medications in,
125–126
Dx codes in, 122–123
Edit menu, 130–131
H&P report, 128
medications in, 123–126
in networked computer
environments, 298–303, 334–340
new, 93
ordering, 183
pop-up text, editing, 126–127
reports for, 128–129, 274
Routing Slips in, 134–137
templates for, 167–169, 308–309
and tests, 183
Tools menu, 132–134
Office visit notes, 128, 247–252
addendums to, 137–138
building, 120–122
follow-up notes as, 118
multiple clinicians in, 119
for networked computer
environments, 298–300, 302
sample, 282
Office Visit Templates, 168–170
Open a Chart, 74
Order entry/management, 22
Order templates, 168, 170–172
OTC (Over the counter)
medications, 80
Other Sensitivities field, 79
Other Treatment (Other Tx), 110, 118
Outbound fax history, 213–214
Over the counter (OTC)
medications, 80
OVs (*see* Office visit)

P

Passwords:
encryption of, 36
standards for, 17–18
user preferences for, 36
Past medical history (PMHX), 79
Patient(s):
adding, to SpringCharts, 271
office visit report to, 128–130
safety of, 8–9, 22
Patient archives, 225–226, 319–320
Patient care, 9, 307

Patient charts, 74–103, 242–247
Actions menu for, 90–92
care tree, 85, 86
Edit menu for, 89–90
face sheet, 76–82, 88
File menu for, 86–88
in networked computer
environments, 294–298,
329–333
New menu for, 93–103
ordering, 183–184
sample, 265–266
and tests, 183–184
toolbar, 76
Patient Data, 222
Patient ID field, 41
Patient information, 39, 41–42, 150,
278, 306
Patient Instruction Manager, 151
Patient Instructions, 9, 132,
150–153, 306
Patient Insurance Information
window, 43
Patient intake sheets, 280
Patient safety, 8–9, 22
Patient Scheduler, 52, 289–290
Patient status, 54
Patient support, 22
Patient Tracker, 33, 52–58, 233–236
archive for, 56–57
CheckOut with, 55–56
color coding in, 54
demographic information in, 55
Location allocations, 54–55
in networked computer
environments, 290–291, 322–324
routing slips, 56
Status allocations, 54–55
tracker groups in, 55
Pending tests, 91, 183
Pending Tests field, 38
Permanent Sign & Lock, 119, 137–138
Personal health records (PHRs), 5
Pharmacy information:
default, 89, 281
sample, 281
Pharmacy Web Services, 95–96
PHI (protected health
information), 17–18
PHRs (personal health records), 5
Physicians:
payments under ARRA to, 11–12
primary care, 284
referring, 80
PI (*see* Present illness)
Plan component (SOAP), 110
PMHX (past medical history), 79
PMS (*see* Practice Management
System)
Point of care, 2